Tuberculosis of the Spine

Sarvdeep Singh Dhatt • Vishal Kumar
Editors

Tuberculosis of the Spine

Springer

Editors
Sarvdeep Singh Dhatt
Department of Orthopaedics
Post Graduate Institute of Medical
Education and Research
Chandigarh, Punjab, India

Vishal Kumar
Department of Orthopaedics
Post Graduate Institute of Medical
Education and Research
Chandigarh, Punjab, India

ISBN 978-981-16-9497-4 ISBN 978-981-16-9495-0 (eBook)
https://doi.org/10.1007/978-981-16-9495-0

This Springer imprint is published by the registered company Springer Nature Singapore Pte Ltd.
The registered company address is: 152 Beach Road, #21-01/04 Gateway East, Singapore 189721, Singapore

Foreword

Writing a foreword to a book by youngsters is often a difficult task, one that is delegated to a senior or retired person, either as a mark of respect or in his capacity of having knowledge on the subject. I write this foreword for this excellent new book authored by two outstanding youngsters, whom I have mentored, with some degree of trepidation, as I am neither retired nor a specialist in the spine. When Dr Sarvdeep Dhatt and Dr Vishal Kumar asked me to do this, I was overwhelmed, as this was an unexpected honour and I think a gesture from their heart. I have seen both these doctors grow from young residents into capable surgeons, with focus on the spine, having gained significant standing in this field in their own right.

The spine is a tough subject to write about, and tuberculosis of the spine is an even more complex issue. When we were studying as postgraduates, the textbooks had diverse opinions about what to do in spinal tuberculosis. In the 1980s, the understanding of the disease process was evolving, and the management had two extremes of thought. One of these was the western thought process, largely practiced by surgeons of British origin in Hong Kong, with surgical interventions on large scales in almost all cases of spinal TB. At the other extreme were poor income countries of the developing world, especially Africa and Asia, where facilities for intervention were very limited. Into this complex scenario, the pre-eminent thought process was led by surgeons like Dr SM Tuli and Dr T Shanmugasundaram, who developed what has now come to be known as the middle path regime. Overtime, the investigative modalities used to diagnose spinal tuberculosis evolved; the disease itself changed its patterns and presentations somewhat, and the indications and timing of interventions became widely recognized. This book is thus timely, and will serve as a tome for the rest of the twenty-first century, as it has taken many steps beyond what is written in the standard textbooks.

The diverse contributors to this book have been able to cover most issues relevant to different parts of the world; the chapter on epidemiology looks at both the western and Asian perspectives. The anatomy of the disease process is explained by anatomists, and the issues related to microbiology are covered by a microbiologist; adding radiologists and nuclear medicine specialists as authors has brought in focused diversity, which is perhaps an essential need for a proper understanding of this complex disease. This makes the book of interest to medical students beyond orthopaedics. The medical and surgical management of spinal TB has been well detailed, but what really stands out is the specific focus on multi-drug resistant strains, as well the evolution of drug eluting ceramics, which maybe a thing of the future. Two special chapters that I have never encountered in any book are the descriptions of TB spine in special conditions like HIV, pregnancy, polytrauma, etc., and the one talking about the "*end point*" of TB spine. All of these combine to make this an outstanding book, which I would recommend not only for doctors in training but even practicing orthopods, who will gain great insights about where we stand today in our fight against this age-old malady.

At the end of the day what matters is the result; the efforts of the 2 authors have borne fruit, and the book "Tuberculosis of the spine" comes across as a well-planned and well written book. Sarvdeep and Vishal need to be complimented for their effort. God bless you both, and I hope there are many more such works to come in the future.

Mandeep S. Dhillon
Prof. & Head, Department of Orthopaedics and PMR
Post Graduate Institute of Medical
Education and Research
Chandigarh, India

Preface

> To study the phenomena of disease without books is to sail an uncharted sea, while to study books without patients is not to go to sea at all.—William Osler

Tuberculosis has often been regarded as "the great masquerader" and this particularly holds true for the Indian Subcontinent and Southeast Asian region which caters the maximum global burden of skeletal tuberculosis though none of the region across the globe is immune to it. Tuberculosis of spine can present with diverse clinical presentations, making it challenging to diagnose and manage at times. Over the past many years, various modalities of diagnosis and treatment have been investigated and evolved including pharmacotherapy, immunomodulation, and surgery. On the other hand, the bacilli seem to be contesting forwards with numerous drug resistant strains. To date, there is no clear consensus regarding streamlined management of this disease and various regimes have been tested and tried throughout the world.

This book looks forward to addressing the current overview of tuberculosis of spine, highlighting diverse presentations, possible diagnostic challenges as well as various management options. It also covers recent advances in diagnostic modalities, surgical management of the disease with a vision of future possible thoughts and innovations. This book can serve as a good, authentic, evidence based compendium for the medical practitioners involved in dealing and managing spinal tuberculosis across the continents. This book has chapters from authoritative authors both from the developed and the developing world and hence the myriad of tuberculosis from time since humane exists is expected to find clue and guide to its diagnostic, therapeutic challenges.

We wish this treatise on tuberculosis serves its goal of being the definitive and guiding text book on spinal tuberculosis.

Thank You Team Springer Nature for giving our pen an immortal place to perpetuate knowledge!

Chandigarh, India — Sarvdeep Singh Dhatt
Chandigarh, India — Vishal Kumar

Contents

About the Editors

Sarvdeep Singh Dhatt is an Professor of Orthopaedics at PGIMER, Chandigarh. He has specialized in Trauma and Complex Spine Surgery. He has won many International awards in this field and done international fellowships from Shoichi Kokubun, Sendai Japan, Memorial Sloan Kettering Cancer Center NY USA, Queen Elizabeth Hospital, Hong Kong, Dartmouth Hitchcock Hospital, USA, Brigham and Women's Harvard Medical School, USA, Leicester General and Kings College Hospital, London, UK, Rigshospitalet National University Hospital, Copenhagen, Denmark and is an Indo American Spine Alliance Visiting Prof, University of Illinois, Chicago, USA. He has to his credit three patents and around 100 publications as well and has authored 3 books. He is also an International Committee member, Eurospine; Member Feedback Committee, North American Spine Society, Joint Secretary, North Zone Orthopaedic Association and Associate Editor, JPMER.

Vishal Kumar, MS, DNB, MAMS, Dip. SICOT, FACS is presently working as an Associate Professor of Orthopaedics at the Postgraduate Institute of Medical Education & Research, Chandigarh, India—a premier institute and a state-of-the-art teaching hospital of the country. His area of interests and specialization is spine and complex trauma. He has fine-tuned his specialist training through several international and national fellowships at centres of international standing and repute including Oxford University Hospitals, Centre for Spinal Studies and Surgery at QMC, Nottingham, University of Leeds, Dartmouth Hitchcock Center, USA, to name a few. He has several indexed publications, edited a textbook of Orthopaedics, and written more than ten chapters in textbooks. He has won more than twenty-five international and national awards including Abdel Hay Masshour SICOT International Award.

Chapter 1
Historical Perspectives of Musculoskeletal Tuberculosis

Ashish Dagar and Dilip K. Sengupta

Abstract The modern strain of *Mycobacterium tuberculosis* might have appeared 20,000–15,000 years ago. India and China account for the first written description of tuberculosis around 3300 and 2300 years ago, respectively. In Ancient Greece, Hippocrates (400–300 BC) described *Phthisis* or *Consumption* as a fatal disease. The term "*Pott's disease*" was coined by Sir Percivall Pott, a British surgeon in 1779. Johann Lukas Schönlein first used the term "tuberculosis" in 1839. Tubercle bacillus was first isolated by Robert Koch. The sanatorium treatment was first described in 1854 by Hermann Brehmer. Menard (1895) described "costo-transversectomy." This approach was further developed by Griffiths, Roaf, and Seddon. Norman Capener (1933) developed the classical "anterolateral decompression." The Frenchmen, Calmette, and Guérin developed BCG vaccine. The first successful Anti-tubercular drug Streptomycin was discovered by Selman Waksman in September 1943. Hodgson in 1960 popularized "The Hong Kong Surgery." Tuli from India in 1975 published successful results of the "middle path regimen." In recent years, "all posterior" approach to the tubercular spine has become popular. In the 1970s and 1980s with the rise of the AIDS epidemic, tuberculosis re-emerged as a potential threat to humanity. The emergence Drug-Resistant strains have led to the complete abrogation of single or dual drug therapy. Multidrug therapies for a prolonged period are the norm now. New antitubercular drugs are being developed, e.g., Bedaquiline, Delamanid, and Pretomanid.

Keywords Musculoskeletal tuberculosis · History of mycobacterium *Mycobacterium tuberculosis* · History of tuberculosis · Spine tuberculosis

---

A. Dagar (✉)
Manipal Hospital, Dwarka, New Delhi, India

D. K. Sengupta
Center for Scoliosis & Advanced Spine Surgery, Dallas, TX, USA

S. S. Dhatt, V. Kumar (eds.), *Tuberculosis of the Spine*,
https://doi.org/10.1007/978-981-16-9495-0_1

Tuberculosis is an infectious, contagious, and multisystemic disease caused by *Mycobacterium tuberculosis* [1]. The genus *Mycobacterium* is believed to have originated around 150 million years ago [2]. Tuberculosis was endemic in animals being caused by *Mycobacterium bovis* or a variant of it, in the paleolithic period [3]. An early strain of *Mycobacterium tuberculosis* might have infected early hominids in East Africa around three million years ago [4]. The modern strain of *Mycobacterium tuberculosis* might have appeared 20,000–15,000 years ago [5, 6]. The first undisputed evidence of *Mycobacterium tuberculosis* was obtained in bone lesions of a 17,000-year-old bison found in Wyoming, USA [7]. The first evidence for tuberculosis in humans was detected in form of bone tuberculosis in a 500,000-year-old skull in Turkey [8].

The oldest known example of spinal tuberculosis dates to 8000 BC in the form of fossil bones [9]. Pott's lesions and tubercular skeletal deformities are reported in Egyptian mummies, dating back to 2400 BC [10, 11]. Tuberculosis was present in American continents long before European colonization as suggested by presence of Pott's deformities in Peruvian mummies [12, 13]. Moreover, tuberculous bacilli was isolated from a psoas abscess which was present in a mummified Inca Child (around 700 BC old) [14].

India and China account for the first written description of tuberculosis around 3300 and 2300 years ago, respectively [15, 16]. "Yakshma," the term used in Indian texts—the Rig Veda, the Atharva Veda; is a reference to tuberculosis [17, 18, 19]. Ancient Hebrew literature also contains references to *Tuberculosis* in form of the word "schachepheth" [20].

In Ancient Greece, Hippocrates (400–300 BC) described Phthisis or Consumption (terms used for describing tuberculosis). He described Phthisis as a disease predominately affecting young population which was invariably fatal in most of the cases. He also defined tubercular lung lesions and resulting symptoms [21]. Hippocrates also described tuberculosis of the spine [19]. In Middle Ages, a new form of tuberculosis was described in which there was involvement of lymph nodes in the cervical region. Because of a common belief that it can be cured by touch of a royal person, it came to be known as "king's evil" [22].

In the sixteenth century, Girolamo Fracastoro was first to clearly define tuberculosis as a contagious disease [23]. In 1679, Francis Sylvius published his work titled "Opera Medica." In this landmark publication, he described pathophysiology of tuberculosis starting from development of tubercles, abscesses, cavitations, and ultimately leading to empyema [24]. The English physician Benjamin Marten first reported the infectious origin of tuberculosis in his publication "A new theory of Consumption" in 1720 [25].

The term "*Pott's disease*" was coined by Sir Percivall Pott, a British surgeon in 1779. He used this term to describe paralysis developing because of tubercular infection of vertebral column [26, 27]. Scottish pathologist Matthew Baille in 1793 used the term "tubercles" to describe caseous necrosis in tubercular abscess [27]. A new form of tuberculosis was described by the French physician Gaspard-Laurent Bayle in 1810. He used the word "miliary" tuberculosis for this clinically fatal presentation of tuberculosis in which there was disseminated systemic involvement [28, 29]. Johann Lukas Schönlein first used the term "tuberculosis" in 1839 [26].

In eighteenth century Western Europe, Tuberculosis was famous as "the robber of youth" as it mainly affected young population with a high mortality rate. It was also referred to as "white plague" as patients affected with tuberculosis appeared white because of pallor resulting from anemia [30, 31]. Tuberculosis was so prevalent in Western civilization that it was termed as "Captain of All These Men of Death."

In 1865, Jeon-Antoine Villemin established infectious nature of the disease by infecting rabbit from a cadaver tissue [32]. Tubercle bacillus was first isolated by Robert Koch (1882) for which he won the Nobel prize in Medicine in 1905 [33, 34]. The Ziehl-Neelsen microscopic acid-fast stain was described by the bacteriologist Franz Ziehl (1859–1926) and the pathologist Friedrich Neelsen (1854–1898) [35].

1.1 Historical Perspectives of Musculoskeletal Tuberculosis Treatment

Ancient Indian text Atharvaveda (1800–1000 BC) described sunshine and "Sipudru," an herbal preparation for the treatment of skeletal tuberculosis [19]. Hippocrates (450 BC) from Greece is the father of Spine Surgery. Hippocrates and Galen (AD 131–201) tried to correct kyphotic deformity due to tuberculosis of the spine with manual pressure, traction (Fig. 1.1), and mechanical appliances [36], but failed [18].

The first successful remedy against TB was first described in 1854 by Hermann Brehmer. He introduced the concept of the sanatorium cure in his doctoral dissertation "Tuberculosis is a curable disease" [37]. He himself was a Tubercular survivor. He cured himself of tuberculosis by isolating himself in Himalayan mountains.

During this era, skeletal (including spinal) tuberculosis was also managed on similar lines—abundant rest/immobilization, fresh air, and high energy/high protein food. Bed rest/Immobilization was usually prolonged and ranged from 1 to 5 years [38]. The idea was to reach the "stage of repair and ankylosis." The outcome of such management was disappointing and most of the patients were scummed to military tuberculosis. The rate of paralysis was high. Development of kyphotic deformity was a norm rather than the exception [39–42].

Limitation of conservative management stimulated different surgical interventions in hope of improved outcomes in skeletal tuberculosis. Peripheral abscesses were managed by aspiration through "antigravity routes" and excision of sinus tracts. Chipault [43] in 1894 described laminectomy as a surgical option for paraplegia due to tuberculosis. However, results were disappointing due to persistence of pain, increase in kyphosis, and worsening neurological deficit. These drawbacks lead to the development of "anterolateral decompression" approaches. Menard (1895) described "costo-transversectomy"—anterolateral extra-pleural approach to spine [44]. This approach was further developed by Griffiths [45], Roaf [46, 47],

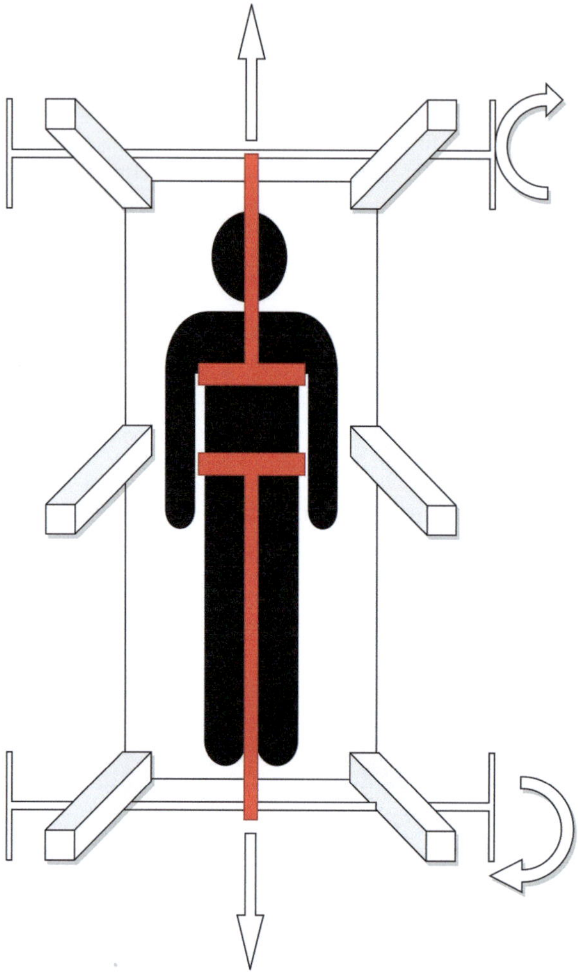

Fig. 1.1 Line Diagram depicting traction appliance designed by Hippocrates to treat tubercular kyphosis

and Seddon [42, 48]. Norman Capener (1933) developed the classical "anterolateral decompression" procedure for spinal tuberculosis, which he coined as the "lateral rhachiotomy" approach [49]. All these surgical approaches were usually riddled with frequent complications such as persistent sinus, nonhealing ulcer formations, secondary pyogenic infection, and death. Calot [50] in 1930 summarized disappointment of surgical results in tuberculosis as "the surgeon who, so far as tuberculosis is concerned, swears to remove the evil from the very root, will only find one result awaiting him—the death of his patient."

Poor results of direct disease site surgical interventions lead to the development of "distant operations," i.e., fusion away from the disease area. Albee [51] and Hibbs [52] introduced posterior spinal fusion, while Brittain [53] introduced extraarticular operations. These operations aimed to provide permanent internal stability (fusion) to the diseased parts. These surgeries although reduced the incidence of ulcer and sinus formation, but the disease activity remained unaffected. The posterior spinal fusion surgeries had nothing to offer to paraplegic patients. Overall results of such procedures were not encouraging [50, 54].

On the Medical front, strides were being taken in the field of the development of vaccines and antitubercular drugs. The Frenchmen, Calmette, and Guérin in the 1900s attenuated a strain (bacille Calmette-Guérin–BCG) of *Mycobacterium bovis*, and used it in immunization [55, 56]. The first successful Antitubercular drug Streptomycin was discovered by Selman Waksman in September 1943 from Cultures of actinomycete—*Streptomyces griseus*. For his outstanding scientific achievement, Waksman was honored in 1952 with the Nobel Prize [57]. Following streptomycin, p-aminosalicylic acid (1949), isoniazid (1952) pyrazinamide (1954), cycloserine (1955), ethambutol (1962), and rifampin (rifampicin; 1963) were introduced as antituberculosis agents.

The availability of antitubercular drugs marked an important milestone in the fight against tuberculosis. There was a renewed interest in direct surgical excision and debridement of disease part because of the encouragement provided by the safety and the efficacy profile of the antitubercular drugs. Because of limited knowledge about antitubercular drug penetration into bone tissue and tubercular abscess, the standard treatment practiced from 1950 to 1960 was "universal excisional surgery" in conjunction with antitubercular drugs [58–61]. Hodgson in 1960 popularized "The Hong Kong Surgery"—anterior radical debridement and reconstruction using rib strut grafts for spinal tuberculosis [59, 62]. The advantage of using effective antitubercular drugs in association with surgical debridement of diseased areas was the disappearance of sinuses, ulcers, and abscesses and the elimination of the danger of postoperative dissemination of tuberculosis.

Over a period, the development of effective multidrug therapy for tuberculosis leads to the realization of the true potential of drug therapy in the repair and regeneration of bony tissue [63]. Apprehensions regarding drug penetration in bony tissue also faded away. These developments led to the evolution of surgical management. Tuli from India in 1975 [64] published successful results of "middle path regimen"—all patients treated with antitubercular chemotherapy, and surgery advised only in patients at risk of neurological deficit or significant kyphosis. He also popularized limited operative debridement—removal of sequestrated vertebrae or discs or the offending tissues compressing the Dural tube [64–66]. The British Medical Research Council (MRC) Working Party on Tuberculosis of the Spine conducted several studies in Korea, Zimbabwe, Hong Kong, and Madras [67–69]. In these studies, the concept of a "middle path regimen" was validated. Indications for surgical intervention also became limited. Surgical interventions became confined to patients who failed to respond to drugs or with complications and to improve quality of function [70].

The use of metal implants in active tubercular infection became popular in the 1990s after a report by Oga et al. [71] that the tubercle bacilli do not adhere to metal and form a biofilm. Instrumentation improved quality of life by providing immediate stability, pain relief, and protection against the development of kyphotic deformity [72, 73]. In recent years, "all posterior" approach to the tubercular spine has become popular. It includes posterior pedicle screw instrumentation combined with either transpedicular decompression or anterior reconstruction through transforaminal or a costo-transversectomy approach [74–77].

1.1.1 Tuberculosis: The Resurrection

In the 1970s and 1980s with the rise of the AIDS epidemic, tuberculosis re-emerged as a potential threat to humanity. Immunodeficient state of patients infected with AIDS virus leads to infection with atypical tuberculous bacilli and development of drug resistance against a large number of antitubercular drugs. The emergence of Multi-Drug Resistance (MDR, i.e., the resistance of the mycobacterium to isoniazid and rifampicin), Extensively Drug Resistance (XDR, i.e., resistant to isoniazid and rifampicin, plus any fluoroquinolone and at least one of three injectable second-line drugs), and Total Drug Resistance (TDR) have led to complete abrogation of single or dual drug therapy. Multidrug therapies for a prolonged period are a norm now. DOTS (directly observed treatment, short-course) strategy was developed by Karel Styblo with the International Union Against Tuberculosis and Lung Disease in the 1970s and was adopted by World Health Organization (WHO) in 1995. New antitubercular drugs are being developed to be used in XDR/TDR cases as a part of multidrug therapy. Examples include Bedaquiline [78], Delamanid [79, 80], and Pretomanid [81, 82].

References

1. Bazin H. Vaccination: A history. Montrouge: John Libbey Eurotext; 2011.
2. Hayman J. Mycobacterium ulcerans: an infection from Jurassic time? Lancet. 1984;2(8410):1015–6.
3. Steele JH, Ranney AF. Animal tuberculosis. Am Rev Tuberc. 1958;77:908.
4. Gutierrez MC, Brisse S, Brosch R, Fabre M, Omaïs B, Marmiesse M, Supply P, Vincent V. Ancient origin and gene mosaicism of the progenitor of Mycobacterium tuberculosis. PLoS Pathog. 2005;1(1):e5.
5. Kapur V, Whittam TS, Musser JM. Is Mycobacterium tuberculosis 15,000 years old? J Infect Dis. 1994;170(5):1348–9.
6. Brosch R, Gordon SV, Marmiesse M, Brodin P, Buchrieser C, Eiglmeier K, Garnier T, Gutierrez C, Hewinson G, Kremer K, Parsons LM, Pym AS, Samper S, van Soolingen D, Cole ST. A new evolutionary scenario for the Mycobacterium tuberculosis complex. Proc Natl Acad Sci U S A. 2002;99(6):3684–9.
7. Rothschild BM, Martin LD, Lev G, et al. Mycobacterium tuberculosis complex DNA from an extinct bison dated 17,000 years before the present. Clin Infect Dis. 2001;33:305–11.
8. Kappelman J, Alcicek MC, Kazanci N, Schultz M, Ozkul M, Sen S. First Homo erectus from Turkey and implications for migrations into temperate Eurasia. Am J Phys Anthropol. 2008;135:110–6.
9. Ayvazian LF. History of tuberculosis. In: Reichman LB, Hershfield, editors. Tuberculosis. New York: Dekker; 1993.

10. Morse D, Brothwell DR, Ucko PJ. Tuberculosis in ancient Egypt. Am Rev Respir Dis. 1964;90:524–41.
11. Zimmerman MR, Bull NY. Pulmonary and osseous tuberculosis in an Egyptian mummy. Acad Med. 1979;55(6):604–8.
12. Allison MJ, Mendoza D, Pezzia A. Documentation of a case of tuberculosis in Pre-Columbian America. Am Rev Respir Dis. 1973;107(6):985–91.
13. Arriaza BT, Salo W, Aufderheide AC, Holcomb TA. Pre-Columbian tuberculosis in northern Chile: molecular and skeletal evidence. Am J Phys Anthropol. 1995;98(1):37–45.
14. Dubos R. The romance of death. Am Lung Assoc Bull. 1982;68:5–6.
15. Cave AJE. The evidence for the incidence of tuberculosis in ancient Egypt. Br J Tuberc. 1939;33:142–52.
16. Brown L. The story of clinical pulmonary tuberculosis. Baltimore MD; 1941.
17. Yeager RL. Opening remarks. Ann N Y Acad Sci. 1963;106:3–4.
18. Bick KM. Classics of Orthopaedics. Philadelphia, PA: JB Lippincott Co; 1976.
19. Duraiswami PK, Tuli SM. 5000 years of orthopaedics in India. Clin Orthop Relat Res. 1971;75:269–80.
20. Daniel VS, Daniel TM. Old Testament biblical references to tuberculosis. Clin Infect Dis. 1999;29(6):1557–8.
21. Hippocrates (460-370 BCE). Book 1–Of the epidemics. In: Adams F, editor. The genuine works of Hippocrates. London: The Sydenham Society; 1849.
22. Murray JF, Rieder HL, Finley-Croswhite A. The King's Evil and the Royal Touch: the medical history of scrofula. Int J Tuberc Lung Dis. 2016 Jun;20(6):713–6.
23. Sabbatani S. Historical insights into tuberculosis. Girolamo Fracastoro's intuition on the transmission of tuberculosis and his opponents. History of an idea. Infez Med. 2004;12(4):284–91.
24. Saeed BW. Malignant tuberculosis. J Ayub Med Coll Abbottabad. 2006;18(3):1–2.
25. Daniel TM. Captain of death: the story of tuberculosis. Rochester, NY: University of Rochester Press; 1997.
26. Daniel TM. Pioneers in Medicine and their Impact on Tuberculosis. Rochester, NY: University of Rochester Press; 2000. pp. 4, 29, 46-48, 50-51, 74-76
27. Dormandy T. The White Death: a history of tuberculosis. London: The Hambledon press; 1999. pp. 2, 4, 13, 34-36, 73-84, 92-94, 101-104, 129-137, 147, 392
28. Garrison FH. An introduction to the history of medicine. Philadelphia & London: W B Saunders & Co; 1921. pp. 109, 288, 411-413, 616
29. Major RH. Classic descriptions of disease. Springfield, USA: Charles C Thomas; 1932. pp. 49-56, 56-57, 58-61, 61-62
30. Daniel TM. The history of tuberculosis. Respir Med. 2006;100(11):1862–70.
31. Segen JC. The dictionary of modern medicine. Park Ridge, NJ: Parthenon; 1992. p. 783.
32. Villemin JA. Etudes sur la tuberculose. Paris: Bailliere; 1868.
33. Gradmann C. Robert Koch and the pressures of scientific research: tuberculosis and tuberculin. Med Hist. 2001;45(1):1–32.
34. Bartolozzi G. Vaccini e vaccinazioni. Terza edizione. Milano: Elsevier; 2012.
35. Ziehl F. Zur F€arbung des tuberkelbacillus. Dtsch Med Wochenschr. 1882;8:451.
36. Guidi G. Chirurgia è graeco latinum conversa. Paris: Petrus Galterius; 1544. p. 552.
37. Daniel TM. Hermann Brehmer and the origins of tuberculosis sanatoria. Int J Tuberc Lung Dis. 2011;15(2):161–2.
38. Jones R, Lovett RW. Orthopaedic surgery. London, UK: Oxford Medical Publications; 1923.
39. Dobson J. Tuberculosis of spine. J Bone Joint Surg Br. 1951;33:517–31.
40. Fellander M. Radical operation in tuberculosis of the spine. Acta Orthop Scand Suppl. 1955;19:1–117.
41. Girdlestone GR. Modern trends in orthopaedics. Series I. London, UK: Butterworth and Co; 1950.
42. Seddon HJ. Pott's paraplegia, prognosis and treatment. Br J Surg. 1935;22:769–99.

43. Chipault A. Etudes de chirugie medullaire. Historique, chirugie operatoire, traitement. Paris: F. Alcan; 1894.
44. Menard V. Cause of paraplegia in Potts's disease. Rev Orthop. 1894;5:47–64.
45. Griffiths DL. Tuberculosis of bones and joints: modern practice in tuberculosis, vol. II. London, UK: Butterworth and Co; 1952. p. 302–33.
46. Roaf R. Tuberculosis of the spine. J Bone Joint Surg Br. 1958;40:3–5.
47. Roaf R, Kirkaldy-Willis WH, Cathro AJM. Surgical treatment of bone and joints tuberculosis. Edinburgh, UK: E and S Livingstone; 1959.
48. Seddon HJ. Pott's paraplegia. In: Platt SH, editor. Modern trends in orthopaedics. Series II. London, UK: Butterworth and Co; 1956. p. 230–4.
49. Capener N. Vertebral tuberculosis and paraplegia. J Bone Joint Surg Br. 1967;49(4):605–6.
50. Calot T. Sur le meilleur traitment localdes tuberculoses doses, articulations et ganglions lymphatique. Acta Chir Scand. 1930;67:206–26.
51. Albee FH. Transplantation of a portion of the tibia into the spine for Pott's disease: a preliminary report. JAMA. 1911;57:885–6.
52. Hibbs RA, Risser JC. Treatment of vertebral tuberculosis by fusion operation. JAMA. 1918;71:1372.
53. Brittain HA. Architectural principles in arthrodesis. 2nd ed. Edinburgh, UK: Livingstone; 1952.
54. Mercer W. Then and now: the history of skeletal tuberculosis. J R Coll Surg Edinb. 1964;9:243–54.
55. Bochalli R. Die Entwicklung der Tuberkuloseforschung in der Zeit von 1878 bis 1959. Stuttgart: Thieme; 1959.
56. Luchino F. BCG vaccination. Am Rev Respir Dis. 1982;125:70–2.
57. Sakula A. Selman Waksman (1888–1973), discoverer of streptomycin: a centenary review. Br J Dis Chest. 1988;82:23–31.
58. Deroy MS, Fisher H. The treatment of tuberculous bone disease by surgical drainage combined with streptomycin. J Bone Joint Surg Am. 1952;34:299–330.
59. Hodgson AR, Stock FE. Anterior spinal fusion for the treatment of tuberculosis of the spine. J Bone Joint Surg Am. 1960;42:1147–56.
60. Orell S. Chemotherapy and surgical treatment in bone and joint tuberculosis. Acta Orthop Scand. 1951;21:109–203.
61. Ostman P. Combined surgical and chemotherapy of abscesses in bone and joint tuberculosis. Acta Orthop Scand. 1951;21:204–10.
62. Hodgson AR, Stock FE, Fang HS, Ong GB. Anterior spinal fusion: the operative approach and pathological findings in 412 patients with Pott's disease of the spine. Br J Surg. 1960;48:172–8.
63. Rajasekaran S. The problem of deformity in spinal tuberculosis. Clin Orthop Relat Res. 2002;398:85–92.
64. Tuli SM. Results of treatment of spinal tuberculosis by middle path regime. J Bone Joint Surg Br. 1975;57:13–23.
65. Kondo E, Yamada K. End results of focal débridement in bone and joint tuberculosis and its indications. J Bone Joint Surg Am. 1957;39:27–31.
66. Wilkinson MC. Tuberculosis of the spine treated by chemotherapy and operative debridement: a long-term follow-up study. J Bone Joint Surg Am. 1969;51:1331–42.
67. Medical Research Council. A 10-year assessment of controlled trials comparing debridement and anterior spinal fusion in the management of tuberculosis of the spine in patients on standard chemotherapy in Hong Kong. Seventh report of the Medical Research Council Working Party on Tuberculosis of the Spine. J Bone Joint Surg Br. 1985;64:393–8.
68. A 15-year assessment of controlled trials of the management of tuberculosis of the spine in Korea and Hong Kong. Thirteenth report of the medical research council working party on tuberculosis of the spine. J Bone Joint Surg Br. 1998;80(3):456–62.
69. A controlled trial of anterior spinal fusion and debridement in the surgical management of tuberculosis of the spine in patients on standard chemotherapy: a study in two centres in South

Africa. Seventh report of the medical research council working party on tuberculosis of the spine. Tubercle. 1978;59(2):79–10544.
70. Rajasekaran S, Khandelwal G. Drug therapy in spinal tuberculosis. Eur Spine J. 2013;22(Suppl 4):587–93.
71. Oga M, Arizono T, Takasita M, Sugioka Y. Evaluation of the risk of instrumentation as a foreign body in spinal tuberculosis. Clinical and biologic study. Spine. 1993;18(13):1890–4.
72. Ha KY, Chung YG, Ryoo SJ. Adherence and biofilm formation of Staphylococcus epidermidis and Mycobacterium tuberculosis on various spinal implants. Spine (Phila Pa). 1976. 2005;30:38–43.
73. Basu S, Chatterjee S, Bhattacharyya MK. Efficacy and safety of instrumentation in caries spine. Indian J Orthop. 2006;40:78–81.
74. Chacko AG, Moorthy RK, Chandy MJ. The transpedicular approach in the management of thoracic spine tuberculosis: a short-term follow up study. Spine. 2005;29(17):E363–7.
75. Sahoo MM, Mahapatra SK, Sethi GC, Dash SK. Posterior-only approach surgery for fixation and decompression of thoracolumbar spinal tuberculosis: a retrospective study. J Spinal Disord Tech. 2012;25(7):E217–23.
76. Zhang H, Sheng B, Tang M, Guo C, Liu S, Huang S, et al. One-stage surgical treatment for upper thoracic spinal tuberculosis by internal fixation, debridement, and combined interbody and posterior fusion via posterior-only approach. Eur Spine J. 2013;22(3):616–23.
77. Zaveri GR, Mehta SS. Surgical treatment of lumbar tuberculous spondylodiscitis by transforaminal lumbar interbody fusion (TLIF) and posterior instrumentation. J Spinal Disord Tech. 2009;22(4):257–62.
78. Rustomjee R, Diacon AH, Allen J, Venter A, Reddy C, Patientia RF, Mthiyane TC, De Marez T, van Heeswijk R, Kerstens R, et al. Early bactericidal activity and pharmacokinetics of the diarylquinoline TMC207 in treatment of pulmonary tuberculosis. Antimicrob Agents Chemother. 2008;52:2831–5.
79. Matsumoto M, Hashizume H, Tomishige T, Kawasaki M, Tsubouchi H, Sasaki H, Shimokawa Y, Komatsu M. OPC-67683, a nitro-dihydroimidazooxazole derivative with promising action against tuberculosis in vitro and in mice. PLoS Med. 2006;3:e466.
80. Gler MT, Skripconoka V, Sanchez-Garavito E, Xiao H, Cabrera-Rivero JL, Vargas-Vasquez DE, Gao M, Awad M, Park SK, Shim TS, et al. Delamanid for multidrug-resistant pulmonary tuberculosis. N Engl J Med. 2012;366:2151–60.
81. Ahmad Z, Peloquin CA, Singh RP, Derendorf H, Tyagi S, Ginsberg A, Grosset JH, Nuermberger EL. PA-824 exhibits time-dependent activity in a murine model of tuberculosis. Antimicrob Agents Chemother. 2011;55:239–45.
82. Diacon AH, Dawson R, Hanekom M, Narunsky K, Maritz SJ, Venter A, Donald PR, van Niekerk C, Whitney K, Rouse DJ, et al. Early bactericidal activity and pharmacokinetics of PA-824 in smear positive tuberculosis patients. Antimicrob Agents Chemother. 2010;54:3402–7.

Chapter 2
History of Tuberculosis Spine (Post-ATT Era)

Dhiraj Sharma and Amarjit Singh Rai

Abstract Throughout history, infectious diseases have plagued those undergoing surgery, but several landmark discoveries in the field of microbiology have significantly impacted on survival. Tuberculosis (TB) has been present for approximately 70,000 years. The discovery of effective TB drug therapy revolutionised the management of this ancient disease and led to an era of treatment re-evaluation. Prior to anti-tuberculosis therapy (ATT), there was no consensus on the management of TB spine and depending on the practitioner it was managed either conservatively or with surgical debridement. Both options yielded unpredictable and often unfavourable outcomes with high morbidity rates. It was not until the discovery of highly effective ATT that the management of spinal TB radically changed. It led to a surgical renaissance whereby surgeons initially performed increasingly invasive, complex surgery for TB spine under the protection of ATT therapy. After an era of reequibrilation, the results from several large trials comparing operative and non-operative showed that ATT was effective at treating spinal TB alone, leading surgeons to gradually narrow their indications for surgical intervention. With time, improvements in surgical instrumentation has led to less reliance on bone grafts, less invasive surgery, and better outcomes for those patients who do require an operation.

Keywords Middle path regime · Spinal tuberculosis · Pott disease

2.1 Introduction

Throughout history, infectious diseases have plagued those undergoing surgery, but several landmark discoveries in the field of microbiology have significantly impacted on survival. 'Germ theory' proposed by Louis Pasteur (1861) was the first to confirm that bacteria cause infectious diseases, and subsequently, Joseph Lister's

D. Sharma · A. S. Rai (✉)
Norfolk and Norwich University Hospitals NHS Trust, Norwich, UK

S. S. Dhatt, V. Kumar (eds.), *Tuberculosis of the Spine*,
https://doi.org/10.1007/978-981-16-9495-0_2

concept of anti-sepsis dramatically improved survival from post-operative sepsis [1, 2]. Alexander Fleming's chance discovery of penicillin was arguably one of the most significant medical breakthroughs. It was so significant that it altered the course of World War II by making battle wounds survivable and significantly reduced surgical mortality from disastrous secondary bacterial infections [3, 4]. TB has been present for approximately 70,000 years and the discovery of highly effective TB drug therapy mirrored the gravitas of Fleming's work and revolutionised the treatment of this ancient disease.

Prior to anti-tuberculosis therapy (ATT), there was no consensus on the management of TB spine and depending on the practitioner it was managed either conservatively or with surgical debridement. Both options yielded unpredictable and often unfavourable outcomes with high morbidity rates [5, 6]. The discovery of Streptomycin in 1944 marked the beginning of a new age for the treatment of tuberculosis: the post-ATT era [7]. This revolutionary treatment enthused an era of experimentation where surgeons sought to implement ATT to its greatest potential [8, 9].

Prior to ATT, surgery on diseased tissue was fraught with complications. Surgery ranged from excision and debridement, to decompression and deformity correction. Posterior laminectomies were commonly performed in the 1900s but were frequently associated with spinal instability and unfavourable outcomes [5]. TB spine predominantly effects the anterior spine, but early surgical techniques and instrumentation meant that posterior approaches could not safely access the anterior column; therefore several surgeons advocated for posterolateral and anterior approaches to the spine as a means of avoiding damage to posterior stabilising structures. The first to perform an alternative approach, Menard (1987), described the 'costotransversectomy' as a means of gaining access to the lateral spine for TB abscess drainage [10]. Later, Müller (1906) described an anterior transperitoneal approach to the lumbar spine, and Ito (1934) advanced this approach, describing extraperitoneal access to the lumbar spine [11, 12]. Although the initial post-operative results were sometimes promising (without microbe source control) patients soon re-developed a debilitating disease burden no matter the surgical approach. Despite surgery, persistent sinuses, secondary infection, and death were common sequelae. Calot aptly described surgery in these circumstance: "the surgeon who, so far as tuberculosis is concerned, swears to remove the evil from the very root, will only find one result awaiting him—the death of his patient" [13].

Under these circumstances, surgeons developed techniques for distant surgery by performing surgery on non-diseased bone. For instance, Albee and Hibbs developed techniques for posterior spinal fusion with the aim of providing spinal stability by bridging diseased vertebrae [14]. Without metal implants for fixation, bone grafts were used for struts to strengthen the vertebral column. As pragmatic as this treatment strategy sounded, without microbe control the deformity and neurological sequelae as a result of the destructive disease process continued and the appeal of this practice soon waned [7].

It was not until the discovery of highly effective ATT that the management of spinal TB radically changed. Streptomycin and para-aminosalicylic acid provided a first glimmer of hope; providing highly effective treatment with outcomes that had never been achieved before [15]. Unfortunately, these advances were soon met with antibiotic resistance. The issue of resistance was quickly recognised, and the importance of microbe eradication, not simply symptom improvement, was appreciated. Triple therapy with Isoniazid (1952), a potent bactericidal, combated resistance and was curative in over 90% of patients [16]. The addition of Rifampin and Pyrazinamide effectively reduced the length of treatment required by approximately 12 months [16–18]. Initially, TB therapy was strictly managed on an inpatient basis. Receiving long courses of TB medication lead to lengthy hospital admissions, so any reduction in treatment time was extremely beneficial to patients and hospital services alike. In the 1950s, a serendipitous discovery was made in Nigeria when hospital bed shortages forced ATT therapy to be given on an outpatient, ambulatory basis. Konstam reported results suggesting that outpatient management was as effective as inpatient therapy and a viable, pragmatic alternative [19]. With each medical advancement, medical management became increasingly well accepted. With the widespread successes of ATT, a period of reequilibration saw surgeons experiment to understand how surgery could be best implemented alongside medical therapy.

2.2 Early ATT and Surgery

ATT was initially implemented as an adjuvant therapy. It was an elixir that acted as a guardian for increasingly complex surgery [20]. Deroy and Fisher reported spinal disease resolution, bone regeneration, and disease that did not relapse [8]. Surgeons could wield their knife happy in the knowledge that patients could make a good recovery, avoiding dreaded disease reoccurrence. This drastic improvement in outcomes re-ignited a surgical enthusiasm and a trend towards 'radical excision'.

Hodgson proposed that early, radical debridement was advantageous because it allowed for smaller volume debridement, whilst avoiding the lengthy operative time associated with advanced disease [21]. The concept of debridement was further fuelled by the early misconception that it helped antibiotics penetrate disease areas better. Wilkinson performed surgery with adjuvant ATT and partly attributed his results to the fact he was able to 'provide access to the antibiotic' [22].

Proponents of aggressive surgery were seeing improved results with ATT, while proponents of a non-surgical approach were seeing drastic improvements in patient outcomes using ATT alone [19, 22–24].

This dichotomy in treatment spurred Tuli (1975) to coin the 'middle-path' regime which aimed to treat all patients with or without neurological deficit with primary ATT and rest [24]. Only those who failed to respond to medical management were considered for surgery. This pragmatic regime showed great promise for the management of spinal TB and paved the way for modern treatment today [25].

> Tuli 2007 [26]: When the potential for remarkable repair and regeneration of the diseased vertebrae (and bones) with multidrug therapy was realized, operative excision and débride-

ment justifiably became less aggressive and were confined (or limited) to removal of sequestrated vertebrae or discs or the offending tissues compressing the dural tube.

The Medical Research Council (MRC) led international trials in 1965 to establish the role of surgery in spinal TB management [27–30]. Patients were split into three cohorts: medical management alone, medical management with debridement, and medical management with debridement and anterior fixation. The 'favourable' outcome status was achieved if a patient had disease resolution and returned to their previous physical activity, without neurological sequelae. The rate of 'favourable' outcomes was equivocal across all three treatment strategies. The results of the MRC trials showed that the majority of patients suffering from spinal TB could be managed successfully with medical treatment. Surgery was an adjuvant to primary medical management.

2.3 Surgical Approaches

Research showed that ATT was an effective first-line treatment for spinal TB. Surgery was an adjunct only indicated in patients who had failed medical therapy presenting with deformity, neurological or functional sequelae such as cord compression and dysphagia.

2.4 Anterior

The anterior approach to the spine was popular because it gave direct access to the diseased bone and avoided disrupting the posterior stabilising structures.

The Hong Kong operation popularised by Hodgson in the 1960s involved radical anterior debridement with the creation of surfaces suitable for strut grafting. The 1978 MRC study in South Africa compared anterior debridement alone with debridement and grafting and reported earlier bony fusion and less severe kyphotic deformities in the group with grafting [31].

Thoracic lesions were typically accessed via thoracotomy and a subpleural approach, and lumbar lesions via a lateral retroperitoneal approach [21, 32–34]. Although anterior approaches to the thoracolumbar spine gave good access to diseased tissue, they placed a significant physiological burden on patients, requiring intensive care recovery and prolonged hospital stays [21, 32–34]. As the evidence for ATT in TB spine gathered, surgeons could only justify operating for specific indications as eluded to by Tuli [24].

Anterior access for most sub-axial cervical lesions was associated with fewer complications. Careful anterior cervical dissection allowed for debridement and reconstruction and was commonly performed via the Smith-Robinson approach (1958), an approach commonly used today [35–37].

Regardless of the lesion level, grafting of debridement defects was required to prevent deformity [27]. Popular autologous graft sites included the rib, iliac crest, and fibula all used with varying success [27, 34, 38]. For large excisional defects of more than two consecutive vertebrae, graft failure occurred at an increased frequency; however, with evolution of spinal instrumentation, multilevel debridement could be supported with artificial cages [39–41]. This option was initially met with trepidation, as there was a fear of metalwork infection and disease reoccurrence. Fortunately however in the presence of ATT, metal work was not found to be associated with higher rates of disease recurrence [38, 41]. Implant associated infections are notoriously difficult to treat owing largely to bacterial adherence and biofilm formation but TB is less likely to form biofilms, which explains why instrumentation in spinal TB is largely accepted today [42].

2.5 Anterior-Posterior

Successes with anterior instrumentation led surgeons to perform combined anterior-posterior instrumentation in patients with severe deformity and in those who were predicted to develop it.

Circumferential surgery was particularly important in the paediatric population. Those undergoing anterior debulking were at particular risk of developing severe kyphosis secondary to the continued growth potential of the intact posterior spine [43–45]. Schultz followed up 117 children who were operated on for spinal TB, and reported that the most severe kyphotic abnormalities were seen in those who underwent anterior fusion alone and in those with disease effecting the thoracic vertebrae [46].

The requirement for circumferential surgery was not limited to children. Adults with significant pre-operative kyphosis and large anterior defects were identified as the most likely to develop severe deformity [37, 47]. Studies by Lee et al. (1968) and Kim et al. (1992) suggested anterior arthrodesis was beneficial in the slowing of deformity progression, but Rajasekaran found that with anterior grafting alone, a majority of patients developed graft failure and worsening kyphosis [48–50]. To tackle this problem, Moon advocated for a two-stage approach, using posterior instrumentation to correct and prevent deformity, before performing anterior debridement and reported excellent deformity control [51].

2.6 Posterior Approach

Traditionally the posterior approach was associated with significant instability and inability to access the anterior column safely. Cotrel and Dubousset in 1988 described posterior instrumentation which would allow for 'universal' posterior surgery [52]. In addition, advances in cross-sectional imaging have meant surgeons are better able to plan surgical approaches to diseased tissue, calculate optimal correction, and monitor disease re-occurrence. With modified posterior approaches, the anterior column could be debrided safely and stabilised. Güven was the first to report results following posterior-only surgery in patients with early disease and reported a 98% cure rate at 10 years [53]. There is good evidence in the literature that although modern posterior-only approaches can be more challenging, surgery through a single posterior incision is safer and able to produce equivocal results when compared to traditional anterior-posterior approaches [54–56].

2.7 Conclusion

After the period of surgical re-adjustment in the post-ATT era, techniques for surgery slowly evolved to become as minimally invasive as anatomy allowed. Advancements in medical instrumentation allowed the spine to be instrumented at each level with pedicled screws, enabling the surgeon to stabilise all three columns of the spine. Placement of pedicle screws is still dependent on surgical technique, but with navigation, cross-sectional imaging and robotic surgery, safer screw placement and correction can be achieved. In addition, advancements in material science to replace several segments of the spine and restore normal anatomy are continuing to improve deformity correction and outcome longevity.

Education early diagnosis, and medical intervention is the first line of treatment. Although National TB Programs have achieved cure rates of 95%., the developing world still sees 8–10% of patients presenting with neurological complications as a sequelae of poor host immunity related to nutrition, poor sanitation and drug resistance [57].

Vaccination has historically led to infectious disease control, eradicating smallpox and drastically impacting tetanus and polio spread, and at the time of writing this, they are proving invaluable in the battle against SARS-COV-2 [1, 58]. Despite these advances, the BCG vaccine remains only mildly effective against TB [59]. Sanatoriums were designed to improve host immunity, and even today, reducing the burden of disease associated with TB spine can only be achieved by tackling poverty and improving population level sanitation, but whilst inequality exists, surgery will continue to tackle the consequences onto whom TB spine is bestowed.

References

1. A short history of vaccination-clinical key [Internet]. [cited 2021 Feb 11]. Available from: https://www.clinicalkey.com/#!/content/book/3-s2.0-B9780323357616000018?scrollTo=%23hl0000363
2. Rutkow I. The rise of modern surgery: an overview. In: Sabiston textbook of surgery [Internet]. 20th ed. Philadelphia, PA: Elsevier; 2017 [cited 2021 Feb 11]. p. 1–19. Available from: https://www.clinicalkey.com/#!/content/book/3-s2.0-B9780323299879000011
3. Fleming A. On the antibacterial action of cultures of a penicillium, with special reference to their use in the isolation of B. influenzæ. Br J Exp Pathol. 1929 Jun;10(3):226–36.

4. Gaynes R. The discovery of penicillin–new insights after more than 75 years of clinical use. Emerg Infect Dis. 2017 May;23(5):849–53.
5. Seddon HJ. Pott's paraplegia: prognosis and treatment. BJS Br J Surg. 1935;22(88):769–99.
6. Mercer W. Then and now: the history of skeletal tuberculosis. J R Coll Surg Edinb. 1964;10:243–54.
7. Schatz A, Bugle E, Waksman SA. Streptomycin, a substance exhibiting antibiotic activity against gram-positive and gram-negative bacteria.∗†. Proc Soc Exp Biol Med. 1944 Jan 1;55(1):66–9.
8. Deroy MS, Fisher H. The treatment of tuberculous bone disease by surgical drainage combined with streptomycin. J Bone Joint Surg Am. 1952 Apr;34-A(2):299–330.
9. Cameron J, a. P, Robinson CLN, Robertson DE. The radical treatment of pott's disease and pott's paraplegia by extirpation of the diseased area and anterior spinal fusion. Am Rev Respir Dis. 1962 Jul 1;86(1):76–80.
10. Menard V. Étude pratique sur le mal de Pott [Internet]. Paris: Hachette Livre BNF; [cited 2021 Feb 13]. Available from: https://www.leslibraires.fr/livre/4771677-etude-pratique-sur-le-mal-de-pott-masson-hachette-livre-bnf
11. Müller W. Transperitoneale Freilegung der Wirbelsaule bei Tuberkuloser Spondylitis. Dtsch Ztschr Chir. 1906;85(128)
12. Ito H, Tsuchiya J, Asami G. A new radical operation for Pott's disease. J Bone Jt Surg. 1934;16(3):499–515.
13. Calot: Surlemeilleurtraitementlocaldestuberculoses...–GoogleScholar[Internet].[cited2020Dec 7]. Available from: https://scholar.google.com/scholar_lookup?journal=Acta+Chir+Scand&title=Sur+le+meilleur+traitement+local+des+tuberculoses+des+os,+articulations+et+ganglions+lymphatiques&author=T+Calot&volume=67&publication_year=1930&pages=206-226&
14. Albee F. The Bone-graft operation for tuberculosis of the spine: twenty years' experience. JAMA. 1930;94(19):1467–71.
15. Iseman MD. Tuberculosis therapy: past, present and future. Eur Respir J. 2002 Jul 1;20(36 suppl):87S–94s.
16. Group BMJP. Various combinations of isoniazid with streptomycin or with P.A.S. in the treatment of pulmonary tuberculosis: seventh report to the medical research council. Br Med J. 1955 Feb 19;1(4911):435–45.
17. Ethambutol in the Initial Treatment of Pulmonary Tuberculosis | U. S. Public Health Service Tuberculosis Therapy Trials1,2 | American Review of Respiratory Disease [Internet]. [cited 2020 Dec 9]. Available from: https://www.atsjournals.org/doi/abs/10.1164/arrd.1973.107.2.177
18. Controlled clinical trial of four 6-month regimens of chemotherapy for pulmonary tuberculosis. Second report. Second East African/British Medical Research Council Study. Am Rev Respir Dis. 1976 Sep;114(3):471–5.
19. Konstam PG, Blesovsky A. The ambulant treatment of spinal tuberculosis. BJS Br J Surg. 1962;50(219):26–38.
20. Infections and Tumors of the Spine- ClinicalKey [Internet]. [cited 2020 Dec 7]. Available from: https://www.clinicalkey.com/?scrollTo=%23hl0001181#!/content/book/3-s2.0-B9780323374620000422?scrollTo=%23hl0000860
21. Hodgson AR, Stock FE. Anterior spine fusion for the treatment of tuberculosis of the spine: the operative findings and results of treatment in the first one hundred cases. JBJS. 1960 Mar;42(2):295–310.
22. Wilkinson MC. Chemotherapy of tuberculosis of bones and joints. J Bone Joint Surg Br. 1954 Feb 1;36-B(1):23–35.
23. Friedman B. Chemotherapy of tuberculosis of the spine. JBJS. 1966 Apr;48(3):451–74.
24. Tuli SM. Results of treatment of spinal tuberculosis by 'middle-path' regime. J Bone Joint Surg Br. 1975 Feb;57(1):13–23.
25. Sandher DS, Al-Jibury M, Paton RW, Ormerod LP. Bone and joint tuberculosis: cases in Blackburn between 1988 and 2005. J Bone Joint Surg Br. 2007 Oct;89(10):1379–81.
26. Tuli SM. Tuberculosis of the spine: a historical review. Clin Orthop. 2007 Jul;460:29–38.

27. A 15-year assessment of controlled trials of the management of tuberculosis of the spine in Korea and Hong Kong. Thirteenth report of the medical research council working party on tuberculosis of the spine. J Bone Joint Surg Br. 1998 May;80(3):456–62.
28. Five-year assessment of controlled trials of short-course chemotherapy regimens of 6, 9 or 18 months' duration for spinal tuberculosis in patients ambulatory from the start or undergoing radical surgery. Fourteenth report of the Medical Research Council Working Party on Tuberculosis of the Spine. Int Orthop. 1999;23(2):73–81.
29. A controlled trial of six-month and nine-month regimens of chemotherapy in patients undergoing radical surgery for tuberculosis of the spine in Hong Kong. Tenth report of the medical research council working party on tuberculosis of the spine. Tubercle. 1986 Dec;67(4):243–59.
30. Five-year assessments of controlled trials of ambulatory treatment, debridement and anterior spinal fusion in the management of tuberculosis of the spine. Studies in Bulawayo (Rhodesia) and in Hong Kong. Sixth report of the Medical Research Council Working Party on Tuberculosis of the Spine. J Bone Joint Surg Br 1978;60-B(2):163–77.
31. A controlled trial of anterior spinal fusion and débridement in the surgical management of tuberculosis of the spine in patients on standard chemotherapy: a study in two centres in South Africa. Seventh report of the medical research council working party on tuberculosis of the spine. Tubercle. 1978 Jun;59(2):79–105.
32. Dietze DD, Fessler RG, Jacob RP. Primary reconstruction for spinal infections. J Neurosurg. 1997 Jun;86(6):981–9.
33. Kirkaldy-Willis WH, Thomas TG. Anterior approaches in the diagnosis and treatment of infections of the vertebral bodies. JBJS. 1965 Jan;47(1):87–110.
34. Anterior Fusion of the spine for infective lesions in adults | The Bone & Joint Journal [Internet]. [cited 2020 Dec 9]. Available from: https://online.boneandjoint.org.uk/doi/abs/10.1302/0301-620X.55B4.715
35. Hsu LC, Leong JC. Tuberculosis of the lower cervical spine (C2 to C7). A report on 40 cases. J Bone Joint Surg Br. 1984 Jan;66(1):1–5.
36. Smith GW, Robinson RA. The treatment of certain cervical-spine disorders by anterior removal of the intervertebral disc and interbody fusion. J Bone Joint Surg Am. 1958 Jun;40-A(3):607–24.
37. Khoo LT, Mikawa K, Fessler RG. A surgical revisitation of Pott distemper of the spine. Spine J. 2003 Mar 1;3(2):130–45.
38. Korkusuz F, Islam C, Korkusuz Z. Prevention of postoperative late kyphosis in Pott's disease by anterior decompression and intervertebral grafting. World J Surg. 1997 Jul;21(5):524–8.
39. Yin XH, Liu ZK, Hao D. The reasons and clinical treatments of postoperative relapse of Pott's disease. Medicine (Baltimore) [Internet]. 2018 Sep 28 [cited 2020 Dec 9];97(39). Available from: https://www.ncbi.nlm.nih.gov/pmc/articles/PMC6181606/
40. Oga M, Arizono T, Takasita M, Sugioka Y. Evaluation of the risk of instrumentation as a foreign body in spinal tuberculosis. Clinical and biologic study. Spine. 1993 Oct 1;18(13):1890–4.
41. Yilmaz C, Selek HY, Gürkan I, Erdemli B, Korkusuz Z. Anterior instrumentation for the treatment of spinal tuberculosis. J Bone Joint Surg Am. 1999 Sep;81(9):1261–7.
42. Ha K-Y, Chung Y-G, Ryoo S-J. Adherence and biofilm formation of staphylococcus epidermidis and mycobacterium tuberculosis on various spinal implants. Spine. 2005 Jan 1;30(1):38–43.
43. Rajasekaran S. Buckling collapse of the spine in childhood spinal tuberculosis. Clin Orthop. 2007 Jul;460:86–92.
44. Rajasekaran S. The natural history of post-tubercular kyphosis in children. Radiological signs which predict late increase in deformity. J Bone Joint Surg Br. 2001 Sep;83(7):954–62.
45. Rajasekaran S, Kanna RM, Shetty AP. History of spine surgery for tuberculous spondylodiscitis. Unfallchirurg. 2015 Dec 1;118(1):19–27.
46. Schulitz KP, Kothe R, Leong JC, Wehling P. Growth changes of solidly fused kyphotic bloc after surgery for tuberculosis. Comparison of four procedures. Spine. 1997 May 15;22(10):1150–5.
47. Kim N-H, Lee H-M, Suh J-S. Magnetic Resonance Imaging for the Diagnosis of Tuberculous Spondylitis. Spine. 1994 Nov;19(21):2451–5.

48. Kim BJ, Ko HS, Lim Y, Seo JG, Zoo SK, Jeon TH. The clinical study of the tuberculous spondylitis. J Korean Orthop Assoc. 1993;28:2221–32.
49. Lee EY, Hahn MS. A study of influences of the anterior intervertebral fusion upon the correctability of kyphosis in the tuberculous spondylitis. J Korean Orthop Assoc. 1968;3:31–40.
50. Rajasekaran S, Soundarapandian S. Progression of the kyphosis in tuberculosis of the spine treated by anterior arthrodesis. J Bone Jt Surg AM. 1987;69:503–9.
51. Moon MS, Woo YK, Lee KS, Ha KY, Kim SS, Sun DH. Posterior instrumentation and anterior interbody fusion for tuberculous kyphosis of dorsal and lumbar spines. Spine. 1995 Sep 1;20(17):1910–6.
52. Cotrel Y, Dubousset J, Guillaumat M. New universal instrumentation in spinal surgery. Clin Orthop. 1980;227:10–23.
53. Güven O, Kumano K, Yalçin S, Karahan M, Tsuji S. A single stage posterior approach and rigid fixation for preventing kyphosis in the treatment of spinal tuberculosis. Spine. 1994 May 1;19(9):1039–43.
54. Zhang HQ, Li JS, Zhao SS, Shao YX, Liu SH, Gao Q, et al. Surgical management for thoracic spinal tuberculosis in the elderly: posterior only versus combined posterior and anterior approaches. Arch Orthop Trauma Surg. 2012 Dec 1;132(12):1717–23.
55. Liu Z, Zhang P, Li W, Xu Z, Wang X. Posterior-only vs. combined posterior-anterior approaches in treating lumbar and lumbosacral spinal tuberculosis: a retrospective study with minimum 7-year follow-up. J Orthop Surg. 2020 Mar 10;15(1):99.
56. Wu W, Lyu J, Liu X, Luo F, Hou T, Zhou Q, et al. Surgical treatment of thoracic spinal tuberculosis: a multicenter retrospective study. World Neurosurg. 2018 Feb 1;(110):e842–50.
57. Kurz SG, Furin JJ, Bark CM. Drug resistant tuberculosis: challenges and progress. Infect Dis Clin N Am. 2016 Jun;30(2):509–22.
58. Oxford–AstraZeneca COVID-19 vaccine efficacy–The Lancet [Internet]. [cited 2021 Feb 14]. Available from: https://www.thelancet.com/journals/lancet/article/PIIS0140-6736(20)32623-4/fulltext?fbclid=IwAR39cr4iOmVyctpuoZ5JdxytsnRdYm6lwsO24Fhb3refju1PcHLC7bTitSs
59. Andersen P, Doherty TM. The success and failure of BCG–implications for a novel tuberculosis vaccine. Nat Rev Microbiol. 2005 Aug;3(8):656–62.

Chapter 3
Epidemiology of Tuberculosis of Spine

Deepak Neradi and Dilip K. Sengupta

Abstract TB has been considered as most lethal disease globally for 3 consecutive years by WHO. It is an age-old disease affecting humans since thousands of years. TB (tuberculosis) typically affects lungs, but it can spread to other sites and cause tuberculosis at extrapulmonary sites (1–3%). Spinal TB accounts for 50% of extrapulmonary TB cases with most common area affected being thoracolumbar junction. Kyphotic spinal deformity is most commonly due to tuberculosis. This chapter deals with epidemiology of TB and spinal TB. We provided data of TB from Western and Asian regions. Incidence and prevalence of spinal TB, MDR (multidrug resistant), and XDR-TB (extensively drug-resistant tuberculosis) in various groups of population are provided.

Keywords Spinal TB · Incidence · Prevalence · Epidemiology · WHO guidelines Success rate

3.1 Introduction

Tuberculosis is a disease of poverty, economic distress, vulnerability, stigma, and discrimination [1]. This disease has almost affected one fourth of the world's population. Globally 8.9–11 million people fell ill with TB, and 1.2 million deaths were noted in HIV-negative TB patients in 2019 WHO labelled few countries as high TB burden countries [2]. Almost 87% of world TB cases belongs to these 30 high TB burden countries. In developing countries, Spinal tuberculosis affects children, whereas in developed nations, it affects elderly people [3]. Spinal TB leads to deformity depending on location and number of vertebrae destroyed. In TB affecting the

D. Neradi
Department of Orthopaedics, PGIMER, Chandigarh, India

D. K. Sengupta (✉)
Center for Scoliosis & Advanced Spine Surgery, Dallas, TX, USA

S. S. Dhatt, V. Kumar (eds.), *Tuberculosis of the Spine*,
https://doi.org/10.1007/978-981-16-9495-0_3

thoracic spine, the most common deformity is kyphosis. Although chemotherapy alone is sufficient to cure the disease, in 20% of patients there is an increase of kyphotic deformity by 10° or more [4]. Adults have lesser deformity at presentation and lesser increase of deformity when compared to children. Incidence of multicentric non-contagious vertebral tuberculosis is 71%. Tuberculosis is the most common opportunistic infection in people infected with HIV worldwide [5].

3.2 TB: Global Perspective

Although TB is a preventable and curable disease, the disease is not yet controlled in a global perspective. Many factors are responsible for this, including increasing population in poor countries, drug abuse, increasing HIV infection, etc. Migration of people to developed countries leads to increase in number of cases in these nations. International migrants increased from 173 million in 2000 to 244 million in 2015, according to United Nations report.

According to WHO's global TB report 2020 [6], TB is one of the top 10 leading causes of death worldwide. It is the leading cause of death from a single infectious agent (ranking above HIV/AIDS). According to this report, the estimated incidence of new cases of TB was 10.0 million (range 8.9–11.0 million), in 2019. In this estimate around 90% of people suffering from TB are adults; males (56%) are affected more than females (32%). Children (<15 years) accounted for 12% of cases. Among the affected, 8.2% were living with HIV. The TB incidences were highest in WHO regions of South-East Asia (44%), followed by Africa (25%), and the Western Pacific (18%), the Americas (2.9%), and Europe (2.5%). Eight countries accounted for two thirds of the global total. Nationwide incidences were highest in India (26%), followed by Indonesia (8.5%), China (8.4%), the Philippines (6.0%), Pakistan (5.7%), Nigeria (4.4%), Bangladesh (3.6%), and South Africa (3.6%) [6]. In 2019, deaths related to tuberculosis were estimated to be 1.2 million in HIV-negative patients and 0.2 million in HIV-positive patients [6].

Tuberculosis can be treated and controlled only if the cases are reported. Under reporting and under diagnosis are the two major causes which hinder disease control. In 2019, the incidence of new cases was 10 million, and people reported as newly diagnosed were 7.1 million showing a large global gap. 50% of this global gap was shared by only five countries, i.e., India (17%), Nigeria (11%), Indonesia (10%), Pakistan (8%), and the Philippines (7%). Also, COVID-19 pandemic affected diagnosis and management of tuberculosis adding burden on disease control. Intensive efforts are mandatory to address under reporting and under diagnosis and reduce the global gap [6].

The incidence of reported tuberculosis globally is on the rise. The reported incidence was 5.7–5.8 million annually during the period 2009–2012, 6.4 million in 2017, 7.0 million in 2018, and 7.1 million in 2019. Most of the increase since 2013 was reported from India and Indonesia, the two countries that rank first and second worldwide. There is an increase in 74% of TB notification rate for newly diagnosed cases in India from 2013 to 2019. In Indonesia, notifications rose from 0.33 million in 2015 to 0.56 million in 2019 (+69% increase) [6]. The silver lining in the horizon is that despite increasing incidence of TB globally, with increasing global population, the actual "incidence rate" of TB (incidence per 100.000 population) is decreasing. The incidence rate of TB in 2019 was 130 per 100,000 population, which includes new and relapse cases, whereas in 2015 it was 142 per 100,000 showing a 9% global reduction of incidence rate. But the reduction in incidence still falls short of WHO milestone for control of TB, discussed later [6].

Control of TB depends not only on diagnosis and reporting of the cases, but treatment coverage, which is defined as "the number of people notified and treated divided by the estimated incidence." Globally, TB treatment coverage increased from 59% (range, 52–67%) in 2015, to 69% (range, 62–77%) in 2018, to 71% (range, 64–79%) in 2019. Four World Health Organization (WHO) regions achieved treatment coverage levels above 75%: the Americas, Europe, South-East Asia, and the Western Pacific. Brazil, China, the Russian Federation, and Thailand are the high burden countries to achieve treatment coverage >80% in 2019, while Central African Republic and Nigeria cannot achieve a coverage of 50% [6]. According to WHO report on TB in 2016 [7], on average, 60% of the East African countries (EAC) has TB treatment coverage. This means that 40% of the population of the EAC has hardly any access to TB treatment. The East African countries with highest and lowest rates of treatment coverage are Rwanda (84%) and Tanzania (37%).

Though the incidence of extrapulmonary tuberculosis (EPTB) is low (3%), there is no significant reduction in its incidence rate when compared to pulmonary TB. In a Korean study the proportion of EPTB cases notified during the period of 2005–2007 was 14%, and it was increased to 20% during the period of 2010–2013 [8]. In another study from Europe, proportion of EPTB cases increased from 16.4% in 2002 to 22.4% in 2011 [9]. Out of the 3% of extrapulmonary TB cases, 10% are of skeletal TB, out of which spinal TB cases make around 50%. The most common location of spinal TB cases is thoracolumbar junction followed by lumbar and then cervical spine. In a review article from India in 2020, Garg and Goyal [10] reported that the most common form of extrapulmonary tuberculosis is spinal tuberculosis accounting to 1–2% of all cases of TB. Among all TB cases, musculoskeletal TB comprises ten percent of which half of them are spinal tuberculosis cases. Spinal TB causes neurological complications, the incidence of which ranges from 10 to 41%.

3.3 TB: US Perspective

In 2014, the incidence rate of TB in the United States was reported as 2.96/100000 people [11]. According to an epidemiological study in the USA conducted during 2002–2011 [12], a total of 75,858 patients were diagnosed with TB. Out of these patients, 2789 were diagnosed as spinal TB. The incidence reduced from 0.07/100000 in 2002 to 0.05/100000 in 2011. The median age of patients was 51 years, out of which 61% were males. There was no difference of incidence among different races. Comorbidities associated with TB patients were hypertension (28.6%), diabetes (11.6%), malnutrition (11.6%), weight loss (11.4%), paralysis (8.1%), and HIV (4%). 22.2% of spinal TB patients had to undergo surgery, out of which 55.6% were males and the median age at surgery was 52 years. The most common location was thoracolumbar region (61.9%). 50% of the patients who underwent surgery were instrumented for ≥3 segments. Posterior approach was used in 38.9%, anterior approach in 26.6%, and combined approach in 34.5% patients. 38.8% patients developed at least one complication during their hospital stay. According to data published by US CDC [13] in 2019 from 60 jurisdictions, the total number of reported TB cases was 8916 with an incidence rate of 2.7/100000. The data also showed that 13 million estimated people in the USA are living with latent TB. The estimated incidence and mortality rate of TB in America region was 0.29 million and 0.03 million, respectively, in 2019. Though the rate of TB in America region is lower among the world, cases are still increasing in this region; this is because of increasing trend of cases in Brazil.

3.4 WHO Plans for Control of TB: WHO End TB Strategy and UN Sustainable Development Goals (SDGs)

In September 2018, many nations assembled at United Nation for a high-level meeting on tuberculosis. Heads of all state members and other leaders committed to end this top infectious disease in the world. This meeting aims at treating at least 40 million people and providing TB preventive treatment for 30 million people from 2018 to 2022. This meeting also aimed in covering 6 million TB people with HIV, 4 million children aged under 5 years who are household contacts of pulmonary TB patients, and 20 million household contacts in older age groups. This meeting also discussed about funding 13 billion US dollars per year for TB management by 2022 and 2 billion US dollars per year for research in TB. After this meeting, the number of people treated for TB increased with over 14 million in 2018 and 2019. When it comes to the provision of TB preventive treatment to the people, there is an increase of 3 million from 2015 to 2019. In 2020, we are at half-way in achieving 2022 targets. Due to COVID-19, there was a sharp drop in TB notification in 2020 indicating its impact on TB services. According to WHO modelling and analysis, 50% reduction in detection over 3 months will lead to 0.4 million more people dying from TB. WHO Director General initiative "Find. Treat. All. #End TB" is being implemented in collaboration with Stop TB partnership and Global Fund to fight AIDS, TB, and malaria. This initiative aims at evaluating 2.9 million population of TB lacking quality care.

During the period of 2014–2015, all member states adopted WHO End TB Strategy and UN Sustainable Development Goals (SDGs) to end the TB epidemic by 2030. This targets to decrease TB incidence by 80%, and TB deaths by 90% by 2030, compared to that in 2015. According to this strategy global reduction of incidence should have been 20% from 2015 to 2020. But globally we achieved only 9% reduction till 2019 compared to 2015. South-East Asia region shows a reduction of 8.7%, Western Pacific regions show a reduction of 6.1%, but the incidence is increasing in the WHO regions of America. According to End TB Strategy and SDG set goals, the decrease in TB-related death from 2015 to 2020 should have been 35%. But globally the reduction achieved so far is only 14% from 2015 to 2019. The reduction in death rate in America region is 6.1%, and in South-East Asia Region is 10% [6].

3.5 TB and HIV and Other Immunosuppressive Disease and Conditions

HIV infection strongly predisposes people to develop spinal TB. According to 2016 WHO list, South Africa ranks top in HIV-TB coinfection with an incidence of 834 cases per 100,000 for total TB cases and 8 to 16 cases per 100,000 for spinal TB cases. The influence of HIV contributed to this high incidence in South Africa. While only 1–2% of TB patients without HIV develop spinal TB, 30% of people with HIV co-infection develop spinal TB [4]. Spinal TB patients with HIV co-infection show greater volume of epidural abscess and lower incidence of vertebral body collapse. ART (Anti-Retroviral Therapy) decrease tuberculosis risk by 65%. Globally, patients with TB and HIV co-infection were 69% in 2019; Africa stands top in TB-HIV co-infection with 86% of TB patients having documented HIV test [14]. Studies mentioned that tuberculosis infection among HIV patients was 10% [15], of which 25% patients had only extrapulmonary disease and spinal tuberculosis accounted for 3.6%.

Population with immunosuppressive diseases or conditions are more susceptible to develop tubercular infection. In a study published in 2004 [16] evaluating SLE patients, the incidence of TB was found to be 3.6%, out of which 45% had extrapulmonary disease. Other studies also demonstrated high incidence of TB in SLE patients [17, 18]. This is because of high cumulative dose of prednisolone. In another epidemiological study evaluating TB and diabetes [19], it showed diabetes increases TB risk by three times. Contrast to other immunocompromised states, in diabetes extrapulmonary disease is less common.

3.6 Diagnosis and Reporting of TB

There are two relatively frequently used indirect methods to diagnose TB infection, tuberculin skin test (Mantoux test) and Interferon Gamma Release Assays. Mantoux test has no diagnostic value as it has low specificity but has some use in latent infection. Other two investigations used in latent TB are interferon-γ (IFN- γ) and enzyme-linked immunosorbent assays. A typical histological feature of TB includes caseous necrosis, epithelioid granuloma, and Langhans giant cells, which may be present in 72%–97% of cases. All these are indirect tests. The most definitive diagnosis of TB involves demonstration of bacteria. Bacteriological diagnosis from the infected tissue may be obtained by AFB culture in 4 weeks, BACTEC culture in 2 weeks, and Gene Xpert MTB/RIF as quickly as in 90mins. WHO in 2017 recommended the use of Xpert MTB/RIF Ultra which has better detection rate in specimens with low number of bacilli. All countries are aiming to increase bacterial confirmation using WHO-recommended diagnostic tests as initial test. This becomes more important to the diagnosis and control of drug-resistant tuberculosis. According to WHO guidelines, detection of Multidrug Resistance and Rifampicin Resistance (MDR/RR) TB requires confirmation of mycobacterium from the specimen and molecular tests to detect drug resistance. India developed three new molecular tests called Truenat MTB, MTB Plus, and MTB-RIF Dx, which can be used in the health care system same as Xpert MTB/RIF and Xpert Ultra.

3.7 Management of Spinal Tuberculosis and Mortality/ Morbidity

WHO End TB Strategy and UN Sustainable Development Goals (SDGs) involve not only diagnosis and reporting of TB, but increase the access of population towards treatment of TB. Management of spinal tuberculosis includes only chemotherapy, debridement surgery, or radical debridement along with fusion. The Medical Research Council of UK compared these three modalities and found no significant differences in functional outcomes. After good results of Anti-Tubercular Therapy (ATT) with drugs alone, Tuli suggested employing “middle path regimen” where patients are treated with chemotherapy and surgery is done only in certain scenarios [20]. Treatment success rate for newly diagnosed people was 85%, and for MDR-TB it was 57% in 2018. Mortality rate of pulmonary TB patients without treatment was 70% in smear positive cases and 20% in smear negative patients. According to the latest report, TB treatment coverage was increased from 59% in 2015 to 71% in 2019. WHO America, Europe, South-East Asia, and Western Pacific regions achieved levels more than 75%. Brazil, China, Russian Federation, and Thailand stand top among the 30 high burden countries in regard to treatment coverage.

3.8 Drug Resistance

Emergence of drug resistance is the major factor hindering control and eradication of tuberculosis. In RR-TB there is resistance only for Rifampicin, and Multidrug Resistance (MDR) is a condition where TB has become resistant to at least two first-line drugs, isoniazid (INH) and Rifampicin. Extensively Drug Resistance (XDR) TB is a condition where there is resistance for fluoroquinolones and second-line injectable drugs along with multidrug resistance. In 2016, 0.6 million new rifampicin-resistant (RR) tuberculosis were reported out of which 0.49 million were multidrug resistance. In 2017, rifampicin resistance was seen in 0.56 million patients, and 82% of them had multidrug resistance. In 2019, about half million people were suffering with rifampicin resistance out of which 78% had multidrug resistance. India (24%) ranks number one, and China (13%) ranks second regarding MDR-TB cases. It was estimated that 9.7% of patients with multidrug resistance had extensively drug-resistant TB (XDR-TB). Multidrug resistance is seen in 4.1% of new TB cases and 19% of previously treated cases in 2016; this number is increased to 3.3% of new TB cases and 17.7% of previously treated cases in 2019. MDR strains are found more in previously treated cases than fresh cases, males are more affected with MDR strains than females (2:1), and farmers accounted for higher percentage of MDR strains (61.6%) [21]. Pyrazinamide showed lowest resistance ratio among first-line drugs with isoniazid and Rifampicin being highest. Ofloxacin showed the highest resistance ratio among second-line drugs. *The reason for the emergence of MDR-TB* strains was attributed to population migration, antibiotic abuse, drug abuse, antibiotic abuse, and reduced compliance. In China, there is an increase of multidrug resistance cases from 1993 to 2000 which remain stable till 2006 and then decreased thereafter. This decline is due to *new diagnostic techniques, increased TB treatment coverage, and increased support from government* towards MDR-TB patients.

Majority of patients with multidrug resistance had resistance to fluoroquinolones due to their extensive use in other respiratory tract infections [22]. In India, 44.8% of patients with multidrug resistance had resistance to at least one second-line drug; this is much higher than China (20.7%) according to this survey. According to WHO report in 2015, 9.7% of MDR-TB patients showed extensive drug resistance (XDR-TB). In India 0.3% to 60% proportion of MDR-TB cases were reported as XDR-TB; all are previously treated cases [23].

3.9 Treatment of Drug-Resistant TB

Treatment success rate in multidrug resistance patients was 77%, and in XDR-TB patients it was 27% in an Asian study [24]. Global treatment success rate for MDR-TB according to latest data is 57%. In countries with high treatment coverage for multidrug resistance (Ethiopia, Kazakhstan, and Myanmar), the success rate is ≥75%.

3.10 Prevention of TB

BCG is the only available vaccine that prevents severe form of tuberculosis in children, but it is not effective in adults. Among countries adopting BCG as part of their standard immunization program, 87 countries reported ≥90% coverage. WHO recommends TB preventive treatment for patients with HIV, family members of confirmed pulmonary TB patients, and clinically risk groups. TB preventive options include 3 months of isoniazid and rifapentine (3HP), 3 months rifampicin and isoniazid (3HR), isoniazid and rifapentine (1HP) for 1 month, daily rifampicin for 4 months (4R), and daily dose of isoniazid (6H) for 6 months or longer.

3.11 Summary

Tuberculosis shows decreasing trends when compared to past years, but the world is still suffering of TB and we couldn't end this disease. Majority of patients belong to WHO regions of South-East Asia (44%), Africa (25%), Western Pacific (18%), and the USA (2.9%). India ranks number one in the world by sharing 26% of global TB burden. WHO designed End TB Strategy to decrease its incidence by 80% and deaths by 90% by 2030 when compared to 2015. UN high-level meeting was held in 2018 which aims to treat 40 million people during 2018–2022 and to provide preventive treatment for 30 million people. Many high TB burden countries are not on the track in achieving 2020 milestones of End TB Strategy. According to the milestone 2020, there should be 20% global reduction of TB incidence when compared to 2015. But we achieved only 9% of reduction by 2019. Only WHO European region is on track in achieving 2020 milestones. Problems in achieving these milestones include emergence of MDR-TB, increasing HIV patients, global migration of patients, and recently COVID pandemic. Due to COVID pandemic many of the financial and human resources had to be allocated from TB program. In 2020, all member states of WHO adopted a global strategy for TB research and innovation to eliminate this epidemic by 2030.

References

1. Janse Van Rensburg A, Dube A, Curran R, Ambaw F, Murdoch J, Bachmann M, et al. Comorbidities between tuberculosis and common mental disorders: a scoping review of epidemiological patterns and person-centred care interventions from low-to-middle income and BRICS countries. Infect Dis Poverty. 2020 Jan 15;9(1):4.
2. High burden for TB list [Internet]. Available from: https://www.who.int/tb/publications/global_report/high_tb_burdencountrylists2016-2020summary.pdf?ua=1
3. Byng-Maddick R, Noursadeghi M. Does tuberculosis threaten our ageing populations? BMC Infect Dis [Internet]. 2016 Mar 11 [cited 2021 Jan 21];16. Available from: https://www.ncbi.nlm.nih.gov/pmc/articles/PMC4787032/
4. Garg RK, Somvanshi DS. Spinal tuberculosis: a review. J Spinal Cord Med. 2011 Sep;34(5):440–54.
5. Castro KG. Tuberculosis as an opportunistic disease in persons infected with human immunodeficiency virus. Clin Infect Dis Off Publ Infect Dis Soc Am. 1995 Aug;21(Suppl 1):S66–71.
6. World Health Organization. Global tuberculosis report 2020 [Internet]. 2020 [cited 2020 Dec 22]. Available from: https://apps.who.int/iris/bitstream/handle/10665/336069/9789240013131-eng.pdf

7. World Health Organization. Global tuberculosis report 2016 [Internet]. 2016 [cited 2020 Dec 22]. Available from: http://www.who.int/tb/publications/global_report/gtbr2016_executive_summary.pdf?ua¼1
8. Lee D. Annual report on the notified tuberculosis patients in Korea. Cheongju Korea Cent Dis Control Prev. 2013;
9. Sandgren A, Hollo V, van der Werf MJ. Extrapulmonary tuberculosis in the European Union and European Economic Area, 2002 to 2011. Euro Surveill Bull Eur Sur Mal Transm Eur Commun Dis Bull. 2013 Mar;21:18(12).
10. Garg D, Goyal V. Spinal Tuberculosis Treatment: An Enduring Bone of Contention. Ann Indian Acad Neurol Jul-Aug. 2020;23(4):441–8.
11. Centers for Disease Control and Prevention: Tuberculosis (TB) Data and Statistics. Centers for Disease Control and Prevention. [Internet]. 2016. Available from: https://www.cdc.gov/tb/statistics/default.htm
12. Ramos RD la G, Goodwin CR, Abu-Bonsrah N, Bydon A, Witham TF, Wolinsky J-P, et al. The epidemiology of spinal tuberculosis in the United States: an analysis of 2002–2011 data. J Neurosurg Spine SPI 2017 Apr 1;26(4):507–512.
13. Centers for Disease Control and Prevention: Tuberculosis (TB) Data and Statistics. Centers for Disease Control and Prevention. [Internet]. 2019. Available from: https://www.cdc.gov/tb/publications/factsheets/statistics/tbtrends.htm
14. Joint United Nations Programme on HIV/AIDS (UNAIDS). UNAIDS data 2017. Geneva UNAIDS; 2017. p. 1–248.
15. Sterling TR, Pham PA, Chaisson RE. HIV infection-related tuberculosis: clinical manifestations and treatment. Clin Infect Dis Off Publ Infect Dis Soc Am. 2010 May;50(Suppl 3):S223–30.
16. Sayarlioglu M, Inanc M, Kamali S, Cefle A, Karaman O, Gul A, et al. Tuberculosis in Turkish patients with systemic lupus erythematosus: increased frequency of extrapulmonary localization. Lupus. 2004;13(4):274–8.
17. Bhattacharya PK, Jamil M, Roy A, Talukdar KK. SLE and Tuberculosis: A Case Series and Review of Literature. J Clin Diagn Res JCDR. 2017 Feb;11(2):OR01–3.
18. Balbi GGM, Machado-Ribeiro F, Marques CDL, Signorelli F, Levy RA. The interplay between tuberculosis and systemic lupus erythematosus. Curr Opin Rheumatol. 2018 Jul;30(4):395–402.
19. Harries AD, Satyanarayana S, Kumar AMV, Nagaraja SB, Isaakidis P, Malhotra S, et al. Epidemiology and interaction of diabetes mellitus and tuberculosis and challenges for care: a review. Public Health Action. 2013 Nov 4;3(Suppl 1):S3–9.
20. Tuli SM. Results of treatment of spinal tuberculosis by "middle-path" regime. J Bone Joint Surg Br. 1975 Feb;57(1):13–23.
21. Huang H, Ding N, Yang T, Li C, Jia X, Wang G, et al. Cross-sectional Whole-genome Sequencing and Epidemiological Study of Multidrug-resistant Mycobacterium tuberculosis in China. Clin Infect Dis Off Publ Infect Dis Soc Am. 2019 Jul 18;69(3):405–13.
22. Lu Z, Jiang W, Zhang J, Lynn HS, Chen Y, Zhang S, et al. Drug resistance and epidemiology characteristics of multidrug-resistant tuberculosis patients in 17 provinces of China. PLoS One. 2019;14(11):e0225361.
23. Prasad R, Singh A, Balasubramanian V, Gupta N. Extensively drug-resistant tuberculosis in India: Current evidence on diagnosis & management. Indian J Med Res. 2017 Mar;145(3):271–93.
24. Li Q, Shi CX, Lu M, Wu L, Wu Y, Wang M, et al. Treatment outcomes of multidrug-resistant tuberculosis in Hangzhou, China, 2011 to 2015. Medicine (Baltimore) [Internet]. 2020;99(30) Available from: https://journals.lww.com/md-journal/Fulltext/2020/07240/Treatment_outcomes_of_multidrug_resistant.59.aspx
25. Viney K, Islam T, Hoa NB, Morishita F, Lönnroth K. The Financial Burden of Tuberculosis for Patients in the Western-Pacific Region. Trop Med Infect Dis [Internet]. 2019; Jun 17 [cited 2021 Jan 21];4(2). Available from: https://www.ncbi.nlm.nih.gov/pmc/articles/PMC6631110/

Chapter 4
Anatomy and Pathophysiology of TB Spine

Chiman Kumari, Daisy Sahni, Rohit Jindal, and Amit Salaria

Abstract The vertebral column, a curved structure consists of 24 individual vertebrae along with intervertebral discs, sacrum (5 fused vertebrae) and coccyx (4 fused vestigial elements). The vertebral canal runs posterior to the bodies of articulated vertebrae, which transmits and protects the spinal cord, spinal nerves along with their coverings and vasculature. There are a series of intervertebral foraminae between the adjacent vertebrae which transmit the spinal nerves and associated vessels. The column receives its blood supply through segmental arteries. The veins form valveless plexuses external and internal to vertebral canal. Any pathology can spread to the vertebrae because of their close contact with the valveless plexuses. The anterior aspect of the column is related to clinically important structures and anterior longitudinal ligament which forms a fascial plane with the pre-vertebral, endo-thoracic fascia and subperitoneal areolar tissue of the posterior abdominal wall. Infection may spread along this fascial plane.

Tuberculosis in humans is caused primarily by *Mycobacterium tuberculosis*, an obligate aerobe. The *Mycobacterium* may remain dormant for a long period of time following primary infection. Tuberculosis of spine is caused by blood-borne spread from the primary site which can be pulmonary, gastrointestinal, or urogenital. The interaction of tubercle bacilli and the host defenses results in local tissue destruction and characteristic pathologic findings of tuberculosis. The spine involvement is characterized by local kyphosis, paravertebral abscesses and involvement of spinal cord.

Keywords Anatomy · Fascial plane · Tuberculosis · Pathophysiology
Plexuses · Spine

C. Kumari · D. Sahni (✉)
Department of Anatomy, PGIMER, Chandigarh, India
e-mail: sahni.daisy@pgimer.edu.in

R. Jindal
Government Medical College and Hospital, Chandigarh, India

A. Salaria
PGIMER, Chandigarh, India

S. S. Dhatt, V. Kumar (eds.), *Tuberculosis of the Spine*,
https://doi.org/10.1007/978-981-16-9495-0_4

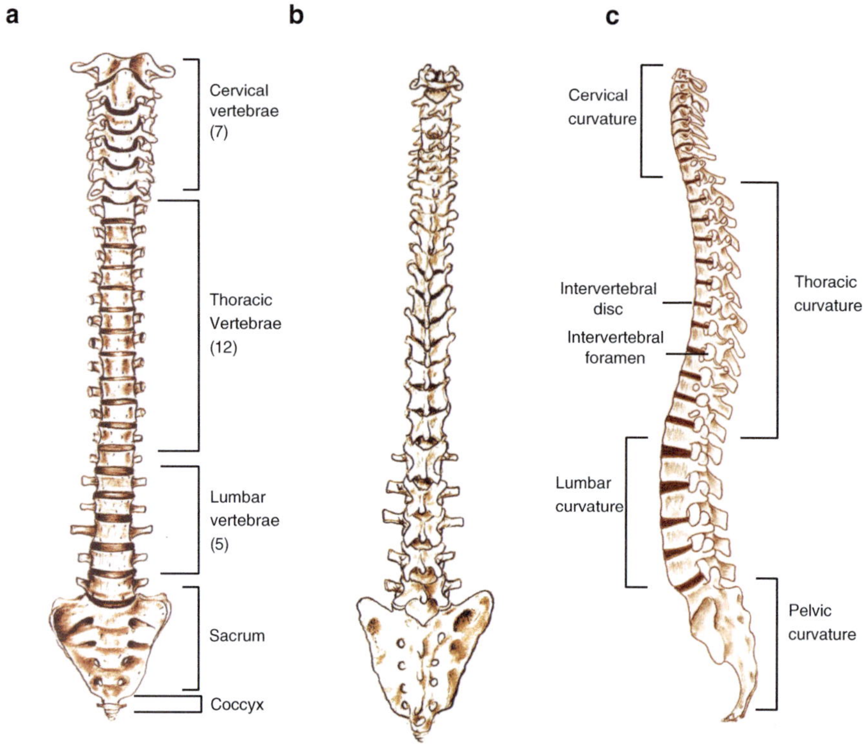

Fig. 4.1 Different views and curvatures of vertebral column (**a**) Ventral, (**b**) Dorsal and (**c**) Lateral

The architecture of the human spine makes it an ideal candidate for balance, mobility and weight transmission of the human body, besides providing protection to the spinal cord lying within the vertebral canal. The spine consists of 33 bony vertebrae (Fig. 4.1) supported by ligaments, joints and muscles. The total length of the adult vertebral column is approximately 60 cm in females and 70 cm in males [1]. The intervertebral discs contribute about one-quarter of its total length [2].

4.1 Structure of a Typical Vertebra

A typical vertebra consists of a ventral body which is linked posteriorly to the neural arch by pedicles on each side. A spinous process projects backwards from the neural arch and on each side there is a transverse process with superior and inferior articular processes, which articulate with similar processes of the adjacent vertebrae.

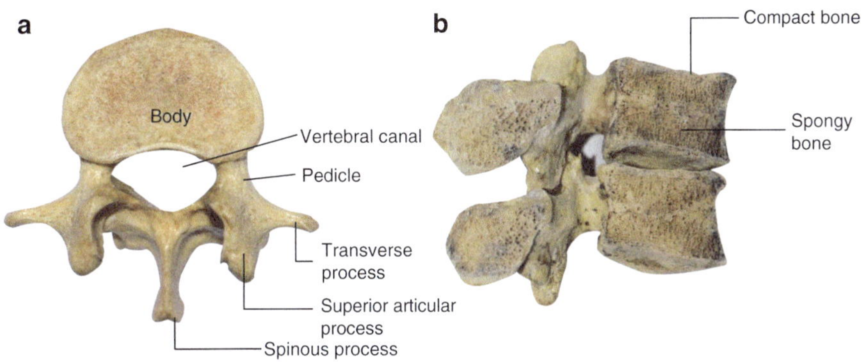

Fig. 4.2 (**a**) Components of a typical vertebra (superior view). (**b**) Sagittal section through two consecutive vertebrae showing inner spongy bone enclosed within compact bone

4.2 Characteristics of Vertebra

The body of a vertebra is composed of vascular spongy bone enclosed by compact bone (Fig. 4.2). The various components of the neural arch vary in size and position in different regions of the vertebral column. The transverse processes of the first cervical vertebra are easily palpable below the mastoid process on both sides. The size of the thoracic transverse processes decreases cranio-caudally and the lumbar transverse processes are comparatively more prominent. The spinous processes are increasingly oblique till mid-thoracic region and overlap with each other and are comparatively horizontal in the lumbar region. The gap between adjacent laminae is maximum between C1-C2, L4–5 and L5-S1 [2].

The anterior aspect of the vertebral column is related to important structures which may be affected in any lesion of vertebrae; in the cervical region, the retropharyngeal spaces while in the thoracic region various structures of the posterior mediastinum can be involved. Similarly, anterior longitudinal ligaments form a fascial plane with the pre-vertebral, endo-thoracic fascia and subperitoneal areolar tissue of the posterior abdominal wall; infection can spread along this fascial plane. Structures of posterior abdominal wall and pelvic cavity are closely related to the vertebral column, which may directly influence the anatomical stability in any pathological changes.

4.3 Vertebral Canal

Vertebral canal extends from the foramen magnum to the sacral hiatus. Its anterior wall is formed by the vertebral bodies, intervening intervertebral discs, and the posterior longitudinal ligaments; the posterior wall is formed by laminae and

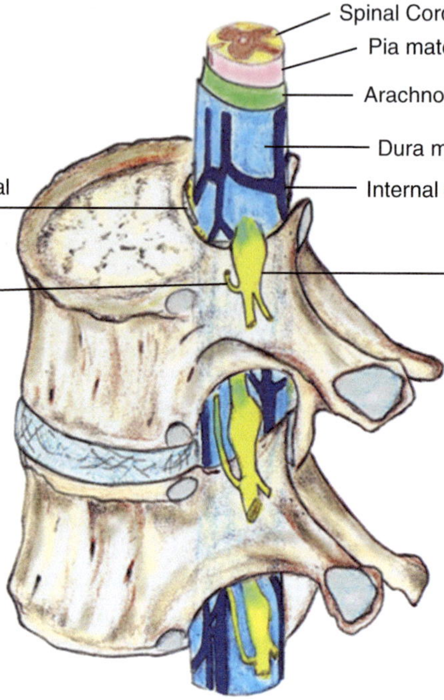

Fig. 4.3 Vertebral canal with its contents

ligamentum flava. Lateral walls consist of intervertebral foraminae. The canal accommodates the spinal cord, cauda equina, meninges, cerebrospinal fluid, adipose tissue, and blood vessels (Fig. 4.3). The shape of the canal in transverse section differs in different regions.

4.4 Intervertebral Foramen (Fig 4.4a, b)

The oval intervertebral foramen is bounded anteriorly by the body and intervening intervertebral disc, above and below by the pedicles of cranial and caudal vertebrae, respectively, and behind by the inferior and superior articular processes of the cranial and caudal vertebrae along with their joints. The foraminae are smaller in the cervical and upper thoracic regions and the size increases caudally. The foramen at L5/S1 level is the narrowest. Structures passing through intervertebral foramen include the spinal nerve trunk along with the meningeal coverings, branches of segmental vessels, and the spino-vertebral nerve (may be more than one). The dura mater fuses with the epineurium of the spinal nerve within or slightly beyond the intervertebral foramen.

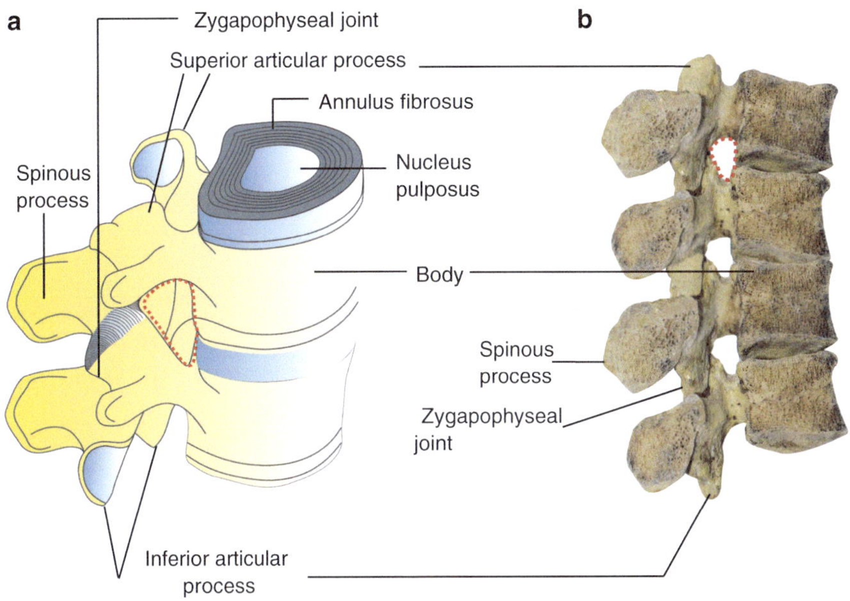

Fig. 4.4 (**a**) Right posterolateral view showing intervertebral foramen (dotted red line). (**b**) Longitudinal section along a part of the vertebral column showing intervertebral foramen from its medial side

4.5 Vertebral Curvatures

The adult vertebral column consists of four sagittal curvatures (cervical, thoracic, lumbar and sacral; Fig. 4.1) in contrast to only two primary curvatures in foetuses. The secondary curvatures (cervical and lumbar) develop as a result of bipedalism as the child grows. The cervical curvature extends to the level of T2 vertebra. The lumbar lordoisis in an adult extends from T12 to sacral promontary [2] and its most anterior point is at the level of L3-L4 or a little below. The anterior concavity of the primary curvatures is due to greater height of the posterior part of the body of vertebrae while the anterior convexity of secondary curvatures is due to the greater anterior height of the intervertebral discs [3].

4.6 Line of Gravity

In the erect posture, the line of gravity extends along the dens of atlas at the level of external auditory meati, anterior to the body of T2, through the centre of the body of T12, posterior part of body of L5, anterior to the sacrum and via hip joints to the lower limbs. The line of gravity may slightly vary in different individuals and with locomotion. The size of the vertebral bodies increases cranio-caudally till S2, where the weight of the body is transmitted from the vertebral column to the pelvic girdle. The articular processes of cervical vertebrae also take part in transmission of body weight [3].

4.7 Joints and Ligaments in the Vertebral Column (Tables 4.1 and 4.2)

The adjacent vertebral bodies are united by anterior and posterior longitudinal ligaments and the fibrocartilaginous intervertebral discs. The surfaces of the body of adjacent vertebrae are covered by sheets of hyaline cartilage (vertebral endplates).

4.8 Intervertebral Disc

The intervertebral discs form bonds between adjacent vertebrae from C2 to sacrum. Each disc consists of an outer fibrous ring—the annulus fibrosus and the inner core—the nucleus pulposus. The annulus fibrosus is made up of fibro-cartilage and collagen. The nucleus pulposus is derived from the embryonic notochord and is

Table 4.1 Ligaments of the vertebral column

Ligament	Attachment	Extent
Anterior longitudinal ligament	• Anterior surface of body of vertebra. • Superficial fibres extend over several vertebrae while the short deep fibres extend over adjacent vertebrae.	Tubercle of atlas to anterior surface of sacrum
Posterior longitudinal ligament	• Posterior surfaces of the vertebral bodies in the vertebral canal. Connects the intervertebral discs.	• C2 to sacral promontory. • Extends cranially as the membrana tectoria from C2 to basi-occiput.
Suprapinous and Interspinous ligaments	Spines of adjacent vertebrae	• Supraspinous ligament continue as ligamentum nuchae from C7 to external occipital protruberance.
Ligamentum flavum	• Laminae of adjacent vertebrae. • Attached to the superior border of the inferior lamina to the inferior region of the ventral surface of superior lamina.	• Junction of axis and C3 to the junction of L5 and sacrum. • Extends as posterior atlanto occipital membrane beyond the posterior arch of atlas cranially to the posterior border of foramen magnum.
Apical ligament	• Tip of dens (C2). • Basiocciput.	
Alar ligament	• Lateral surface of dens. • Tubercle of basiocciput.	

Table 4.2 Joints of vertebral column

Joint	Component bony element	Type of joint
Between adjacent vertebral bodies	• Adjacent vertebral bodies. • Intervertebral disc lies in between the layer of hyaline cartilage of each adjacent vertebra.	Symphyses
Zygapophyseal joint	Superior articular processes of caudal vertebra with the adjacent inferior articular processes of cranial vertebra	Synovial
Interspinous joint	Between adjacent spines	Syndesmoses
Interlaminar	Adjacent laminae are joined by ligamentum flavum	Syndesmoses
Intertransverse joint	Adjacent transverse processes joined by intertransverse ligaments	Syndesmoses
Atlanto axial joint	Two lateral joints medial to the foramen transversarium and a median joint between anterior dens and anterior arch of the atlas	Synovial
Atlanto occipital Joint	• Between condyles of basiocciput and lateral masses of atlas. • Anterior and posterior arches of atlas are joined to the anterior and posterior margins of the foramen magnum by respective atlanto-occipital membranes.	Synovial

situated in the centre in the thoracic region and more posteriorly in the cervical and lumbar regions. Its hydraulic property maintains its height and resistance to axial loads. Since all the components of the disc are interrelated to each other, any dysfunction in one component shifts the work load to the other. In older age, as the height of the nucleus decreases, more load is borne by the annulus, which leads to its tear resulting in herniation.

4.9 Vascular Supply

The nutrition to the vertebral column and its contents are furnished by the segmental arteries of the respective regions. The arteries are accompanied by corresponding veins.

4.10 Arterial Supply

Pre- and post-central branches enter the vertebral body from the anterior and posterior surfaces while the *post-laminar* branches penetrate the posterior surface and *pre-laminar branches* penetrate the anterior surface of the respective lamina (Fig. 4.5) [4]. The segmental arteries are branches of vertebral, deep cervical, posterior intercostal, lumbar and lateral sacral arteries. These segmental arteries give branches to the spinal cord, roots of spinal nerves, vertebrae, their ligaments and joints, dura mater and the epidural tissue. The dorsal branches of the segmental

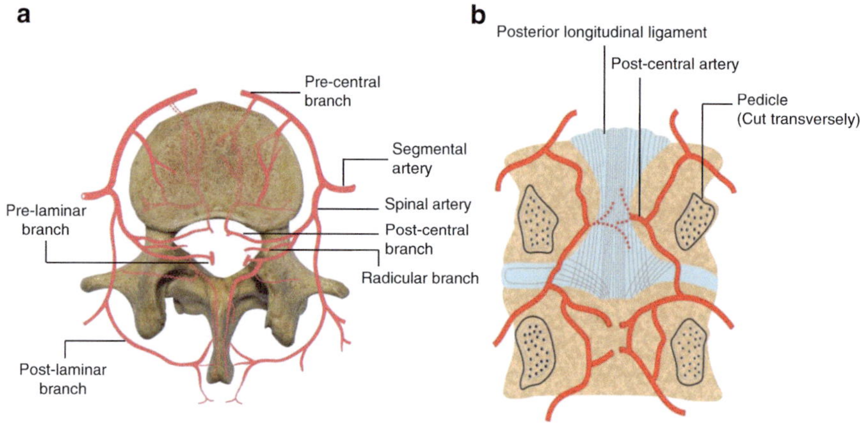

Fig. 4.5 (**a**) Arterial supply of a vertebra. (**b**) Post-central arteries anastomose with each other within the vertebral canal

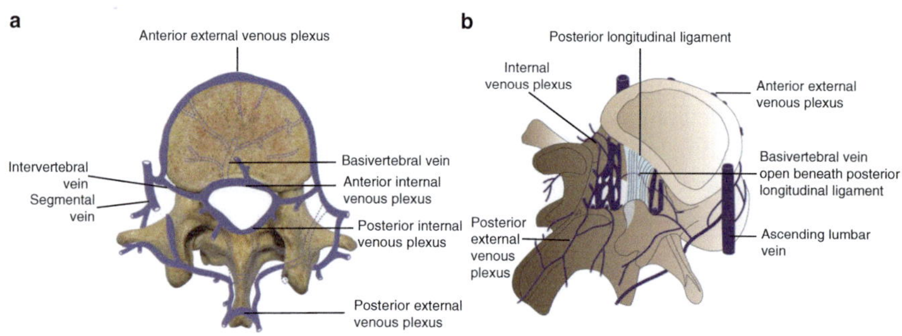

Fig. 4.6 (**a**) Venous drainage of vertebral column. (**b**) Note that the basivertebral vein drains into connecting channels beneath the posterior longitudinal ligament within the vertebral canal

arteries provide the nutrient arteries to the vertebrae. The post-central branches divide into two nutrient arteries, each travel to adjacent vertebrae. These nutrient arteries anastomose with each other and with that of opposite side beneath the posterior longitudinal ligament to supply spongy bone, marrow cavity and peripheral area of the annulus fibrosus.

4.11 Veinous Drainage

Intricate plexuses are formed by the draining veins of the vertebral column along its entire length, which are present external and internal to the vertebral canal. These venous channels are present longitudinally as well as circumferentially (Fig. 4.6).

4.12 External Vertebral Venous Plexus

The anterior and posterior external vertebral plexuses are more developed in the cervical region and anastomose freely with each other. The anterior vertebral venous plexus receives tributaries from the vertebral bodies and communicates with the basivertebral and internal vertebral veins. The posterior vertebral venous plexuses which are present around the neural arch communicate with the vertebral, posterior intercostal and lumbar veins.

4.13 Internal Vertebral Venous Plexus

The anterior and posterior internal venous plexuses are present within the epidural fat, around the wall of the vertebral canal. These are joined by one or more transverse veins. At the level of the foramen magnum, internal plexus is connected through a dense network of veins with the vertebral veins, emissary veins of the occipital bone, venous plexus of hypoglossal canal, basilar venous plexus, sigmoid sinus and occipital sinus.

The external and internal vertebral venous plexuses are connected to each other by veins that pass through the intervertebral foramen.

4.14 Basivertebral Vein

This horizontal pair of veins drain the spongy part of the vertebral body, into external and internal vertebral venous plexuses. These are enlarged in elderly people.

4.15 Intervertebral Vein

The anterior and posterior internal venous plexuses drain into the intervertebral vein which passes through the intervertebral foramen along with the spinal nerve. The intervertebral veins drain into the vertebral, posterior intercostals, lumbar and lateral sacral veins and the blood finally drains into the caval or the azygos system.

The venous plexuses are valveless. They freely communicate with the dural venous sinuses, veins of the neck and the pelvis. Hence, any increase in pressure in the body cavities or any of the connecting veins, may get transmitted into these plexuses or cerebrospinal fluid (CSF) within the cranial cavity. This may result in congestion of the affected areas. The spinal cord is spared in venous engorgement of these plexuses as the radicular veins have valves. These plexuses can act as an alternative route of venous return to heart in case of venous obstruction in neck or body cavities.

The vertebrae being one of the closest connections of these valveless venous plexuses, unimpeded to and fro blood flow can spread any infection or neoplastic emboli from related areas to the vertebrae. Due to the same reason, spread of septic emboli may occur from one vertebra to another vertebra through this intricate valveless plexuses.

4.16 Lymphatic Drainage

The lymphatics pass along with the corresponding blood vessels. They drain into the deep cervical, posterior intercostal, aortic, sacral and internal iliac groups of lymph nodes.

4.17 Innervation (Fig. 4.7)

The components of the vertebral column get their innervation from branches of dorsal rami of spinal nerves along with sinovertebral nerve (usually more than one) and sympathetic fibres which pass via the grey rami communicantes or directly from thoracic sympathetic ganglia.

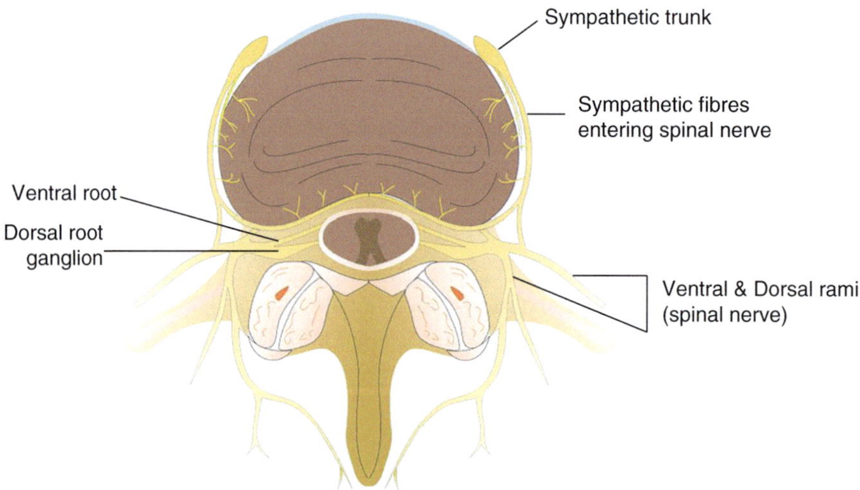

Fig. 4.7 Innervation of a vertebra

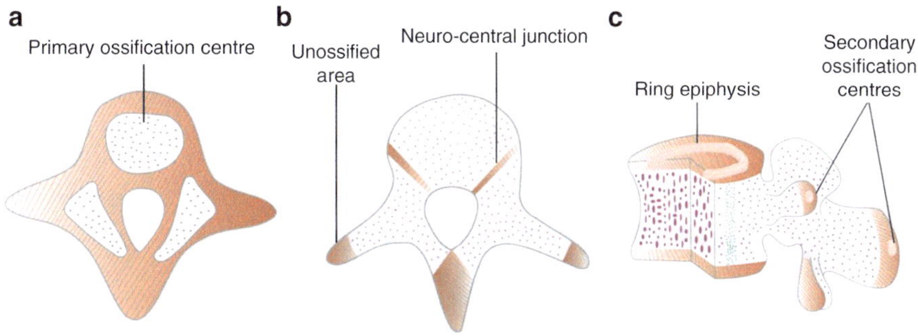

Fig. 4.8 Cartilaginous ossification in a typical vertebra. (**a**) Primary ossification centres in foetal life (one at centrum, two at neural arch). (**b**) Vertebra at the time of birth (the areas in brown remain unossified). (**c**) Typical vertebra at the time of puberty (the areas in brown remain unossified). Secondary ossifications centres appear at puberty

4.18 Growth and Development of Vertebra (Fig. 4.8)

Vertebra develops by cartilaginous ossification. There are three primary and five secondary (at puberty) ossification centres. Fusion takes place by 18–25 years.

The growth of a vertebra has similarities with the growth of epiphyseal plate of long bone [5]. Hence, a growing vertebra will also be highly vascular [6]. So, in the developing stage of a vertebra, haematogenous dissemination of infectious emboli to vertebrae may be common.

4.19 Pathophysiology of Spinal Tuberculosis

Rohit Jindal and Amit Salaria

4.19.1 Introduction

The worldwide annual incidence of tuberculosis is about ten million and tuberculosis remains one of the leading causes of death and disability [7]. Osteoarticular involvement is seen in about 8–15% cases of extrapulmonary tuberculosis and spinal tuberculosis constitutes nearly 50% of all cases of skeletal tuberculosis [8].

4.19.2 Causative Organism of Tuberculosis

Bacillus of the *Mycobacterium tuberculosis* complex (MTBC) causes tuberculosis. MTBC is a group of highly related organisms consisting of around sixty species of which *M. tuberculosis* is by far the most common causative agent of human infections. *M. africanum, M. bovis, M. microti* and some other mycobacteria have also been implicated in human infections [9]. Atypical or Nontuberculous mycobacteria (NTM) are also known as mycobacteria other than tuberculosis (MOTT) and these can cause disease resembling tuberculosis, more often in immunocompromised hosts [10].

The bacilli are aerobic, non-motile, non-sporing, non-encapsulated and slow growing. The cell wall contains high content of mycolic acids which is responsible for acid fastness resulting in characteristic red rod-shaped bacilli on Ziehl–Neelsen staining (Fig. 4.9).

Different components of the mycobacterium possess different biological activities which contribute to the virulence, pathogenesis, immune response and response to treatment of the disease [11]. The cell wall is essential for bacterial viability and integrity and is responsible for much of the pathogenesis and resistance towards common antibiotics [12]. The tubercular protein induces delayed hypersensitivity and induces formation of epithelioid and giant cells [11]. Besides these other glycolipids and lipopolysaccharides produced by mycobacteria play essential roles in interaction of the mycobacterium with the host in the course of infection [13].

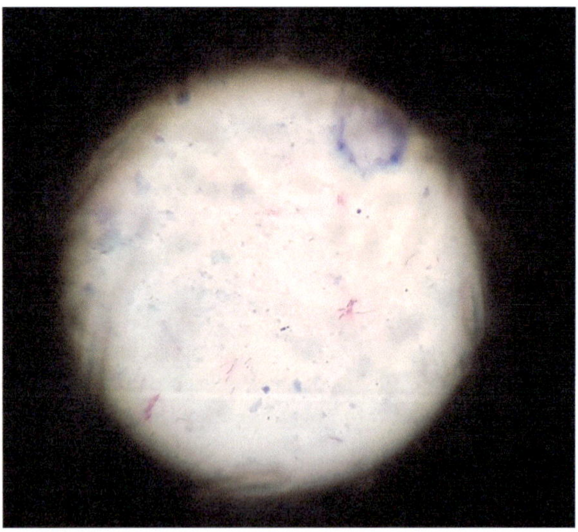

Fig. 4.9 Acid-fast bacilli were seen on Ziehl–Neelsen staining (oil immersion 100X). *Picture courtesy: Dr. Lipika Gautam* and *Dr. Nidhi Singla*

4.19.3 Risk Factors for Infection and Transmission

M. tuberculosis spreads from human to human primarily by airborne route. Droplet nuclei about 5–10 microns in size are generated during the act of coughing, sneezing or talking in an infected patient and these remain suspended in environment for several hours depending upon the environment [14]. When inhaled they can cause *M. tuberculosis* infection in humans. Another less important cause of transmission is digestive transmission of *M. bovis* primarily through unpasteurized cow's milk, where the bacilli are lodged in intestines or tonsils, and direct cutaneous or mucous inoculation is the rarest form of transmission. The factors related to transmission are summarized in Table 4.3.

4.19.3.1 Development and Course of Tuberculosis Infection

The risk of progression from exposure to the development of active disease is a complex interplay of bacillus and host immunity. The immune system is able to eradicate all viable bacilli in only a miniscule number of cases but is able to contain the infection in majority of the cases and the bacillus becomes walled off in caseation granulomas [15]. Rapid progression to tuberculosis disease, either pulmonary, extrapulmonary or generalized tuberculosis can occur in approximately 5% of patients within the first 2 years after infection. Most of the patients with tuberculosis disease have reactivation of latent infection. This activation of disease is caused mostly by reactivation of the dormant tubercle bacilli acquired from primary infection and less frequently may be caused by reinfection. The risk of progression to disease is much higher in HIV-positive and other immune-compromised individuals

Table 4.3 Factors related to transmission of tuberculosis

Factors related to Index Case	1. Bacillary load in the index case. (a) Smear positive most contagious. (b) Smear negative /culture positive less contagious. (c) Culture negative and EPTB non-contagious. (d) Patients with latent infections but no active pulmonary disease are non-contagious. 2. Virulence of the tubercle bacilli.
Environment	1. Close proximity to an infectious case. 2. Small room /settings with poor ventilation. (a) Overcrowding.public transportation settings, workplaces, healthcare facilities, mines and prisons (b) Low socioeconomic status.
Duration of exposure	1. Household contacts. 2. Healthcare workers.

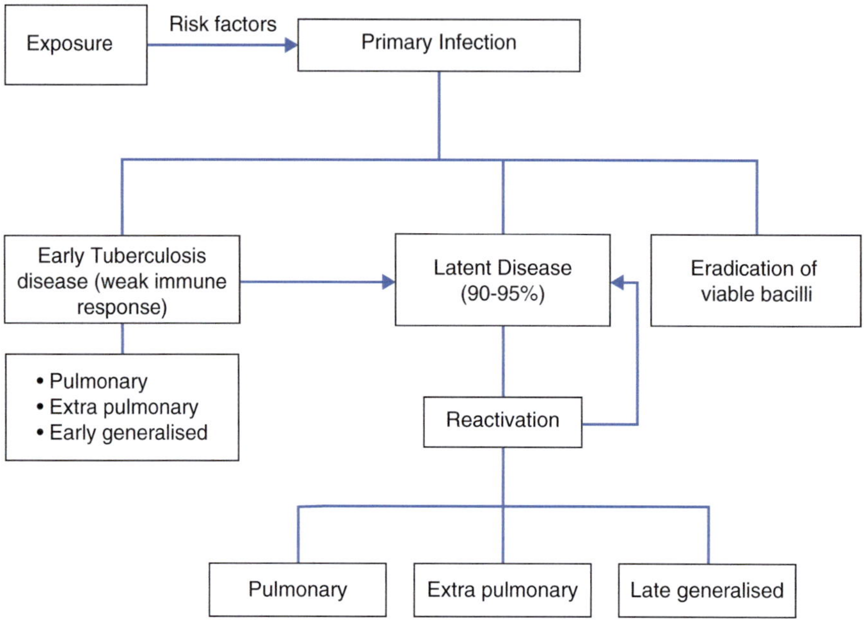

Fig. 4.10 Progression from exposure to disease in tuberculosis

[16] and in persons using immunomodulators such as tumour necrosis factor (TNF)-alpha inhibitor [17]. Diabetes, alcohol use, malnutrition (both micro- and macro-deficiency), tobacco smoking, prolonged corticosteroid therapy and chronic renal failure are also associated with higher rates of tuberculosis [18–21]. There is some evidence that suceptibility to tuberculosis may have a genetic basis but the influence of these genetic associations is not clear (Fig. 4.10) [22].

4.19.4 Pathogenesis

After entry into the body, *Mycobacterium tuberculosis* encounters a series of host defence mechanisms with final outcome depending on the balance between bacillary growth and extent of host immunity. Cell-mediated immunity plays a key role in the pathogenesis of tuberculosis in unexposed immune-competent hosts. Host immune response leads to characteristic pathological features of tuberculosis like caseating granulomas and cavitation (Figs. 4.11 and 4.12).

Following inhalation of *Mycobacterium tuberculosis*, depending on their intrinsic microbicidal capability alveolar macrophages ingest the pathogen and destroy them. *Mycobacterium bacilli* often evade this initial destruction by alveolar macrophages and instead of continuing to multiply inside the macrophages leading to their destruction and recruitment of more macrophages, blood monocytes and other inflammatory cells to the primary disease site. The bacilli grow exponentially but

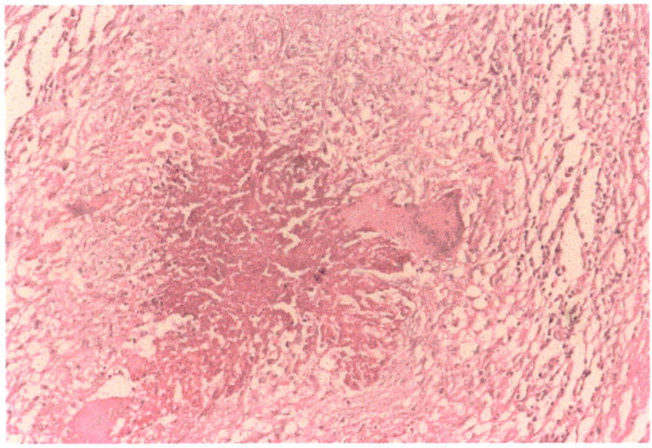

Fig. 4.11 Photomicrograph showing epithelioid cell granuloma with central caseation necrosis (H&E, x200). *Photograph courtesy: Dr. RPS Punia, GMCH Chandigarh*

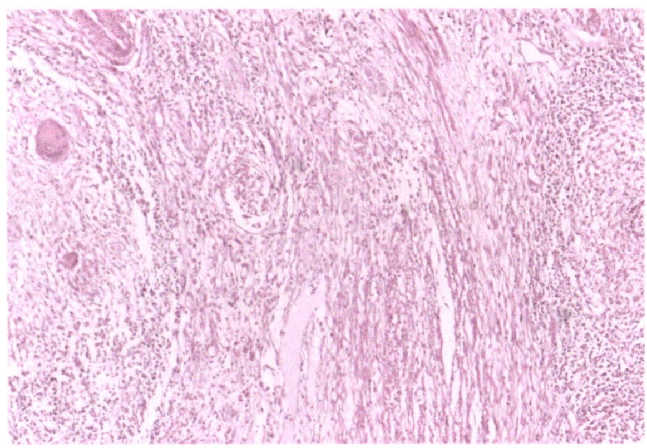

Fig. 4.12 Photomicrograph showing multiple epithelioid cell granulomas along with Langhans type of giant cells (H&E, ×100). *Photograph courtesy: Dr. RPS Punia, GMCH Chandigarh*

there is little tissue destruction. This stage leads to activation of specific cells by antigen-specific T cells and these specific monocytoid cells differentiate into two types of giant cells, epithelioid and multinucleated Langhans' type giant cells. This process is the stage of granuloma formation and is aimed at containing the infection and preventing its further spread in the body. This latent stage is disrupted under conditions of decreased immune competence giving rise to endogenous reactivation of dormant foci resulting in post-primary tuberculosis characterized by caseation necrosis [23].

4.19.5 Mechanisms and Patterns of Involvement of Spine

Tuberculosis can affect each and every organ of the body by haematogenous and lymphatic dissemination from the primary focus. Seeding can occur at the time of primary infection or during reactivation. Spinal tuberculosis may spread by haemetogenous route from a primary focus either in the pulmonary region or in the genito-urinary system, tonsils or gastro-intestinal tract or from adjacent para-aortic lymph nodes [24]. The pattern of vertebral vascular supply dictates the common areas of involvement in spinal tuberculosis [25]. The tubercular bacilli reach the spine through the arterial route or the Batsons venous plexus [26].

Commonly, the richly supplied 'paradiscal' subchondral upper and lower end-plates are primarily involved as the intervertebral disc is avascular in adults [27, 28]. The intervertebral disc is secondarily involved in adults whereas in children it can be primarily involved due to it being vascularized in children [27]. The 'central' type of vertebral body involvement, skipped lesion in the vertebral column and vertebral disease associated with tubercular meningitis, are thought to be due to spread of infection along the Batsons peri-vertebral plexus of vein [26, 27]. 'Anterior type' of involvement of vertebral bodies can occur due to extension of an abscess beneath the anterior longitudinal ligaments and the periosteum leading to loss of periosteal blood supply to anterior and lateral surfaces of many contagious vertebra [28]. The involvement of 'posterior' elements including spinous processes, laminae, transverse processes, articular processes (synovial), and pedicles is relatively rare with a reported incidence of 3–5% for isolated posterior involvement [29].

Tuberculosis infection in the spine typically produces a marked exudative reaction with marked hyperaemia. The infection destroys the epiphyseal cortex, the intervertebral disc, and the adjacent vertebrae. It may spread beneath the anterior longitudinal ligament to reach neighbouring vertebrae. The vertebral body becomes soft and gets easily compressed to produce either wedging or total collapse. The lower part of the dorsal and upper part of the lumbar spine are most commonly involved [26, 28]. With healing, the exudate is resorbed, osteoporosis decreases and density of body gradually increases to normal. When the intervertebral discs have been completely destroyed, the adjacent bodies fuse with each other. Spinal tuberculosis can lead to progressive bony destruction and kyphosis, formation of cold abscess and spinal cord involvement secondary to canal encroachment or stretching of the cord over longstanding severe kyphosis.

4.19.5.1 Cold Abscess

Cold abscess composing of caseous material, bony debris and tubercle bacilli is formed due to marked exudative reaction and collection of liquefaction material. It follows the path of least resistance and trickles in between the fascial planes and along the nerves and vessels and collects at the distant sites depending upon the region involved. In the cervical region may form at the anterior triangle, posterior triangle or retropharyngeal space or even track down to mediastinum (Fig. 4.13). Thoracic involvement leads to mediastinal collections in the pre and paravertebral regions and sometimes along the chest wall. A large paravertebral abscess in the thoracic spine, may appear in the radiographs as a fusiform or bulbous paravertebral abscess (Fig. 4.14). Thoracolumbar and lumbar spine involvement leads to psoas

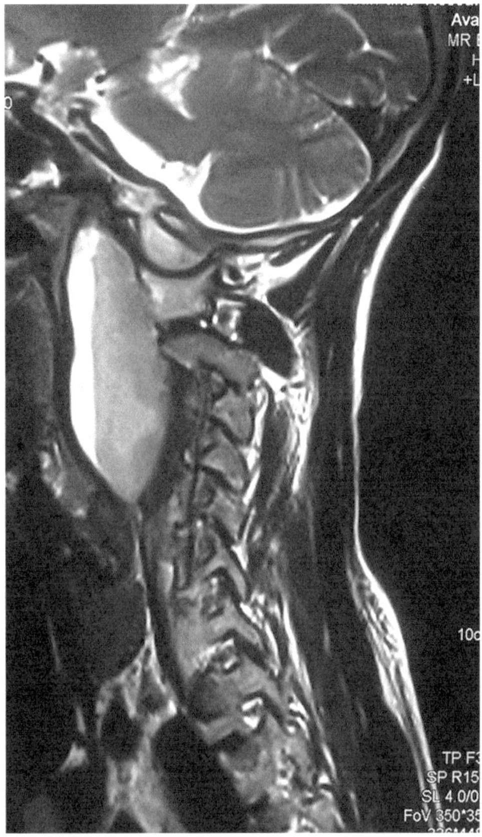

Fig. 4.13 MRI showing large retropharyngeal abscess in tuberculosis of upper cervical spine

abscess which may present at the iliac fossa or medial aspect of the thigh (Fig. 4.15). Although the cold abscess feels warm the temperature is not raised as much as seen in pyogenic abscess, hence the name cold [28]. Occasionally, these cold abscesses may burst to end in single or multiple discharging sinuses. The tuberculous discharge is typically serousanginous and the ulcer develops due to bursting of the cold abscess. The ulcers are shallow, maybe multiple, generally oval in shape which might coalesce to have irregular cresentric borders. The edges are typically reddish-blue with undermined edges. The floor of the ulcer is lined by pale granulation tissue with scanty serosanginuous discharge [30].

4.19.5.2 Paraplegia

Neurological involvement in spinal tuberculosis may be caused either during the active phase or in the healed phase. During active phase, the posterior extension of the tubercular debris consisting of caseous material, granulation tissue, sequestrated

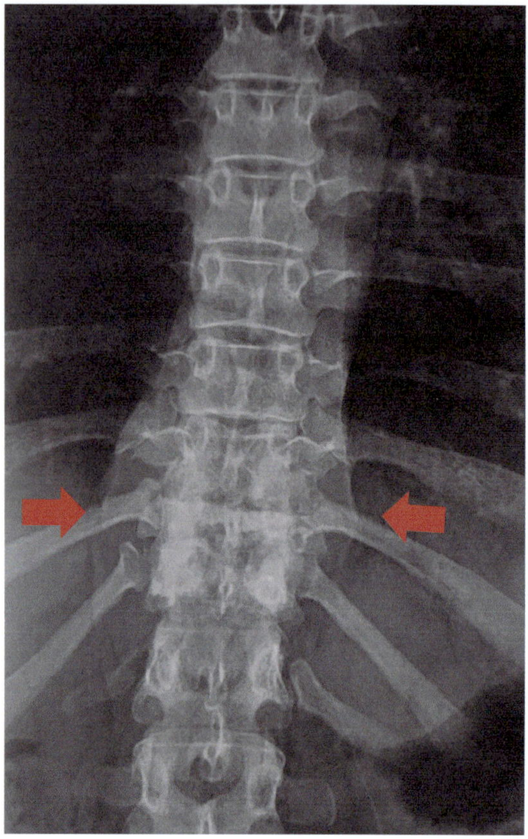

Fig. 4.14 X-ray showing large paravertebral abscess in tuberculosis of D10 and D11 vertebrae

disc or bony fragments can cause narrowing of spinal canal [31]. Inflammatory oedema of the cord is also thought to play a part in development of deficit [32]. This so-called early onset paraplegia has a generally favourable prognosis [28, 33]. Neurological involvement is common when the dorsal spine is involved because of the relatively smaller cord/canal ratio in the dorsal region and the abscess remains confined under tension and is thereby forced into the spinal canal [28]. Rarely cord infarction due to endarteritis, periarteritis and thrombosis of the branches of spinal artery and spinal tumour syndrome can also cause neurological deficit [26, 28]. Pathological dislocation or subluxation can also cause neurological involvement [31, 34, 35]. Late-onset paraplegia usually occurs after several years of persistence of the disease in the vertebral column and the causes are usually mechanical like localized internal gibbus and severe kyphotic deformity. It has been suggested that a disease healing in kyphosis greater than 60 degrees for more than 10 years [36] causes stretching the spinal cord over an internal anterior bony projection, producing gliosis and atrophy [34]. Degenerative spinal stenosis, ossification of ligamentum flavum and resulting cord compression at compensatory hyper-lordotic and/or hypermobile segment can also cause late-onset deficit [37, 38, 39].

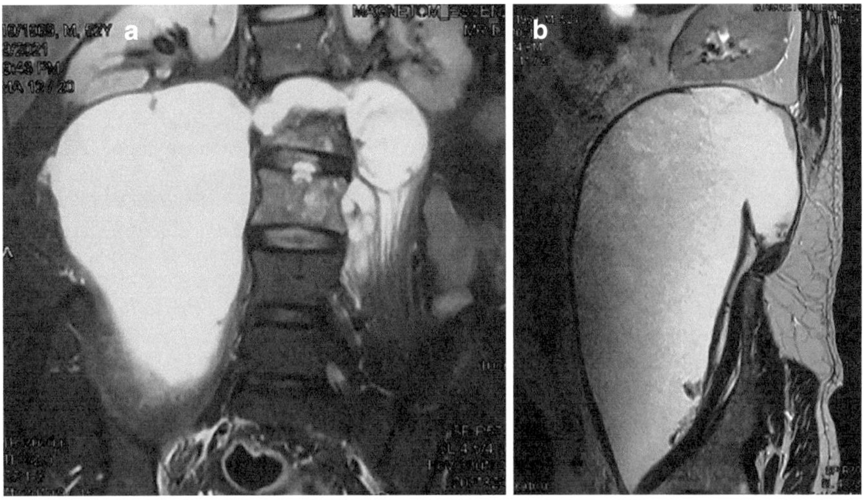

Fig. 4.15 Large psoas abscess. (a) Coronal view, (b) Sagittal view in a case of L1 and L2 tuberculosis

4.19.5.3 Kyphotic Deformity

Kyphotic deformity develops due to preferential involvement of anterior elements of vertebral column in majority of cases of spinal tuberculosis. The severity of the deformity is determined by the extent of initial vertebral body destruction, age of the patient and the vertebral level involved [40]. The presence of any two features amongst separation of the facet joints, retropulsion, lateral translation and toppling in children may point to a final severe deformity (Spine at Risk Signs). In children, the deformities may continue to progress even after the healing of the disease [41]. In adults, more severe deformities are seen when the cervico-thoracic or thoraco-lumbar junction is involved or pre-treatment level of deformity is greater than 30 degrees [40]. Approximately 3% of conservatively treated patients may end up with a deformity greater than 60 degrees which besides cosmetic deformity may result in costopelvic impingement, cardiorespiratory insufficiency as well as late-onset neurological deficit because of stretching of spinal cord [36].

References

1. Baron E, Tunstall R. Back. In: Standring S, editor. Gray's Anatomy: The Anatomical Basis of Clinical Practice. London: Elsevier; 2021. p. 814–55.
2. Harrison RJ. Bones. In: Romanes GJ, editor. Cunningham's Textbook of Anatomy. New York: Oxford Medical Publications; 1995. p. 75–174.
3. Hamilton WJ, editor. Textbook of Human Anatomy. 2nd ed. London: The Macmillan Press Ltd; 1976.

4. Rosse C, Gaddum-Rosse P, editors. Hollinshed's Textbook of Anatomy. 5th ed. New York: Lippincott-Raven Publishers; 1997. p. 107–75.
5. Larsen EH, Nordentoft EL. Growth of the Epiphyses and Vertebrae. Acta Orthop Scand. 1962;32(1–4):210–7.
6. Leonard MK Jr, Blumberg HM. Musculoskeletal Tuberculosis. In: Schlossberg D, editor. Tuberculosis and Nontuberculous Mycobacterial Infections. Washington, DC: American Society for Microbiology; 2017. p. 371–92.
7. World Health Organization. Global tuberculosis report 2017. http://www.who.int/tb/publications/global_report/en/. Accessed Dec 14, 2020.
8. Millet JP, Moreno A, Fina L, del Baño L, Orcau A, de Olalla PG, et al. Factors that influence current tuberculosis epidemiology. Eur Spine J. 2013;22(S4):539–48.
9. Sharma A, Bloss E, Heilig CM, Click ES. Tuberculosis Caused by *Mycobacterium africanum*, United States, 2004–2013. Emerg Infect Dis. 2016 Mar;22(3):396–403.
10. Rahama O, Thaker H. Atypical mycobacteria: an important differential for the general physician. Clin Med. 2013;13(5):504–6.
11. Bhatia R. The Mycobacterium. In: Sharma SK, Mohan A, editors. Tuberculosis. 2nd ed. Jaypee Publishers: New Delhi; 2009. p. 102–8.
12. Brennan P, Crick D. The Cell-Wall Core of Mycobacterium tuberculosis in the Context of Drug Discovery. Curr Top Med Chem. 2007;7(5):475–88.
13. Angala SK, Belardinelli JM, Huc-Claustre E, Wheat WH, Jackson M. The cell envelope glycoconjugates of Mycobacterium tuberculosis. Crit Rev Biochem Mol Biol. 2014;49(5):361–99.
14. Churchyard G, Kim P, Shah NS, Rustomjee R, Gandhi N, Mathema B, et al. What We Know About Tuberculosis Transmission: An Overview. J Infect Dis. 2017 Oct 1;216(Suppl 6):S629–35.
15. Narasimhan P, Wood J, Macintyre CR, Mathai D. Risk factors for tuberculosis. Pulm Med. 2013:1–11.
16. Corbett EL, Watt CJ, Walker N, et al. The growing burden of tuberculosis: global trends and interactions with the HIV epidemic. Arch Intern Med. 2003;163(9):1009–21.
17. Winthrop KL. Risk and prevention of tuberculosis and other serious opportunistic infections associated with the inhibition of tumor necrosis factor. Nat Clin Pract Rheumatol. 2006;2(11):602–10.
18. Baker M, Harries A, Jeon C, Hart J, Kapur A, Lonnroth K, et al. The impact of diabetes on tuberculosis treatment outcomes: a systematic review. BMC Med. 2011;9:article 81.
19. Cegielski JP, McMurray DN. The relationship between malnutrition and tuberculosis: evidence from studies in humans and experimental animals. International Journal of Tuberculosis and Lung Disease. 2004;8(3):286–98.
20. Bates MN, Khalakdina A, Pai M, Chang L, Lessa F, Smith KR. Risk of tuberculosis from exposure to tobacco smoke: a systematic review and meta-analysis. Arch Intern Med. 2007;167(4):335–42.
21. Romanowski K, Clark EG, Levin A, Cook VJ, Johnston JC. Tuberculosis and chronic kidney disease: an emerging global syndemic. Kidney Int. 2016;90(1):34–40.
22. Moller M, de Wit E, Hoal EG. Past, present and future directions in human genetic susceptibility to tuberculosis. FEMS Immunol & Med Microbiol. 2010;58(1):3–27.
23. Mitra DK, Rai AK. Immunology of tuberculosis. In: Sharma SK, Mohan A, editors. Tuberculosis. 2nd ed. New Delhi: Jaypee Publishers; 2009. p. 109–21.
24. Dass B, Puet T, Watanakunakorn C. Tuberculosis of the spine (Pott's disease) presenting as "compression fractures.". Spinal Cord. 2002;40(11):604–8.
25. Wiley AM, Trueta J. The vascular anatomy of the spine and its relationship to pyogenic vertebral osteomyelitis. J Bone Joint Surg (Br). 1959;41(4):796–808.
26. Agrawal V, Patgaonkar PR, Nagariya SP. Tuberculosis of spine. J Craniovertebr Junction Spine. 2010 Jul-Dec;1(2):74–85.
27. Garg RK, Somvanshi DS. Spinal tuberculosis: a review. J Spinal Cord Med. 2011;34(5):440–54.

28. Tuli SM. Tuberculosis of the Skeletal system. 4th ed. New delhi: Jaypee Brother Med Publishers; 2010.
29. Narlawar RS, Shah JR, Pimple MK, Patkar DP, Patankar T, Castillo M. Isolated tuberculosis of posterior elements of spine: magnetic resonance imaging findings in 33 patients. Spine. 2002;27(3):275–81.
30. Das S. A manual on clinical surgery. 13th ed. Kolkatta: Dr S Das's Publications; 2018.
31. Hodgson AR, Skinsnes OK, Leong CY. The pathogenesis of Pott's paraplegia. J Bone Joint Surg Am. 1967;49:1147–56.
32. Jain AK, Jena A, Dhammi IK. Correlation of clinical course with magnetic resonance imaging in tuberculous myelopathy. Neural India. 2000;48:132–9.
33. Hodgson AR, Stock FE. Anterior Spine Fusion for the Treatment of Tuberculosis of the Spine The Operative Findings and Results of Treatment in the First One Hundred Cases. J Bone Joint Surg Am. 1960;42(2):295–310.
34. Jain AK. Tuberculosis of the spine: a fresh look at an old disease. J Bone Joint Surg Br. 2010 Jul;92(7):905–13.
35. Jain AK, Kumar J. Tuberculosis of spine: neurological deficit. Eur Spine J. 2013;22(Suppl 4):624–33.
36. Tuli SM. Current concepts: severe kyphotic deformity in tuberculosis of the spine. International Orthop (Sicot). 1995;19:327–31.
37. Luk KD, Krishna M. Spinal stenosis above a healed tuberculous kyphosis. A case report. Spine. 1996;21(9):1098–101.
38. Chen Y, Lu X-H, Yang L-L, Chen D-Y. Ossification of Ligamentum Flavum Related to Thoracic Kyphosis After Tuberculosis. Spine. 2009;34(1):E41–4.
39. Subramani S, Shetty AP, Kanna RM, Shanmuganathan R. Ossified 33. ligamentum flavum causing neurological deficit above the level of post-tuberculous kyphotic deformity. J Clin Orthop Trauma. 2017;8:174–7.
40. Rajasekaran S. Kyphotic deformity in spinal tuberculosis and its management. Int Orthop. 2012;36(2):359–65. https://doi.org/10.1007/s00264-011-1469-2.
41. Rajasekaran S. The natural history of post-tubercular kyphosis in children: radiological signs which predict late increase in deformity. J Bone Joint Surg. 2001;83B:954–62.

Chapter 5
Clinical Presentation, Features, and Examination of a Case of Suspected Tuberculosis

Shankar Acharya and Vishnu Prasad Panigrahi

Abstract India is a country where tuberculosis (TB) is an epidemic disease, and osteoarticular TB is common. The spine is affected by almost 50 percent of those afflicted with osteoarticular TB. Early suspicion, timely diagnosis, and treatment may prevent neurological deficits and other complications like spine deformity or instability. The onset of symptoms is usually insidious and classical constitutional symptoms may be minimum or absent. A high index of suspicion and early investigations, including blood tests, X-rays, and MRI are essential for early diagnosis. A cold abscess may present occasionally without any symptoms and rarely with acute neurological deficit.

Keywords Skeletal Tuberculosis · Potts spine · Constitutional Symptoms Deformity · Cold Abscess · Neurological Deficits

5.1 Introduction

Skeletal system involvement is seen in 1–2% of total cases of TB and about 10% of extrapulmonary TB [1, 2]. Spinal TB accounts for more than 50% of skeletal TB and commonly affects the productive age group, thus becoming a burden to the family and country. It is more common in developing countries where many still live in low socioeconomic conditions with poor nutrition, overcrowding, and lack of proper hygiene. There is no gender difference in the susceptibility to TB. Due to rising life expectancy along with increasing rates of diabetes mellitus, cancer chemotherapy, HIV, and increasing use of immunosuppressive medication, TB is now commonly seen in the elderly [3, 4].

S. Acharya (✉) · V. P. Panigrahi
Department of Spine Surgery, Sir Gangaram Hospital, New Delhi, India
e-mail: chairman.orthospine@sgrh.com

S. S. Dhatt, V. Kumar (eds.), *Tuberculosis of the Spine*,
https://doi.org/10.1007/978-981-16-9495-0_5

The symptoms of spinal TB are usually subtle. Patients may present with classical symptoms of weight loss, evening rise of temperature, loss of appetite, back pain not resolving with physiotherapy, or sometimes may not have any symptoms at all. The importance of taking a detailed history and a thorough examination of the spine and other joints cannot be emphasized enough. A family history of tuberculosis, or contact with a patient having active tuberculosis, the habits, socioeconomic conditions could be pointers for an early diagnosis. By the end of clinical evaluation, one should be able to locate the pathology and identify evolving complications that may require further investigations and management.

5.2 Signs and Symptoms

According to a case series, in approximately 90% of patients with spinal TB, the location is in the lower thoracic and upper lumbar vertebrae [5]. Overall, the thoracolumbar junction is most commonly involved, followed by lumbar and cervical regions [6, 7]. The thoracolumbar region is frequently involved due to biomechanical transition from a rigid thoracic spine to a mobile lumbar spine, making it prone to microtrauma, which might aid the seeding of TB bacilli. The TB bacilli usually reach the vertebral body via hematogenous route from a primary site like the lungs or genitourinary system, etc. [8, 9]. There is a rich arterial plexus in the subchondral region of each vertebra which facilitates the seeding of TB bacilli in the paradisical region. As the same segmental artery supplies two adjacent vertebrae, usually both are involved. Batson's venous plexus is a valve-less system connecting the spine with intra-abdominal and intra-thoracic cavities. The TB bacilli spread via Batson's plexus may lead to central lesions in the vertebral body and also the involvement of non-contiguous vertebrae, while dissemination beneath the anterior or posterior longitudinal ligaments leads to involvement of multiple contiguous vertebrae [10, 11]. According to a recent case series utilizing FDG-PET SCAN for monitoring treatment response, the percentage of non-contiguous vertebral involvement in skeletal TB was 63.6% [12].

The clinical picture usually depends on multiple factors like age, location of disease, duration, etc. The immune status, co-morbidities, and development of complications like a cold abscess, secondary infection, deformity, and neurological sequelae further complicate the neurological picture [13]. Chronic low back pain is the most common symptom, which is insidious in onset, gradually progressive, dull aching in nature, usually non-radiating [6]. Sometimes there may be an association with constitutional symptoms like malaise, decline in appetite, and loss of weight. There may be a history of healed pulmonary tuberculosis or of other regions in the past or exposure to a person with pulmonary tuberculosis.

Night pain is characteristic of this condition. If present, it wakes up the patient from sleep. The sudden excruciating pain is attributed to a loss of protective muscle spasm, which unmasks the instability of the spine. Night pain is also attributed to inflammation and venous engorgement in the supine position [14]. Back pain in

Table 5.1 Stages of tuberculosis spine: (Kumar 1988)

Stage	Description	Clinical	Radiological	Duration
I	Pre-destructive	Dull back pain, muscle spasm	Straightening of spine	<3 months
II	Early destruction	Increased muscle spasm, Night pain	Diminished disc space, paradisal erosion, kyphosis <10°	2–4 months
III	Advanced destruction and collapse	Additional Deformity	Two or more vertebrae with collapse. Kyphosis (11°–30°)	3–9 months
IV	Neurological involvement	Motor or sensory weakness	Cord compression/ cord changes Kyphosis (31^{0}–60^{0})	Variable
V	Residual deformity	Variable	Reactivated / healed with deformity	>3–5 years

skeletal TB is especially refractory to conservative measures. Radicular pain can be a presenting feature when a root is compressed due to abscess formation or a bony fragment. Radicular pain referred to the abdomen can mimic cholecystitis, pancreatitis, appendicitis, and renal diseases, which can lead to a delay in diagnosis and sometimes unnecessary investigations and procedures.

On examination, there is muscle spasm, which can present as torticollis in the cervical spine, prominent paraspinal muscle in the thoracolumbar spine, and a sciatic list due to unilateral spasm. Local tenderness over the involved region can be elicited. Patients are very cautious moving about while supporting the diseased part. Some signs of skeletal TB are "Head Supporting Sign" in cervical TB and "Tripod sign" [15] in thoracolumbar spine involvement. Spinal TB is classified by Kumar (1988) based on clinical and radiological findings [15] (Table 5.1).

5.3 Presenting with Neurological Deficit

Sir Percival Pott, in 1779, described paraplegia in a patient with tuberculous spondylitis with a kyphotic deformity [16]. Involvement of neurology in spinal TB varies from 23% to 76% [17]. Paraparesis is common in the thoracic and cervical spine but rare below L1 as the spinal cord ends at L1 and the canal is very spacious here [18, 19]. Neurological symptoms can be as subtle as gait disturbances to complete bladder and bowel incontinence. In developing countries, patients usually present after the appearance of weakness. Patients initially present with a clumsy and slow gait due to a combination of pain and weakness. Cervical cord compression presents with weakness in all four limbs. Thoracic cord compression presents as weakness of both lower limbs with or without bladder and bowel involvement, while lumbar spine involvement usually presents with lower motor neuron symptoms.

Paraparesis can occur during active disease (early-onset <2 yrs) or in late healed stages (late-onset) [20]. With active disease, the cause is either direct compression by an abscess, inflammatory tissue, sequestrum, instability, or intrinsic causes like

Table 5.2 Classification of paraplegia in TB spine (Tuli, modified by Jain (2005)

Stage	Complaints	Motor	Sensory	Autonomic
I	Nil	Plantar extensor/ ankle clonus ASIA Motor score – 100	Nil	Nil
II	Able to walk with support	ASIA Motor score Tetra paresis (60–100) Paraparesis (80–100)	Lateral column Involvement	Nil
III	Confined to bed Can move limbs	ASIA Motor score Tetra paresis (0–30) Paraparesis (50–80)	Lateral column Involvement	May be present
IV	No limb movement	ASIA Motor score Tetra paresis (0) Paraparesis (50)	Both lateral and posterior column involvement	May be present
V	Flexor spasms	Flaccid paralysis	Complete loss	Complete loss of bladder and bowel control

inflammation, meningitis, infective thrombi, or vascular insult due to endarteritis. Paraplegia in healed disease is due to the stretching of the spinal cord over the internal gibbus, bony ridges, scarring, or disease reactivation [21–23]. Paraplegia in healed TB is better prevented than treated [24].

Typically, motor power is lost early in the spinal cord compression followed by sensory and autonomic deficit [9, 25]. In a typical anterior lesion, compression starts anteriorly and gradually progresses to the posterior. Initially, spasticity develops, which the patient may not recognize. It can be detected on clinical examination by brisk deep tendon reflexes and extensor plantar response. Gradually, due to increasing compression, anterior columns get involved leading to a loss of motor power. With further compression, lateral spinothalamic tracts are involved leading to loss of pain, temperature, and crude touch. With the involvement of posterior columns, complete loss of sensation occurs, and by this time, disturbances in bladder and bowel set in. When the compression is prolonged, spasticity is replaced by flaccidity and flexor spasms. Paraplegia due to TB has been classified according to Tuli and later modified by Jain is clinically relevant [26] (Table 5.2). Lesions located near the conus medullaris or cauda equina may present with early bladder and bowel involvement and have mixed features of upper motor neuron and lower motor neuron lesions with asymmetric loss of sensations.

5.4 Presentation with Cold Abscess

Paravertebral abscesses are observed in at least 50% of cases of spinal TB [15, 27]. A cold abscess, as the name signifies, lacks features of inflammation such as color, dolor, and rubor and its presence signify active disease. Cold abscesses usually have a well-defined border with smooth and regular margins, and in most of them, a fluctuation can be elicited. If the abscess is large, the overlying skin is usually stretched and shiny. Superficial abscesses slowly destroy the subcutaneous and dermal tissue, causing a discharging sinus. The pus within the abscess is usually at body temperature and is pale yellow or white. It has no pungent odor typical of pyogenic or fungal infection and contains caseous material with debris and sequestrated bone. Tubercular sinuses take a long time to resolve but gradually heal with a thin scar when the underlying disease process is controlled. Secondary infection can lead to typical signs of inflammation which heals with an ugly fibrotic scar adherent to the underlying tissue. The culture of pyogenic organisms from the pus does not rule out tuberculosis.

Paravertebral abscesses, after destroying the surrounding areolar tissue, tend to travel along the path of least resistance such as along muscle, subpleural, subperitoneal, perivascular, perineural, and fascial planes and can present as a superficial abscess far away from the primary focus (Fig. 5.1).

In the cervical spine, retropharyngeal abscesses can emerge as swellings in the anterior or posterior triangles of the neck, the axilla, or the subscapular region. Retropharyngeal abscess leads to a loss of the normal pharyngo-vertebral crepitus that is normally felt when the larynx is gently moved from side to side against the vertebral column. It can also present as a life-threatening condition with stridor or can produce hoarseness and dysphagia [28]. Spread along the brachial plexus can present as an abscess in the arm or forearm.

In the thoracic region, a cold abscess is localized as a fusiform paravertebral swelling. Sometimes it can track along the arcuate ligament or the opening of the diaphragm. It can also track along the intercostal vessels and present as a swelling in the chest wall [29].

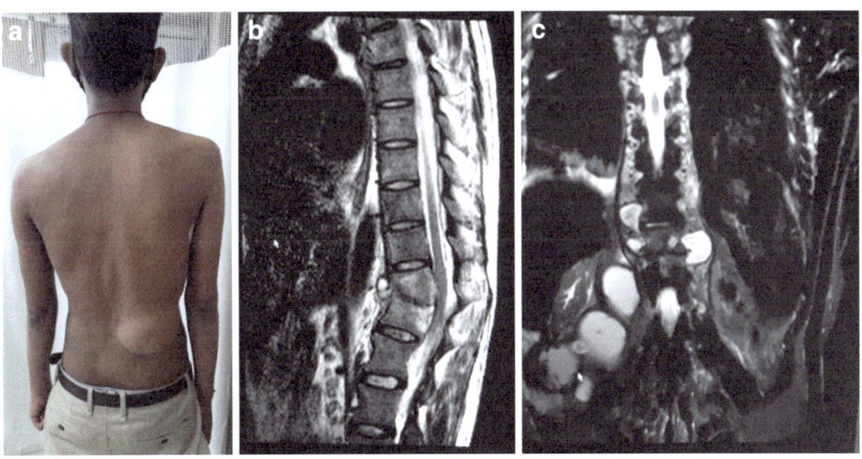

Fig. 5.1 (**a**) CKD patient presenting with cold abscess in right loin with intact neurology. (**b**) T2 sagittal MRI showing T11-T12 spondylodiskitis. (**c**) T2 coronal MRI, large inflammatory mass in right paraspinal region extending till dermis

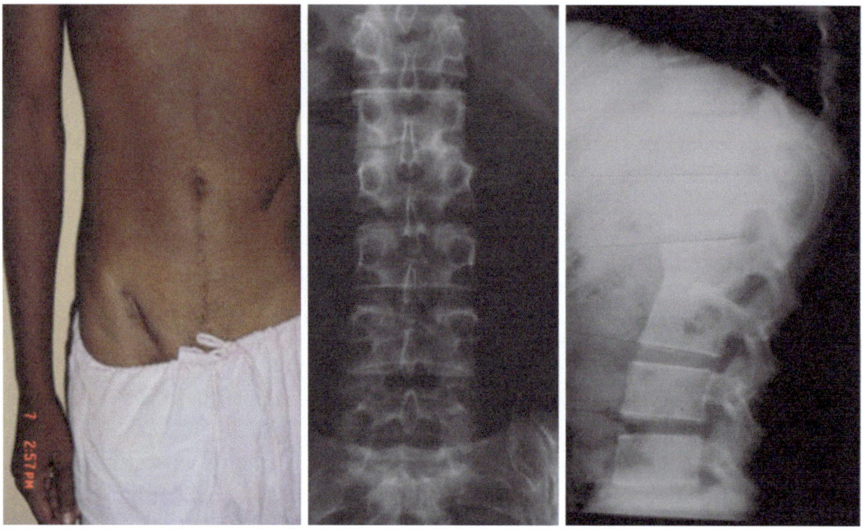

Fig. 5.2 23 yr. male with L1-L2 healed tuberculosis with multiple healed sinuses

In the lumbar spine, a cold abscess is usually seen in the Petit's triangle or groin. It can track along the psoas muscle and cause a pseudo-flexion deformity of the hip. Sometimes it can track along femoral or gluteal vessels and can appear as a mass in the Scarpa's triangle or as a gluteal abscess, respectively. If it tracks along the obturator vessels, it is seen in the adductor region [30]; if the sciatic nerve is involved, then the abscess may appear in the gluteal region, the posterior thigh, and sometimes even the popliteal fossa (Fig. 5.2).

Extension to distant sites can mislead the examiner away from the source of TB focus, so understanding the spread of the pus is important. The focus in the cervical spine may present as an abscess in the mediastinum or elbow, and thoracic spine involvement can spread through the diaphragmatic orifice into the lumbar region. Lumbar spine focus can present as an abscess in the thigh, calf, and sometimes even in the ankle.

5.5 Presentation with Spine Deformity

Patients can present with deformity during the active stage or the healed stage. Deformity can occur following surgical debridement or even many years later in the elderly when osteoporosis weakens the bony architecture. TB initially involves the anterior column, and progressive destruction results in kyphotic deformity and finally instability. Following the destruction of the intervertebral disc, cancellous

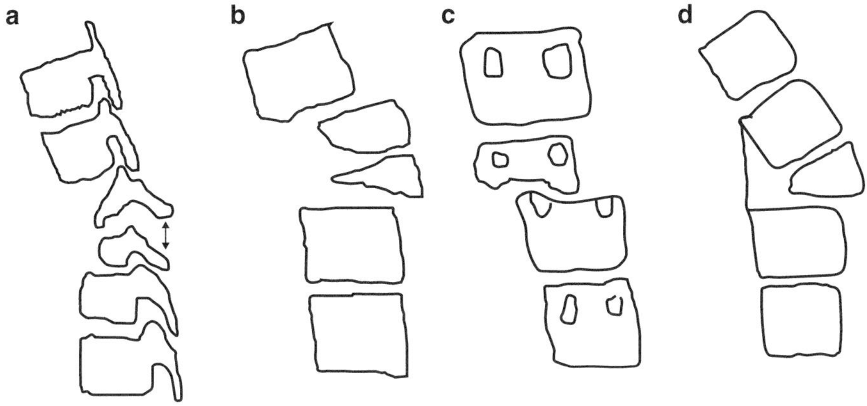

Fig. 5.3 (**a**) Separation of facets. (**b**) Retropulsion. (**c**) Lateral translation. (**d**) Toppling

bones come into contact with each other, and if treatment is started at this stage, the lesion heals without significant deformity. With the delay in treatment, further destruction occurs, leading to progressive deformity. Clinically the presentation depends on the number of vertebrae involved, i.e., *knuckle* (1 vertebra), *gibbus* (2 vertebrae), and *rounded kyphosis* (>3 vertebrae) [31]. Further collapse will cause retropulsion of the vertebral body leading to cord compression and neurological deficit [15].

In growing children, regular follow-up is required until maturity, especially if there are *spine at risk* signs like lateral *translation, retropulsion, subluxation, and toppling* [32] (Fig. 5.3). Children with facet destruction during active disease are prone to develop severe deformity during the growth phase. Severe deformities can lead to poor quality of life, cardiopulmonary compromise, and neurological deficit [1]. Kyphosis does not cause many problems in the cervical and lumbar spine as compared to the thoracic and thoracolumbar spine, due to inherent lordosis.

5.6 Suspecting Cranio-Vertebral (CV) junction TB

CV junction TB is rare, accounting for 0.3–1% of all tuberculous spondylitis [33]. It is very important to rule out this serious condition when a patient complains of prolonged neck pain, particularly in endemic areas. Delay in diagnosis can be life-threatening due to cardiorespiratory shutdown. Clinicians should be very suspicious and rule out atlanto-axial instability, lateral subluxation of dens, and basilar invagination. Delays can lead to quadriplegia or even death (Fig. 5.4).

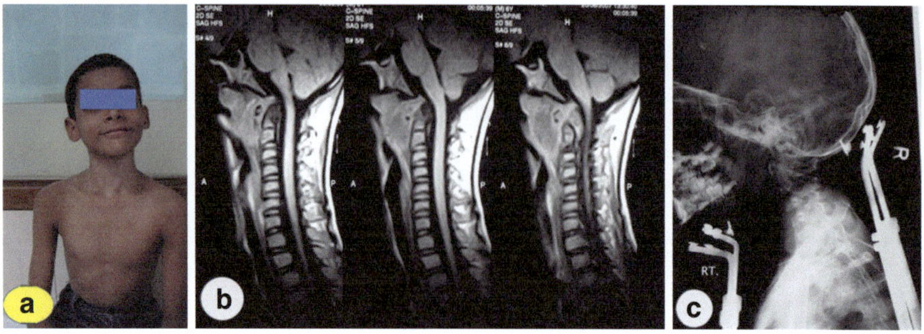

Fig. 5.4 CV junction tuberculosis: (**a**) with torticollis. (**b**) T2 saggital view. (**c**) with HALO immobilisation

5.7 Suspecting Sub-axial Cervical Spine TB

Cervical spinal TB accounts for only 3–5% of spinal TB [34, 35]. They present with mechanical neck pain and stiffness, which do not resolve as expected with conservative measures. The pain is associated with local tenderness, and sometimes the patient supports the head to prevent any motion. Neck movements are restricted, and there may be associated with torticollis. Occasionally presents with atypical features like hoarseness of voice or dysphagia due to a retropharyngeal abscess. They can even present with life-threatening stridor. Neglected cases can present with neurological involvement or features of myelopathy.

5.8 Suspecting Thoracic Spine TB

Patients often present with diffuse pain in the midback or upper back with local deep thrust tenderness. Hunchback deformity is seen in advanced cases, particularly in children (Fig. 5.5). Dermatologic pain along the supply of a particular intercostal nerve should raise the suspicion of a pathological lesion rather than a mechanical one. In developing countries, the patients often present after the onset of neurological sequelae.

5.9 Suspecting Lumbar Spine TB

Lumbar spine TB is often misdiagnosed as mechanical or degenerative or osteoporotic fractures. Most often, degenerative changes (type 1 Modic changes) are overdiagnosed as tuberculosis in countries where TB is endemic. Sometimes radicular pain from lumbar spine TB can present as abdominal pain, and patients are subjected to many unnecessary investigations [36].

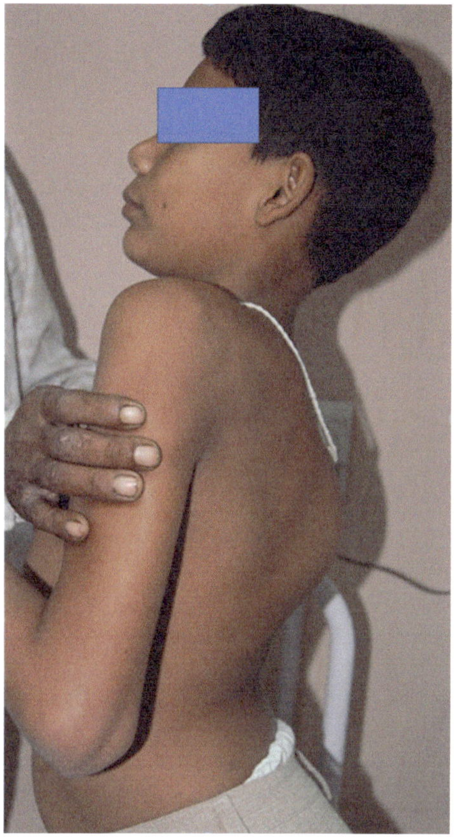

Fig. 5.5 Hunchback deformity

5.10 Suspecting Sacroiliac Joint TB (SJT)

SJT comprises approximately 5–10% of all skeletal TB [37]. Diagnosis is usually delayed due to the nonspecific nature of the disease [38]. It usually starts in the synovium and then involves the joint. Patients usually present with low back pain and buttock pain. The typical presentation is pain while climbing the stairs. In advanced stages with extensive destruction and instability, the patient complains of remarkable pain and difficulty in walking [39]. Unilateral symptoms should differentiate this from ankylosing spondylitis and transient synovitis. Abscesses can spread either anteriorly or posteriorly. Sacral roots can get irritated and cause pain along with their distribution. Examination reveals tenderness over the sacroiliac joint. Stress tests like pelvic compression test, FABER test (flexion, abduction, and external rotation), and Gaenslen's tests will be positive. Hip range of motion will be terminally painful. SJT usually ends with bony ankylosis. Rarely destruction leading to instability may need debridement and fusion.

5.11 Suspecting Intradural/Intramedullary Tuberculoma

Very rare presentation, reported as two in 100,000 cases of all TB infection [40]. Should be differentiated from neoplasms. The presentation is with progressive neurological deficit without any back pain or other signs. On examination, there is a motor loss, sensory deficits, and brisk reflexes. Plantar reflex is extensor with bladder bowel involvement. These patients have a poor prognosis of neurologic recovery due to intrinsic damage.

5.12 Signs and Symptoms in Pediatric Spinal TB

Children are more affected than adults, though these days clear patterns may not be there. When a child presents to the spine clinic with back pain, it is very important to have a high degree of suspicion because there may be rapid progression due to an immature skeleton, flexibility, and activity levels [41]. Vertebral bodies in children have more cartilage which gets rapidly destroyed with active disease and mechanical loading. Asymmetric loading of ring apophysis leads to the development of new deformity or progression of the already formed deformity and can lead to a neurological sequela [42].

Children should be followed at regular intervals, both clinically and radiologically, till skeletal maturity even after being declared healed because residual deformity can progress due to a growing spine and physical activities. Rajasekharan (2001) in his follow-up series mentioned four "spine at risk signs" for progression of deformity, they are *retropulsion, subluxation, lateral translation, or toppling*. In a report of 61 children with kyphotic deformity with more than 5 years follow-up, deformity progressed in 39%, was static in 17%, and decreased in 44%. One-third of children exhibited unacceptable progression with more than 2 of 4 spine-at-risk signs. Children aged <7 years or having involvement of >3 vertebral bodies or disease located in the lower thoracic or thoracolumbar junction are more prone to progression [33, 43].

5.13 Elderly with Suspected Tuberculosis

With increasing life expectancy, more and more elderly are diagnosed with spinal TB [44]. Special problems in the elderly include compromised health, comorbidities, and drug interactions. The aged population is at three times more risk of developing drug reactions and six times more prone to death and 20 times more risk of the wrong diagnosis [45]. Risk factors for an increased incidence of spinal TB include malignancy, diabetes mellitus, poor nutrition, immunosuppression, chronic hospitalization, etc. Approximately 90% of the time, the disease is due to reactivation of primary [46]. While examining an elderly look for signs of disseminated TB, TB meningitis, or other system involvement [47]. Back pain in the elderly is commonly overlooked due to associated degenerative disease.

5.14 Atypical Presentation

Any features apart from axial pain, constitutional symptoms, kyphosis, or typical radiological features are considered as atypical [48]. Skip lesions, concentric collapse, neural arch involvement in isolation, ivory vertebrae are some atypical patterns. Other rare presentations include disc prolapse, cold abscess without bone involvement, meningeal, neural, and perineural tissue involvement [49, 50]. Multisegmented involvement is defined as the involvement of two non-contiguous vertebrae without destruction of vertebra or disc in-between. Batson's plexus is considered responsible. Seen in up to 20% of cases according to a case series by Goldman [51]. There is no relation with HIV, chronicity, or multi-drug resistant TB with non-contiguous involvement [52].

In the past, tuberculosis was thought to be a disease of the low socioeconomic group and malnourished individuals but in the last two decades, more and more people living in healthy environments and elite classes are affected with atypical features leading to diagnostic errors. The increase in an immunocompromised state like HIV, malignancy, chemotherapy, diabetes, elderly, and other chronic illness is also one of the reasons for increasing incidences of atypical presentation.

5.15 Presentation in Immunosuppressive Individuals

Mycobacterium is an intracellular bacterium found in the healthy individual but can cause clinical disease when the host's local or systemic immunity goes down, such as in HIV infection, organ transplant, radiotherapy, chemotherapy, immunosuppressive drugs like infliximab, etc. [53, 54]. Skeletal TB is ten times more common in HIV patients compared to the general population. They present with atypical features like polycentric with multiple site abscesses and widespread destruction [55, 56]. Still, they have very little pain. They may have co-existent pulmonary and other extrapulmonary site lesions. Their sinuses rarely heal. They are more likely prone to drug resistance.

5.16 Suspecting Tuberculosis Complicating Spine Surgery

Though rare, tuberculosis can cause surgical site infection in predisposed individuals like those with a history of pulmonary TB in the past or immunosuppression. Occasionally osteoporotic collapse with TB can coexist and biopsy and a high index of suspicion is required. History of pulmonary TB or recent contact with TB patient should be carefully evaluated. A biopsy is needed for diagnosis. Inadvertent vertebroplasty or kyphoplasty may lead to a flare-up [57].

5.17 Under and Over-Diagnosed (Differential Diagnosis)

Because of its varied nature of clinical features and radiological presentations, (*great mimicker),* there is always a risk of the wrong diagnosis. Under-diagnosis is usually encountered in the elderly while overdiagnosis is encountered very frequently in India. According to a study, around 25% of various diseases were radiologically diagnosed as TB [58]. The commonly misdiagnosed entities are brucella spondylodiscitis, pyogenic spondylodiscitis, degenerative changes (Modic changes), rheumatoid arthritis, spinal metastasis, ankylosing spondylitis (pseudoarthrosis), plasmacytoma, lymphoma, etc. (Table 5.3). Hence it is important to have tissue diagnosis and drug sensitivity testing before starting anti-TB medication.

Degenerative spondylosis can be sometimes over-diagnosed as TB spondylitis, particularly in endemic areas. Imaging studies and regular clinical follow-up can help in differentiating both. And clinical and radiological deterioration should be highly suspicious of underlying pathology [59].

Disco-vertebral lesion or Andersson's lesion or sterile discitis of ankylosing spondylitis can sometimes lead to diagnostic difficulties. Morning stiffness, sacroiliac joint involvement and are the pointers. Further blood tests and imaging findings help in coming to a diagnosis [60]. Rheumatoid arthritis can mimic cervical spine TB. History of polyarthralgia and involvement of small joints are clinical clues [61].

Neoplasms like lymphomas, multiple myeloma, and metastatic lesions can pose a challenge in diagnosis both clinically and radiologically. Usually, neoplasms have multifocal lesions and less paraspinal involvement. Primary malignant neoplasms like Ewing's sarcoma, osteosarcoma, chordoma, chondrosarcoma, and

Table 5.3 Differentiating features between spinal tuberculosis and common mimics

Features	Spinal TB	Pyogenic spondylodiscitis	Spinal metastasis	Brucella spondylodiscitis
Common region	Thoracolumbar	Lumbar	Thoracic	Lumbar
Predilection	Disc and bodies Major soft tissue lesions	Disc and bodies Less soft tissue involvement	Pedicles, lamina, posterior body wall	Disc and bodies Minimal soft tissue involvement
Risk factors	Exposure to TB	Diabetes, immunosuppression	Systemic malignancy	Unpasteurized milk
Clinical Pointers	Chronic back pain, constitutional symptoms	Acute severe back pain, fever	Night pains, constitutional symptoms.	Fever, backache, malaise

fibrosarcoma should be kept in mind with an atypical presentation. Sometimes tuberculosis and malignancy coexist because of immunosuppression due to malignancy or chemoradiotherapy. Benign lesions like osteoid osteoma, GCT, histiocytosis, plasmacytoma, aneurysmal bone cyst, etc. can also mimic spinal tuberculosis [62–64].

Pyogenic spondylitis can be differentiated clinically by its rapid course, high-grade fever, more predilection to lumbar and cervical regions, less kyphosis, and severe systemic illness [65, 66]. This should be confirmed by relevant investigations. Brucella spondylitis is suspected when there is a history of handling animal products or consuming unpasteurized milk. The lumbar spine is usually involved and is associated with constitutional symptoms. Radiological evidence is further helpful. Spondylodiscitis with atypical mycobacteria is difficult to treat, has a very slow clinical course. And can lead to progressive deformity and severe neurologic sequelae [67].

Benign vertebral compression fractures can be differentiated from TB by the absence of constitutional symptoms, typical history, and a short duration of symptoms. Confirmation can be done by MRI that shows no inflammatory edema in the vertebral body and abscesses which are so typical of TB.

Summary

- Presentation of spinal tuberculosis is insidious, usually without constitutional symptoms.
- High index of suspicion and appropriate investigations are vital for early diagnosis and favorable prognosis.
- Delayed presentation leads to complications like deformity, neurological deficits, etc.
- Thoracolumbar region is most commonly involved.
- Rise in incidence of TB spine in elderly.
- Mostly spinal TB affects anterior column but atypical forms exists.
- TB is a great mimicker; tissue diagnosis and determination of drug sensitivity are vital before starting treatment.

Acknowledgments We would like to thank Dr. Chand Sahai, senior Anesthesiologist, as part of our surgical team and for correcting grammatical mistakes in the manuscript.

References

1. Gautam MP, Karki P, Rijal S, Singh R. Pott's spine and paraplegia. JNMA J Nepal Med Assoc. 2005 Jul-Sep;44(159):106–15.
2. Tuli SM, editor. Textbook-Tuberculosis of the skeletal system(Bones, Joints, Spine and Bursal sheaths). 3rd ed. New Delhi: Jaypee Brothers; 2004.

3. Isada CA. Spinal tuberculosis deserves a place on the radar screen. Cleve Clin J Med. 2004 Jul;71:537–9.
4. Alavi SM, Sharifi M. Tuberculous spondylitis: risk factors and clinical/paraclinical aspects in the south west of Iran. J Infect Public Health. 2010 Dec 1;3(4):196–200.
5. Wang H, Li C, Wang J, Zhang Z, Zhou Y. Characteristics of patients with spinal tuberculosis: seven year experience of a teaching hospital in Southwest China. Int Orthop. 2012;36:1429–34.
6. Pertuiset E, Beaudreuil J, Liote F, et al. Spinal tuberculosis in adults: a study of 103 cases in a developed country, 1980-1994. Medicine (Baltimore). 1999;78:309–20.
7. Kulchavenya E. Extrapulmonary tuberculosis: are statistical reports accurate? Ther Adv Infect Dis. 2014;2:61–70.
8. Tuli SM. Tuberculosis of the shoulder. In: Tuberculosis of the Skeletal System. New Delhi, India: JayPee Brothers Medical; 1993.
9. Boachie-Adjei O, Squillante RG. Tuberculosis of the spine. Orthop Clin North Am. 1996;27(1):95–103.
10. Jain AK. Tuberculosis of the spine: a fresh look at an old disease. The Journal of bone and joint surgery. British volume. 2010 Jul;92(7):905–13.
11. Quiñones-Hinojosa A, Jun P, Jacobs R, Rosenberg WS, Weinstein PR. General principles in the medical and surgical management of spinal infections: a multidisciplinary approach. Neurosurg Focus. 2004 Dec 15;17(6):E1.
12. Dureja S, Sen IB, Acharya S. Potential role of F18 FDG PET-CT as an imaging biomarker for the noninvasive evaluation in uncomplicated skeletal tuberculosis: a prospective clinical observational study. Eur Spine J. 2014 Nov 1;23(11):2449–54.
13. Wibaux C, Moafo-Tiatsop M, Andrei I, et al. Changes in the incidence and management of spinal tuberculosis in a French university hospital rheumatology department from 1966 to 2010. Joint Bone Spine. 2013;80:516–9.
14. Kanna RM, Shetty AP, Rajasekaran S. Spinal tuberculosis: pathogenesis, clinical features, and investigations. AOSpine Masters Series, Volume 10: Spinal Infections. 2018 Jun 15.
15. Kumar K. Tuberculosis of spine: natural history of disease and its judicious management. J Western Pac Orthop Assoc. 1988;25:1–8.
16. Dobson J. Percivall Pott. Ann R Coll Surg Engl. 1972;50:54–65.
17. Kotil K, Alan MS, Bilge T. Medical management of Pott disease in the thoracic and lumbar spine: a prospective clinical study. J Neurosurg Spine. 2007 Mar 1;6(3):222–8.
18. Hsu LC, Cheng CL, Leong JC. Pott's paraplegia of late onset. The cause of compression and results after anterior decompression. J Bone Joint Surg. 1988 Aug;70(4):534–8.
19. Nene A, Bhojraj S. Results of nonsurgical treatment of thoracic spinal tuberculosis in adults. Spine J. 2005 Jan 1;5(1):79–84.
20. Jain AK, Kumar J. Tuberculosis of spine: neurological deficit. Eur Spine J. 2013;22(Suppl 4):624–33.
21. Hodgson AR, Skinsnes OK, Leong CY. The pathogenesis of Pott's paraplegia. J Bone Joint Surg Am. 1967;49:1147–56.
22. Subramani S, Shetty AP, Kanna RM, Shanmuganathan R. Ossified ligamentum flavum causing neurological deficit above the level of post-tuberculous kyphotic deformity. J Clin Orthop Trauma. 2017;8:174–7.
23. Luk KD, Krishna M. Spinal stenosis above a healed tuberculous kyphosis. A case report Spine. 1996 May 1;21(9):1098–101.
24. Jain AK, Dhammi IK, Jain S, Mishra P. Kyphosis in spinal tuberculosis – prevention and correction. Indian J Orthop. 2010 Apr;44(2):127–36.
25. Kumar K. A clinical study and classification of posterior spinal tuberculosis. Int Orthop. 1985;9:147–52.
26. Jain AK, Sinha S. Evaluation of systems of grading of neurological deficit in tuberculosis of spine. Spinal Cord. 2005 Jun;43(6):375–80.
27. Lifeso R. Atlanto-axial tuberculosis in adults. J Bone Joint Surg. 1987 Mar;69(2):183–7.

28. Bhargava SK, Gupta S. Large retropharyngeal cold abscess in an adult with respiratory distress. J Laryngol Otol. 1990;104:157–8.
29. Faure E, Souliamas R, Riquet M, et al. Cold abscess of the chest wall: a surgical entity? Ann Thorac Surg. 1998;66:1174–8.
30. Mallick IH, Thoufeeq MH, Rajendran TP. Iliopsoas abscesses. Postgrad Med J. 2004;80:459–62.
31. Rajasekaran S, Shanmugasundaram TK. Prediction of the angle of Gibbus deformity in tuberculosis of the spine. J Bone Joint Surg Am. 1987;69:503–9.
32. Rajasekaran S. The natural history of post-tubercular kyphosis in children: radiological signs which predict late increase in deformity. The Journal of bone and joint surgery. British volume. 2001 Sep;83(7):954–62.
33. Behari S, Nayak SR, Bhargava V, Banerji D, Chhabra DK, Jain VK. Craniocervical tuberculosis: protocol of surgical management. Neurosurgery. 2003 Jan 1;52(1):72–81.
34. Hsu LC, Leong JC. Tuberculosis of the lower cervical spine (C2 to C7). A report on 40 cases. The Journal of bone and joint surgery. British volume. 1984 Jan;66(1):1–5.
35. Turgut M. Spinal tuberculosis (Pott's disease): its clinical presentation, surgical management, and outcome. A survey study on 694 patients. Neurosurg Rev. 2001 Apr 1;24(1):8–13.
36. Meena S, Barwar N, Gupta T, Chowdhury B. Spinal tuberculosis presenting as abdominal pain: rare presentation of a common disease. Oman Med J. 2014 Mar;29(2):e069.
37. Garg RK, Somvanshi DS. Spinal tuberculosis: a review. J Spinal Cord Med. 2011 Sep 1;34(5):440–54.
38. Pouchot J, Vinceneux P, Barge J, Boussougant Y, Grossin M, Pierre J, Carbon C, Kahn MF, Esdaile JM. Tuberculosis, of the sacroiliac joint: clinical features, outcome, and evaluation of closed needle biopsy in 11 consecutive cases. Am J Med. 1988 Mar 1;84(3):622–8.
39. Papadopoulos EC, Papagelopoulos PJ, Savvidou OD, Falaga ME, Sapkas GS, Fragkiadakis EG. Tuberculous sacroiliitis. Orthopedics. 2003 Jun 1;26(6):653–7.
40. Rhoton EL, Ballinger WE Jr, Quisling R, Sypert GW. Intramedullary spinal tuberculoma. Neurosurgery. 1988 Apr 1;22(4):733–6.
41. Shetty A, Kanna RM, Rajasekaran S. TB spine–Current aspects on clinical presentation, diagnosis, and management options. Semin Spine Surg. 2016;28:150.
42. Jain AK, Sreenivasan R, Mukunth R, Dhammi IK. Tubercular spondylitis in children. Indian J Orthop. 2014 Mar;48(2):136–44.
43. Rajasekaran S. Buckling collapse of the spine in childhood spinal tuberculosis. Clin Orthop Relat Res. 2007;460:86–92.
44. World Health Organization. Global tuberculosis report 2013. World Health Organization; 2013.
45. Teale C, Goldman JM, Pearson SB. The association of age with the presentation and outcome of tuberculosis: a five-year survey. Age Ageing. 1993 Jul 1;22(4):289–93.
46. Yoshikawa TT. Tuberculosis in aging adults. J Am Geriatr Soc. 1992 Feb;40(2):178–87.
47. Sood R. The problem of geriatric tuberculosis. J Indian Acad Clin Med. 2000;5:157.
48. Babhulkar SS, Tayade WB, Babhulkar SK. Atypical spinal tuberculosis. J Bone Joint Surg Br. 1984;66:239–42.
49. Pande KC, Babhulkar SS. Atypical spinal tuberculosis. Clin Orthop Relat Res. 2002;398:67–74.
50. Ahmadi J, Bajaj A, Destian S, Segali HD, Zee CS. Spinal tuberculosis: atypical observations at MR imaging. Radiology. 1993;189:489–93.
51. Goldman AB, Freiberger RH. Localized infectious and neuropathic diseases. InSeminars in roentgenology 1979 Jan 1 (Vol. 14, No. 1, pp. 19–32). WB Saunders.
52. Polley P, Dunn R. Noncontiguous spinal tuberculosis: incidence and management. Eur Spine J. 2009 Aug 1;18(8):1096–101.
53. Erkens CG, Kamphorst M, Abubakar I, Bothamley GH, Chemtob D, Haas W, Migliori GB, Rieder HL, Zellweger JP, Lange C. Tuberculosis contact investigation in low prevalence countries: a European consensus.
54. Brassard P, Kezouh A, Suissa S. Antirheumatic drugs and the risk of tuberculosis. Clin Infect Dis. 2006 Sep 15;43(6):717–22.

55. An HS, Vaccaro AR, Dolinskas CA, Cotler JM, Balderston RA, Bauerle WB. Differentiation between spinal tumors and infections with magnetic resonance imaging. Spine. 1991 Aug;16(8 Suppl):S334–8.
56. Rades D, Bremer M, Goehde S, Joergensen M, Karstens JH. Spondylodiscitis in patients with spinal cord compression: a possible pitfall in radiation oncology. Radiother Oncol. 2001 Jun 1;59(3):307–9.
57. Lai PJ, Liao JC, Chen LH, Lai PL. Tuberculous spondylitis after percutaneous vertebroplasty: a case series of 9 cases. Biom J. 2019 Aug 1;42(4):285–92.
58. Kumaran SP, Thippeswamy PB, Reddy BN, Neelakantan S, Viswamitra S. An institutional review of tuberculosis spine mimics on MR imaging: Cases of mistaken identity. Neurol India. 2019;67:1408–18.
59. Smith AS, Blaser SI. Infectious and inflammatory processes of the spine. Radiol Clin N Am. 1991 Jul;29(4):809–27.
60. Bron JL, de Vries MK, Snieders MN, van der Horst-Bruinsma IE, Van Royen BJ. Discovertebral (Andersson) lesions of the spine in ankylosing spondylitis revisited. Clin Rheumatol. 2009 Aug 1;28(8):883–92.
61. Del Grande M, Del Grande F, Carrino J, Bingham III CO, Louie GH. Cervical spine involvement early in the course of rheumatoid arthritis. In Seminars in arthritis and rheumatism 2014 Jun 1 (Vol. 43, No. 6, pp. 738–744). WB Saunders.
62. Patnaik S, Jyotsnarani Y, Uppin SG, Susarla R. Imaging features of primary tumors of the spine: A pictorial essay. Ind J Radiol Imag. 2016 Apr;26(2):279.
63. Shankar J, Jayakumar P, Vasudev M, Ravishankar S, Sinha N. The usefulness of CT perfusion in differentiation between neoplastic and tuberculous disease of the spine. J Neuroimaging. 2009 Apr;19(2):132–8.
64. Yeom JA, Lee IS, Suh HB, Song YS, Song JW. Magnetic resonance imaging findings of early spondylodiscitis: interpretive challenges and atypical findings. Korean J Radiol. 2016 Oct 1;17(5):565–80.
65. Lee KY. Comparison of pyogenic spondylitis and tuberculous spondylitis. Asian Spine J. 2014 Apr;8(2):216.
66. Jung NY, Jee WH, Ha KY, Park CK, Byun JY. Discrimination of tuberculous spondylitis from pyogenic spondylitis on MRI. Am J Roentgenol. 2004 Jun;182(6):1405–10.
67. Petitjean G, Fluckiger U, Schären S, Laifer G. Vertebral osteomyelitis caused by non-tuberculous mycobacteria. Clin Microbiol Infect. 2004;10:951–3.

Chapter 6
Diagnostic Modalities in TB Spine: Clinical Laboratory Diagnosis and Technological Advancements

Rajat R. Verma and Shivan Marya

Abstract Tuberculosis (TB) remains a major global health burden. There still remains a large gap between the notified and estimated incident cases. Extrapulmonary TB represents 15% of all TB cases, and the diagnosis is more challenging due to the paucity of the organism. Smear microscopy is often insensitive, and culture methods are prolonged.

Spinal tuberculosis is a destructive form of tuberculosis. It accounts for approximately half of all cases of musculoskeletal tuberculosis. Spinal tuberculosis is more common in children and young adults. Characteristically, there is destruction of the intervertebral disk space and the adjacent vertebral bodies, collapse of the spinal elements, and anterior wedging leading to kyphosis and gibbus formation.

The gold standard method of diagnosis of tuberculosis is the growth of Mycobacterium in culture specimens from the infected tissue and is considered the single most confirmatory diagnostic test for spinal TB. However, due to its very poor sensitivity, histopathological studies demonstrating classical granulomas and staining of smears to identify acid fast bacilli (AFB) are considered as reference standards for all other diagnostic modalities. Apart from indirect serological markers of inflammation, immunological tests have also been used with varied results. Molecular diagnostics are frequently being used because of its rapidity.

The engineering of antigens/antibody nanocarriers represents an exciting front in the field of diagnostics, potentially flagging the way toward development of better diagnostics for TB.

Keywords Spinal tuberculosis · Extrapulmonary TB · Molecular diagnostics Nanotechnology

R. R. Verma (✉)
Department of Complex Spine Surgery, Salford Royal Hospital, Stott Lane, Salford, Lancashire, UK
e-mail: rajat.verma@nca.nhs.uk

S. Marya
Salford Royal Hospital NHS Foundation Trust, Salford, Lancashire, UK

S. S. Dhatt, V. Kumar (eds.), *Tuberculosis of the Spine*,
https://doi.org/10.1007/978-981-16-9495-0_6

6.1 Introduction

Tuberculosis is an ancient disease with evidence of it in records dating back to Egyptian times. Sir Percival Pott first described tuberculosis of the spine in 1779, hence it is also referred to as 'Potts disease' or 'Potts spine' [1].

The incidence and prevalence vary between countries and paucity of data makes an accurate assessment even more challenging. Extrapulmonary TB was reported in 15% of new TB cases in the WHO global report from 2019. Osteoarticular TB accounted for 11.3% of these extrapulmonary sites with spinal TB accounting for the vast majority, reported to be up to 50% [2–6].

There is a global resurgence of tuberculosis secondary to the HIV epidemic resulting in a large group of immunodeficient individuals. Currently, much of the resources and efforts have been focused on managing pulmonary TB, which continues to be a significant public health concern. In comparison, there is less guidance available on the management of skeletal TB and majority of the data comes from studies done in pulmonary manifestation of the disease [7–10]. The risk of developing tuberculosis is estimated to be 15–21 times greater in people co-infected with HIV than among those without HIV infection. HIV and TB form a lethal combination, each speeding the other's progress. In 2019, about 208,000 people died of HIV-associated TB. In the WHO African Region, where the burden of HIV-associated TB is highest, 86% of TB patients had a documented HIV test result [11].

Although there have been major advances in early diagnosis and improved management of cases over the past four decades, the rising prevalence of immunodeficient survivors and the emergence of multidrug resistance (MDR) has resulted in resurgence of TB as a public health menace [11].

The first component of the WHO post-2015 strategy is early diagnosis of tuberculosis, including universal drug-susceptibility testing, and systematic screening of contacts and high-risk groups [12].

Scaling up the use of WHO-recommended diagnostics (e.g. rapid molecular tests) as the initial diagnostic test for TB should be promoted to increase the bacteriological confirmation of the disease. In 2019, 57% of pulmonary cases were bacteriologically confirmed, a slight increase from 55% in 2018. In the developed countries with widespread access to the most sensitive diagnostic tests, approximately 80% of pulmonary TB cases are bacteriologically confirmed [13].

Tuberculous infection of the spine behaves differently from pulmonary TB. Haematogenous spread of the Mycobacterium tuberculosis into the cancellous bone of the vertebral bodies results in Spinal tuberculosis. The primary infection site comes from either a pulmonary focus or other extrapulmonary foci, such as the lymph nodes [14–17]. Tubercular osteomyelitis is caused predominantly by spread via the paravertebral venous route, and destruction usually starts in the anterior-inferior part of vertebral body with spread under the anterior spinal ligament to adjacent inferior vertebra. Anterior involvement is mostly due to the spread of abscess under the ligaments and periosteum. Contrary to pyogenic osteomyelitis, the disk is typically spared due to lack of bacterial enzymes, until later in the disease course [18]. Predisposing factors for spinal TB include many categories, such as previous TB infection, malnutrition, alcoholism, diabetes mellitus and human immunodeficiency virus infection [14, 19, 20].

The treatment of TB is very challenging due to multiple mycobacterial populations in the disease locus with different growth kinetics and metabolic characteristics. *Mycobacterium tuberculosis* is a strict aerobe and thrives in regions with higher tissue oxygen, such as the lungs. In the osseous tissue, the organism can multiply but not to the same extent. Bony tuberculosis is generally paucibacillary, with dormant mycobacteria that are not easy to kill and they may retain viability even after chemotherapy. An accurate diagnosis of skeletal tuberculosis (TB) is essential to enable its timely and effective treatment. In spinal TB, treatment at the pre-destructive stage by the standard drugs leads to healing in about 95% of patients without significant deformities or neurological complications. However, once symptoms progress to neurological deficits, a significant number of patients may never recover neurological function [4].

6.2 Difficulty in Diagnosis

Diagnosis of spinal tuberculosis is based on clinical and radiological clues, with supporting histological and/or microbiological features. However, even when there is strong clinical suspicion of spinal TB, diagnosis is not straightforward: clinical findings suffer from lack of specificity, and the results of tests assessing TB infection (tuberculin skin test or IFN-g release assays) may not be specific [21]. Spinal TB is paucibacillary, and the sites of infection may not be easily accessible for the collection of specimens suitable for microscopy, histology, culture or molecular tests [6, 22]. Despite this, the isolation of mycobacteria from clinical samples is useful both for confirmation of diagnosis and for determination of drug susceptibility. Due to the insidious clinical features of spinal TB, diagnostic delay is often prolonged (mean 6.5 months from presentation, with a time range from 3 to 12 months) [23].

In the UK, there were 4713 new cases of pulmonary TB diagnosed in 2019, with and incidence of 8.4 per 100,000. Of these 156 (3.3%) patients had TB Spine [24]. In comparison, the number of new cases of pulmonary TB in India in 2019 was 24,04,976 with an incidence of 159 per 100,000 [25]. Despite the vast difference in incidence rates, in the UK, there was an average delay of 75 days from onset of symptoms to starting antitubercular treatment. The primary reason for this was a delay in diagnosis. It is evident from this data that delay in diagnosis is not necessarily related to incidence rates and healthcare resources, which are considerably more favourable in the West.

Both patient and medical factors contribute to a delay in diagnosis, and it has been estimated that there is an average delay of 1 year between onset of symptoms and patient presentation alone [26]. The diagnostic difficulties will be elaborated in the following sections, however, it must be emphasized that establishing an early diagnosis of TB spine is instrumental in preventing complications of deformity and neurological deficit from developing, and thereby improving patient outcomes from this disease. If detected in a timely manner, TB of the spine can often be managed with antitubercular therapy without necessitating surgical intervention [27]. Despite all the advances in technology, the diagnosis revolves around a high clinical index of suspicion based on the history and examination findings that is supplemented with biochemical and radiological evidence.

Currently, no form of extrapulmonary tuberculosis can count on a single reliable rule-out test (i.e. test with minimal or absent false-negative results). The diagnosis of EPTB is thus often made by the integration of several non-specific clues from various investigations [28].

6.3 Conventional Diagnostic Tests

In order to establish a confirmed diagnosis of tuberculosis, it requires the demonstration of presence of *Mycobacterium tuberculosis* bacilli by either microbiological, cytopathological or histopathological techniques [29].

The classical approach to the diagnosis of tubercular infections involves the isolation and identification of mycobacterial colonies growing on Lowenstein-Jensen medium. This however takes a significant period of time, hence more recent recommendations describe using a combination of phenotypic (direct) and molecular assay (indirect) to allow for the more rapid identification of the presence of mycobacterium [30].

6.4 Microscopy

Mycobacteria are also referred to as acid fast bacilli (AFB) due to the property of its cell wall resulting from a high lipid content. This binds to Fuchsin dye, preventing it from escaping from the cell when exposed to acid alcohol.

The presence of acid fast bacilli (AFB) on microscopy, combined with history of constitutional symptoms of tuberculosis and evidence of pulmonary lesions on chest X-rays, helps establish an early diagnosis. In addition to helping establish a diagnosis, acid fast smears also help monitor response to treatment. The main limitation of smears is that a minimum of 10,000 AFB per ml of sample is required for them to be detected, which is often not the case in paucibacillary diseases such as spinal TB [31].

There are various microscopy illumination techniques, and WHO evaluation showed that the diagnostic accuracy of light emitting diode (LED) microscopy is comparable to that of conventional fluorescence microscopy with much less expense [32].

The techniques used for acid fast staining are [31]:

- *Carbol fuchsin stains:* a mixture of fuchsin with phenol (carbolic acid).
  - Ziehl–Neelsen (hot stain).
  - Kinyoun (cold stain).
- *Fluorochrome stains:* Auramine O, with or without a second fluorochrome, rhodamine.

6.4.1 ZN Staining (Hot)

In this smear, Mycobacteria are stained red and the background light blue. It is referred to as hot staining as heat is used to help improve the penetration of carbol fuchsin into the bacilli. The smear is then treated with 20% H_2SO_4 for de-colouring and subsequently counter stained using methylene blue. Due to their high lipid content in the cell wall, tubercular bacilli resist decolourisation by H_2SO_4 hence are referred to as acid fast. Ziehl–Neelsen staining has the advantages of being a reliable, reproducible and inexpensive technique also helps monitor response to antitubercular treatment. The disadvantages of this technique, however, are that it has low sensitivity (40%) and is unable to differentiate between different types of Mycobacteria [33, 34].

6.4.2 Kinyoun (Cold)

This technique employs the use of an increased concentration of phenol as compared to ZN staining, thereby eliminating the need to use heat for penetration of carbol fuchsin. Similar to ZN staining, the Mycobacteria appear red on a light blue background [30].

6.5 Auramine Flourochrome

Fluorochrome staining carries an advantage of being able to scan a significantly larger area of the smear in comparison to Ziehl–Neelsen staining. This results in both an increased sensitivity to detect bacilli and reduction of time required to scan the smear.

6.5.1 Culture

Culture techniques are able to detect significantly fewer tubercle bacilli (10–100/ml of sample) as compared to microscopy. Further, the bacilli isolated can be used to identify the species and for drug sensitivity testing. Hence, the detection of tuberculosis bacilli on culture is considered the 'gold standard' to establish a diagnosis of tuberculosis. The disadvantage of traditional culture techniques is the time taken in order to detect visible growth, which can be up to 4–8 weeks with LJ media.

The different culture media used to grow MTB can be classified into:

i. *Solid Media.*

   a. *Egg Based*—Contents include whole eggs or egg yolk, potato flour, salts and glycerol that are solidified by inspissation. They have a long shelf life and support the growth of most of mycobacteria. The most commonly used egg-based media is the Lowenstein-Jensen (LJ) media.
   b. *Agar Based*—These media are chemically better defined in comparison to egg-based media. As a result, colonies may be visible significantly faster than egg-based media in 10–12 days.
   c. *Selective Media*—Antimicrobial agents that suppress contaminating bacteria are used to make these media are more selective for allowing the growth of mycobacteria alone. Hence, they are used in conjunction with a non-selective egg or agar medium. Examples of selective media include the Gruft modification in which nalidixic acid and penicillin are added to LJ media or the Mitchison selective 7H11 medium to which carbenicillin, polymyxin B, trimethoprim and amphotericin B are added.

ii. *Liquid Media.*

   Liquid based or broth media can be used for early isolation of mycobacteria and subculturing. Some of the frequently used broth media are Middlebrook 7H9, BACTEC 12B and Dubos Tween albumin broth.

   a. *Mycobacteria Growth Indicator Tube (MGIT)*—The MGIT contains a fluorescence-quenching-based oxygen sensor (silicon rubber impregnated with a ruthenium pentahydrate) which is added to modified Middlebrook 7H9 media in order to help detect the growth of tubercle bacilli.
   b. *BACTEC 460 TB System*—It is a semi-automated system that uses 14C-labelled palmitic acid as carbon source in the medium. In the presence of bacilli, this is metabolized to release $14CO_2$, which is detected by the instrument. The average time to detect bacilli in a smear-positive specimen is 9–14 days in case of tuberculosis. However, the disadvantages of this technique include inability to observe colony morphology, difficulty in identifying mixed cultures, overgrowth by contaminants, cost and radioisotope disposal [35].
   c. *Automated Continuous Monitoring Systems*—The BACTEC 9000 MB system also uses a fluorescence quenching-based oxygen sensor similar to that as

the MGIT system to detect growth. The MB/BacT ALERT 3D system employs a colorimetric CO2 sensor in each bottle and reflected light to monitor the presence and production of CO2 dissolved in the culture media. As the bacilli grow, CO2 is produced which diffuses through the membrane to the sensor and dissolves in water resulting in the accumulation of hydrogen ions. The amount of CO2 produced is proportional to the growth of microorganism in media, resulting in collection of Hydrogen ions and reduction in the pH of the sensor. This causes the colour to change from dark to light green or yellow.

6.6 Serological Tests

It is known that IgM levels are an indicator of activity level of tuberculosis and have been shown to decline over a 3 month period after initiating therapy. In contrast, IgG levels show an increasing trend over the same time interval, hence are not diagnostic in value however are representative of chronic or healed disease [36]. IGRA (Interferon Gamma Release Assay) is an ELISA test to detect the presence of the cytokine Interferon Gamma that is produced as a part of the cell-mediated inflammatory response by the body to the tubercular antigen [37]. QuantiFERON-TB Gold is one such test that has been shown to have sensitivity of 84% and specificity of 95% in correctly detecting IFN gamma in patients with spinal TB with vertebral body collapse.

Though Enzyme-Linked Immunosorbent Assay (ELISA) has improved the detection of these antibodies, it does not help differentiate between pulmonary and extrapulmonary TB or active and latent disease.

6.7 Technological Advances in Diagnosis of Spinal TB

As outlined in the previous sections, diagnosis of Spinal TB is crucial prior to starting antibiotic therapy to prevent the development of drug resistance. There exists some disparity in the literature regarding the gold standard for diagnosing Spinal TB. Some authors feel a positive culture is essential to make an 'absolute diagnosis', whereas others suggest spinal tuberculosis is a paucibacillary disease hence traditional Lowenstein Jenson media cultures and Zeihl Nelson staining is not the gold standard for diagnosis [38]. The main drawbacks of culture and sensitivity for acid fast bacilli are that they require live organisms to yield a positive result, have a long incubation period, and sensitivity decreases significantly in patients who are already on antitubercular therapy [36].

The advancements to traditional diagnostic modalities discussed in the previous section are aimed at improving the sensitivity and specificity of detection of TB bacilli and reduce the time required. The advancements are:

6.8 Molecular Testing Methods

There is a movement in clinical laboratories away from the conventional time consuming and tedious test for species identification of Mycobacteria recovered in culture, e.g. nucleic acid probes have been produced to identify MTB, *Mycobacterium avium intracellulare, M. kansasii* and *M. gordonae*. There are four major applications used in clinical laboratories:

1. Use of DNA probes for culture confirmation of isolates recovered from clinical specimens.
2. Use of DNA sequencing for identification of mycobacteria.
3. Use of nucleic acid amplification tests (NAAT) for direct detection of MTB from clinical specimens.
4. DNA fingerprinting and strain typing of mycobacterium species.

6.9 Nucleic Acid Probes

The first nucleic acid based technology used to identify mycobacteria in positive cultures with very high accuracy, sensitivity and specificity. In this technique, ribosomal RNA (rRNA) present in the cells and in culture in high quantities acts as a genetic target. The radio-labelled (acridine ester) single-stranded DNA probes hybridize with rRNA forming stable DNA-RNA complexes. After the inactivation of an unhybridized probe, light generated is recorded by an instrument that is proportional to the amount of probe present. A predetermined threshold is used to determine positivity. This technique requires two hours.

6.10 In Situ Hybridization

This technology uses an oligonucleotide probe labelled with fluorescein, and the interpretation is made by direct observation using fluorescence microscopy. It is popularly known as fluorescence in situ hybridization (FISH).

6.11 Nucleic Acid Amplification (NAA) Methods

PCR technique is now widely used in the research and diagnostic fields. This technique is based on the amplification of specific DNA sequences to a large number of copies that can be detected by separation on gel electrophoresis. The amplification is achieved by using synthetic oligonucleotide primers complementary to specific DNA sequence. This process leads to a million-fold amplification of target

DNA. The target most frequently amplified is the IS 6110 repetitive element which is present in multiple copies (up to 20) in most strains of M. tuberculosis. The effectiveness of PCR for tuberculosis depends on experience and accuracy of the personnel conducting the assay.

Real-time PCR is a technique that reduces the detection time and also quantifies the amount of M TB present in the clinical sample. The whole process of amplification and detection takes place in a single reaction vessel in a closed system. Thus it reduces the risk of amplicon contamination in the laboratory. Since this technique is completely automated, there is no need of post-amplification processing and electrophoresis for the detection of amplicons [39].

6.11.1 Xpert MTB/RIF Test

The Xpert MTB/RIF test (Cepheid, Sunnyvale, California) is an automated Polymerase chain reaction test that simultaneously detects TB and checks for Rifampicin resistance in less than 2 hours [35]. To perform the test, tissue samples taken at the time of biopsy are combined with a lysis reagent and a mixture is made by rapidly oscillating the two together. The mixture obtained is then allowed to stand and 2 ml of it is drawn and processed in the GeneXpert machine. Results from this are available in approximately 90 minutes [40].

The advantages of this system [39, 40] are:

- Rapid results—the results are obtained within 2 hours as compared with results of cultures which take 4–6 weeks.
- Fully automated system—minimal training and technical knowledge is required to run the test, thereby making it a lot less operator dependent as compared with cultures and microscopy.
- Simultaneous detection of rifampicin resistance—MDR TB is a growing problem with increasing resistance to Isoniazid and Rifampicin. The GeneXpert system detects mutations in gene sequences present in TB bacilli that are resistant to rifampicin, which provides rapid information about multidrug resistance.
- Ability to detect smaller amounts of TB bacilli—Conventional cultures typically require the presence of 10,000 colony forming units (CFU's) per ml to be able to detect it, however as the GeneXpert system amplifies the nucleic acid of the pathogen, it has been shown to require the presence of only 130 CFU/ml. This is believed to have a significant impact on diagnosing paucibacillary tuberculosis like Spinal TB.
- Differentiate between typical and atypical mycobacterium.

Recently there have been studies performed in South Africa [40] and India [41] that compared the sensitivity and specificity of Xpert MTB/RIF test to conventional diagnostic modalities (microscopy, culture, histopathology) for Spinal Tuberculosis. Both studies independently concluded that GeneXpert testing had a better sensitivity and specificity to diagnose Spinal TB as compared to conventional methods.

Further both studies found that the GeneXpert system accurately detected all cases of MDR TB in their respective series of patients.

As with any test the Xpert MTB/RIF test has some disadvantages too [40, 41]:

- Detecting non-viable pathogens—as the test works by amplifying the nucleic acid from the pathogen, it can also detect the presence of non-viable pathogens and thereby give an erroneous false-positive result.
- Missing mono drug resistance—Most MDR TB pathogens are resistant to both INH and Rifampicin. The GeneXpert can only detect Rifampicin resistance and presume that if there is no rifampicin resistance, there will be no resistance to INH either. Occasionally, however, cases of mono resistance to INH have been reported, and it is evident that these cases would be missed by the GeneXpert as they are still sensitive to Rifampicin.
- Single gene target—this test amplifies a single gene target in *Mycobacterium tuberculosis bacilli*, however, this may be absent in a proportion of the TB bacilli, thereby resulting in a false-negative result.

6.11.2 Multiplex PCR

The multiplex PCR is aimed at amplifying two or more gene targets of mycobacterium. The Xpert MTB/RIF and other PCR studies amplify a single gene (usually IS6110), however studies from India have shown that there is a proportion of TB bacilli in which the IS6110 target is absent, hence would result in false-negative results.

In such instances, the Multiplex PCR that amplifies both IS6110 and MPB 64 genes present in mycobacterium has been shown to have a superior sensitivity and specificity [42, 43]. It has been demonstrated that in order to reduce the cost of this investigation, both the genes can be amplified together from a single tissue sample [43].

6.12 Nanotechnology

Despite all advances in TB diagnosis landscape, there is no accurate, rapid, inexpensive, point-of-care assay available for M. tuberculosis detection, well-matched for children, extrapulmonary TB (EPTB) and HIV-associated TB [28]. Nanotechnology aims to fill this void by providing a fast, efficient and cheap point-of-care test that uses particles sized 1–100 nm. It appears to be promising in the diagnosis of infectious diseases like TB due to the ability of nano diagnostic techniques to achieve consistent and rapid conclusions using simple and portable devices by using various body fluids, such as blood, sputum or urine samples from patients [44].

The nano diagnostic techniques being developed for diagnosing TB include [28]:

a. *Gold Nanoparticle-Based TB Diagnostic Techniques.*

   Gold NPs utilize DNA probes (oligonucleotide derived from the gene sequence of the M. tuberculosis RNA polymerase subunit) coupled with the NPs for the colourimetric detection of M. tuberculosis. At a wavelength of 526 nm, if the complementary DNA is present, the nanoprobe solution remains pink in colour (no DNA probe aggregation), while the solution turns purple (due to nanoprobe aggregation at a high NaCl concentration) in the absence of complementary DNA in the samples.

b. *Gold Nanoparticle-Mediated Dipstick.*

   Colloidal Gold NPs were coated with the M. tuberculosis antigen using alkanethiols derivatives, and when mixed with serum containing antibodies, it resulted a red colour that is visible to the naked eye

c. *Silica Nanoparticle-Based Detection.*

   Indirect immunofluorescence microscopy has been developed by utilizing nanoparticle coupled with fluorescent dye for the detection of M. tuberculosis

d. *Quantum Dots-Based Detection System.*

   In this system, one probe binds to the 23S rRNA gene of the mycobacterium very precisely and a second probe precisely recognizes IS900 conserved sequence in mycobacterium, which was treated on sulphurous acid chromium quantum dots. As a result, a sandwich is formed after hybridization with target gene sequences of mycobacterium DNA, isolated from suspected samples of TB patients. Subsequently, quantum dot-magnetic bead conjugates are exposed to ultraviolet (UV) light, which emits red fluorescence (visible to the naked eye).

e. *Biosensor-Based Detection.*

   This is based on the detection of short nucleotide sequences of M. tuberculosis DNA. The different types of sensors are mass/piezoelectric, biochemical, electrical, and optical sensors.

Overall there is no perfect test for diagnosing Spinal TB and as mentioned before it often requires a combination of history, examination findings (which may be nonspecific) with imaging (MRI is more sensitive than radiographs) and laboratory diagnosis.

References

1. Chauhan A, Gupta BB. Spinal tuberculosis. Indian Acad Clin Med. 2007;8:110–4.
2. Naim-ur-Rahman. Atypical forms of spinal tuberculosis. J Bone Joint Surg Br. 1980;62-B:162–5.
3. Talbot JC, Bismil Q, Saralaya D, Newton D, Frizzel RM, Shaw DL. Musculoskeletal tuberculosis in bradford–a 6-year review. Ann R Coll Surg Engl. 2007;89:405–9.
4. Tuli SM. Historical aspects of Pott's disease (spinal tuberculosis) management. Eur Spine J. 2012;22:529–38.

5. World Health Organization. WHO report on the proposed post-2015 TB Strategy and targets. Available from: http://apps.who.int/gb/ebwha/pdf_files/EB134/B134_12-en.pdf?uaZ1.
6. Golden MP, Vikram HR. Extrapulmonary tuberculosis: an overview. Am Fam Physician. 2005;72(9):1761–8.
7. Kotil K, Alan MS, Bilge T. Medical management of pott disease in the thoracic and lumbar spine: a prospective clinical study. J Neurosurg Spine. 2007;6:222–8.
8. Cormican L, Hammal R, Messenger J, Milburn HJ. Current difficulties in the diagnosis and management of spinal tuberculosis. Postgrad Med J. 2006;82:46–51.
9. Pandita A, Madhuripan N, Hurtado RM, Dhamoon A. Back pain and oedematous schmorl node: a diagnostic dilemma. BMJ Case Rep. 2017;2017 https://doi.org/10.1136/bcr-2017-219904.
10. World Health Organization. Global tuberculosis report 2019. World Health Organization; 2019.
11. World Health Organization. TB facts. Available at: http://www.who.int/mediacentre/factsheets/fs104/en/
12. World Health Organization. .https://www.who.int/tb/publications/2015/end_tb_essential.pdf?ua=1
13. WHO Global TB Report 2020. https://apps.who.int/iris/bitstream/handle/10665/336069/9789240013131-eng.pdf
14. McLain RF, Isada C. Spinal tuberculosis deserves a place on the radar screen. Cleve Clin J Med. 2004;71(537–539):543–9.
15. World Health Organization. High-priority target product profiles for new tuberculosis diagnostic. Report of a consensus meeting. Available from: https://apps.who.int/iris/bitstream/handle/10665/135617/WHO_HTM_TB_2014.18_eng.pdf?sequence=1
16. Boachie-Adjei O, Squillante RG. Tuberculosis of the spine. Orthop Clin North Am. 1996;27:95e103.
17. Schirmer P, Renault CA, Holodniy M. Is spinal tuberculosis contagious? Int J Infect Dis. 2010;14:e659e66.
18. Lee KY. Comparison of pyogenic spondylitis and tuberculous spondylitis. AsianSpine J. 2014;8:216–23.
19. Raviglione MC. Tuberculosis. In: Kasper D, Fauci A, Hauser S, Longo D, Jameson J, Loscalzo J, editors. Harrison's principles of internal medicine. 19th ed. New York, NY: McGraw-Hill; 2015.
20. Ansari S, Amanullah MF, Ahmad K, Rauniyar RK. Pott's spine: diagnostic imaging modalities and technology advancements. N Am J Med Sci. 2013;5:404e11.
21. Sester M, Sotgiu G, Lange C, et al. Interferon-gamma release assays for the diagnosis of active tuberculosis: a systematic review and meta-analysis. Eur Respir J. 2011;37(1):100–11.
22. Norbis L, Miotto P, Alagna R, Cirillo DM. Tuberculosis: lights and shadows in the current diagnostic landscape. New Microbiol. 2013;36(2):111–20.
23. Fuentes Ferrer M, Gutierrez Torres L, Ayala Ramirez O, et al. Tuberculosis of the spine. A systematic review of case series. Int Orthop. 2012;36(2):221–31.
24. Public Health England. Tuberculosis in England: 2020 report (presenting data to end of 2019) [Internet]. 2020 [cited 2020 Dec 28]. Available from: https://assets.publishing.service.gov.uk/government/uploads/system/uploads/attachment_data/file/943356/TB_Annual_Report_2020.pdf
25. Central TB Division Government of India. India TB Report 2020 [Internet]. 2020 [cited 2020 Dec 28]. Available from: https://tbcindia.gov.in/WriteReadData/l892s/India TB Report 2020.pdf
26. Sternbach G. Percivall Pott: tuberculous spondylitis. J Emerg Med [Internet]. 1996;14(1):79–83. Available from: http://www.sciencedirect.com/science/article/pii/0736467995020535
27. Shetty A, Kanna R, Rajasekaran S. TB spine–current aspects on clinical presentation, diagnosis, and management options. Seminars in Spine Surgery 2016;28(3):150–162.
28. Gupta AK, Singh A, Singh S. Diagnosis of tuberculosis: nanodiagnostics approaches. Nano Bio Medicine. 2019:261–83.

29. Sharma SK, Mohan A. Tuberculosis: from an incurable scourge to a curable disease–journey over a Millennium. Indian J Med Res. 2013;137:455e493.
30. Winn W, Allen S, Janda W, et al. Koneman's Color atlas and textbook of diagnostic microbiology. 6th ed; 2006. p. 1064e1124.
31. Kapil A. Ananthanarayan & Paniker's textbook of microbiology. 9th ed. chennai: Universities Press (india) Pvt Ltd; 2013. p. 352.
32. Purohit M, Mustafa T. Laboratory diagnosis of extrapulmonary tuberculosis (EPTB) in resource- constrained setting: state of the art, challenges and the need. J Clin Diagn Res. 2015;9:EE01eEE06.
33. Liu KT, Su WJ, Perng RP. Clinical utility of polymerase chain reaction for diagnosis of smear-negative pleural tuberculosis. J Chin Med Assoc. 2007;70:148e151.
34. Haldar S, Bose M, Chakrabarti P, et al. Improved laboratory diagnosis of tuberculosis and the Indian experience. Tuberculosis. 2011;91:414e426. 42. Derese Y, Hailu E, Assefa T, et al. Comparison of PCR with standard culture of fine needle aspiration samples in the diagnosis of tuberculosis lymphadenitis. J Infect Dev Ctries. 2012;6:53e57.
35. Pfyffer GE, Palicova F. Mycobacterium: general characteristics, laboratory detection, and procedures. In: Versalovic J, Carroll KC, Funke G, Jorgensec JH, Landry ML, Warnock DW, eds. Mannual of clinical microbiology. 10th ed. ASN press; 2011:472e502.
36. Jain AK, Jena SK, Singh MP, Dhammi IK, Ramachadran VG, Dev G. Evaluation of clinico-radiological, bacteriological, serological, molecular and histological diagnosis of osteoarticular tuberculosis. Indian J Orthop. 2008 Apr;42(2):173–7.
37. Garg RK, Somvanshi DS. Spinal tuberculosis: a review. J Spinal Cord Med [Internet]. 2011;34(5):440–54. https://doi.org/10.1179/2045772311Y.0000000023.
38. Khanna K, Sabharwal S. Spinal tuberculosis: a comprehensive review for the modern spine surgeon. Spine J. 2019;19(11):1858–70.
39. Centers for Disease Control and Prevention. A new tool to diagnose tuberculosis: the Xpert MTB/RIF Assay [Internet]. [cited 2021 Jan 1]. Available from: https://www.cdc.gov/tb/publications/factsheets/pdf/xpertmtb-rifassayfactsheet_final.pdf
40. Held M, Laubscher M, Zar HJ, Dunn RN. GeneXpert polymerase chain reaction for spinal tuberculosis: an accurate and rapid diagnostic test. Bone Joint J. 2014 Oct;96-B(10):1366.
41. Solanki AM, Basu S, Biswas A, Roy S, Banta A. Sensitivity and specificity of gene Xpert in the diagnosis of spinal tuberculosis: a prospective controlled clinical Study. Glob spine J. 2020 Aug;10(5):553–8.
42. Sharma K, Meena RK, Aggarwal A, Chhabra R. Multiplex PCR as a novel method in the diagnosis of spinal tuberculosis–a pilot study. Acta Neurochir (Wien) [Internet]. 2017 Mar 21;159(3):503–7. https://doi.org/10.1007/s00701-016-3065-0.
43. Sharma K, Sharma A, Sharma SK, Sen RK, Dhillon MS, Sharma M. Does multiplex polymerase chain reaction increase the diagnostic percentage in osteoarticular tuberculosis? A prospective evaluation of 80 cases. Int Orthop. 2012 Feb;36(2):255–9.
44. Wang Y, Yu L, Kong X, Sun L. Application of nanodiagnostics in point-of-care tests for infectious diseases. Int J Nanomedicine. 2017;12:4789–803.

Chapter 7
Microbiological Diagnosis of Spinal Tuberculosis

Kusum Sharma and Megha Sharma

Abstract Timely diagnosis of spinal tuberculosis is imperative to initiate appropriate therapy and to prevent long-term sequalae-like deformities. The clinical and radiological features have several mimickers, and microbiological evidence of *Mycobacterium tuberculosis* or its products form the basis of definite diagnosis. The chapter concisely presents all the aspects associated with microbiological diagnosis of spinal tuberculosis ranging from the desired samples that should be sent for investigation, pros and cons of conventional techniques of staining and culture, and the modalities targeting the protein or nucleic acid of M. tuberculosis. Among the nucleic acid amplification tests, which now serve as important first-line tests for diagnosis, a brief description of each ranging from conventional polymerase chain reaction to isothermal amplification to commercial systems is presented in this chapter. Finally, brief summary of gene sequencing and methods for testing drug susceptibility for spinal tuberculosis are also discussed.

Keywords Nucleic acid amplification test · Drug resistant tuberculosis of spine MALDI TOF

7.1 Introduction

Spinal tuberculosis (STB) is the most common form of osteoarticular tuberculosis, constituting nearly half of the cases [1]. It is an ancient disease as tuberculosis of the bones has been documented from the mummies in Egypt [2]. STB is a worldwide concern; while developed countries face the challenges of emergence of disease in immunocompromised patients, the developing countries battle with problems of diagnostic delay and drug resistant strains [1, 3]. It is important to diagnose STB in the early inflammatory phase so as to prevent spinal deformity and neurological

K. Sharma (✉) · M. Sharma
Department of Medical Microbiology, Postgraduate Institute of Medical Education and Research, Chandigarh, India

S. S. Dhatt, V. Kumar (eds.), *Tuberculosis of the Spine*,
https://doi.org/10.1007/978-981-16-9495-0_7

sequelae. Nearly 47.5% of inadequately treated patients develop spinal deformity and the mortality is 8.6% [4]. The clinical and radiological features of STB overlap with other infectious and non-infectious diseases of the spine [5]. Further, empiric therapy with anti-tubercular treatment given for prolonged duration adds to unnecessary toxicity, poor compliance and drug resistance [3]. Hence, microbiological diagnosis is of STB is of paramount importance, preferably with rapid turn-around time and simultaneous detection of resistance.

7.2 Samples To Be Sent for Microbiological Investigations

In order to improve the diagnostic yield, it is important that optimal specimen is sent for microbiological investigation. The early inflammatory stage is the best time for sampling as the yield of organism is highest and timely initiation of therapy can greatly improve prognosis. The intricate anatomical organization around the spine poses specific challenges for collecting an adequate sample, and interventional radiology is often employed for targeted sampling. In a study evaluating yield of microbiological investigations using different sample types, it was found that in comparison to vertebral bodies, it was the soft tissue samples (consisting of paraspinal/psoas abscesses and intervertebral discs) that had better yield than vertebral bodies [6]. The yield of detection increases if multiple samples from different sites are sent rather than one isolated sample. Caution is advised if a bone marrow aspiration from the iliac crest is scheduled from a patient of active tuberculous spondylitis as there is a risk of *M. tuberculosis* contamination on the aspirated material [7].

7.3 Microbiological Investigations

The microbiological investigations available for STB can be broadly divided into conventional investigations, proteomics detection and nucleic acid amplification tests.

1. Conventional Staining

   Staining using special stain of Ziehl–Neelsen for *Mycobacterium tuberculosis* is the first investigation sent for STB, owing to its rapid reporting. It is based on the principle that an intact cell wall of tubercle bacilli contains mycolic acid and a variety of other lipids and fatty acids that are negatively charged and hence bind strongly to the basic dye carbol fuschin in the presence of a mordant (phenol or heat). Once this bond is established, it resists decolorization even with strong acids, hence called acid-fast. Finally a counterstain is added to bring about a bluish-green contrast in the background enabling easy visualization of the brightly stained pinkish-red beaded bacilli. The turn-around time for ZN smear is usually within hours, starting from sample decontamination to smear reporting. However, the smear lacks sensitivity. The usual sensitivity of ZN smear ranges from 10–30% for extrapulmonary samples, and a higher sensitivity of 52% was observed when the FNAC sample was collected under computed tomography- or fluoroscopy guidance [8]. Diffre et al. [9] also suggested that fluoroscopy-guided aspiration should be conducted for improving the culture yield from pyogenic vertebral osteomyelitis.

The other staining technique used for *M. tuberculosis* is the auramine staining. This fluorescent dye enables easy visualization of the fluorescing bacilli against a dark ground under the fluorescent microscope, thereby allowing rapid scanning of smears.

2. Mycobacterial Culture

Isolation of tubercle bacilli on culture remains the gold standard for diagnosing STB. Solid culture, done either on egg-based media or agar-based media, enables getting a pure culture and differentiating colonies on the basis of morphology. The Lowenstein-Jensen medium slant is the most commonly used egg-based solid medium. It takes around 2 to 8 weeks for the colonies to show on this medium, a period too long to be clinically relevant. Nonetheless, the isolation of tubercle bacilli on solid media is important for morphological identification and to obtain a pure growth for further processing like susceptibility testing and extracting good amount of DNA.

The other solid media include agar-based Middlebrook 7H10 and 7H11, while 7H12 is a liquid broth for culturing *M. tuberculosis*. The liquid cultures offer shorter turn-around time, however, they only denote turbidity of the medium, which could arise due to contamination also; hence a confirmation is required. The reported sensitivity of LJ culture, Middlebrook 7H10 and liquid broth-based culture medium for detecting *M. tuberculosis* in extrapulmonary samples have been reported to be 44%, 39% and 51%, respectively [10]. Liquid culture also took half the time in reporting as compared to solid cultures (13 vs. 26 days) [10].

Automation has changed the way mycobacterial cultures were put traditionally. At least two commercial systems for mycobacterial culture are available, the BACTEC 460 and MGIT (Mycobacterial Growth Indicator Tube) 960. These systems allow continuous monitoring of tubes containing enriched broth and inoculated with clinical samples. As soon as the growth of organism reaches a sufficient threshold, the system gives a beep, and the culture bottle can then be harnessed for isolating the organism without risk of cross-contamination. Further, drug susceptibility testing can also be undertaken using such systems.

3. Proteomics

Considering the risky procedure of sample collection in STB and inherent lengthy procedure of culture methods, alternative tests using minimally invasive samples and allowing rapid results have also been developed. A recent study analyzing immunological markers for diagnosing STB reported that chemokine receptor CXCR3 was found to be a reliable marker as it was found only in cases of STB and absent in healthy controls [11]. The CXCR3 was measured in tissue samples using immunohistochemistry and from the blood samples of patients using ELISA. The levels of IFN-gamma, CXCR3 and CXCL10 were significantly higher in the peripheral blood of patients of STB and could serve as important diagnostic markers with high sensitivity and specificity [11].

Another study analyzing specific biomarkers using matrix-assisted laser desorption ionization time-of-flight mass spectroscopy (MALDI TOF-MS) reported two novel auxiliary markers, CFHR1 and CFHR2, for diagnosing tuberculosis of the bone [12].

MALDI TOF was also instrumental in proteomic analysis of the bony remains of Romans from the third century and diagnosing bone tuberculosis from them [13].

4. Nucleic Acid Amplification Tests

NAATs involve the use of primers targeted against the specific genes of *M. tuberculosis* and amplifying those genes to several thousand times till it become detectable by means like gel electrophoresis, hybridization or in-built software. NAATS greatly increase the sensitivity of detection since they can detect a single cell of the organism theoretically. They provide rapid results and are suitable for clinical decision-making in case of STB [14].

(a) The most common format of NAATs is polymerase chain reaction (PCR), wherein the three steps of denaturation, annealing and extension bring about the amplification of the nucleic acid in the presence of heat-stable enzyme Taq polymerase and a thermocycler providing different temperatures needed for each step. PCRs can be further divided as conventional PCR, nested PCR, multiplex PCR and real-time PCR. In conventional PCR, usually a single gene is targeted using one set of primers following a given amplification protocol.

In nested PCR, the amplified product from one reaction is subjected to next PCR using different gene target so as to increase the sensitivity and specificity.

In multiplex PCR, a combination of target genes, standardized according to the amplification protocol is used simultaneously in the same reaction mixture. This enables the detection of those cases that are missed by a single target. E.g. IS6110 is the most commonly used gene target for *M. tuberculosis* worldwide due to its multicopy presence in the genome, however, it can be either missing or be present as few copies in as many as 15–40% of the Indian population. It may, thus, miss onto those cases if used as the gene target in isolation. Multiplex PCR, using a combination of genes, has shown efficacy over uniplex PCR for diagnosing STB [15].

Real-time PCR—This format of PCR is software-driven and enables viewing of the amplification in real-time. The software generates a graphical representation of the amplified product in a semi-quantitative way. There is no need for post-amplification processing, thus minimizing the risk of contamination and subsequent steps of gel electrophoresis. The interpretation of real-time PCR is done on the basis of cycle threshold (Ct) value that gives an estimation of the bacterial load. Unlike conventional PCRs, which take nearly 3–4 hours in reporting, real-time PCR enables detection of *M. tuberculosis* DNA within 30 minutes and its quantification within 60–70 minutes.

(b) Loop-Mediated Isothermal Amplification.

LAMP assay utilizes a different format for amplifying the nucleic acid. Here, instead of the relying on a thermocycler that would manage temperature changes, the whole process of amplification is brought about at a uniform temperature, hence called isothermal. This is achieved by using special loop primers and Bst polymerase enzyme that allow continuous amplification at single temperature using strand displacement chemistry [16]. Further, the amplification is visualized either through naked eye or by addition of a fluorescent dye that intercalates with double-stranded DNA. Due to these features, LAMP technique is more suited for resource-limited settings as it cuts down the cost of sophisticated equipment like thermocycler and gel documentation system. LAMP could serve as a useful tool for diagnosis of STB at peripheral healthcare settings where the opportunity exists for early identification of cases. Results are obtained within 60–70 minutes. A single study evaluating LAMP assay using different gene targets for diagnosis of osteoarticular tuberculosis reported a sensitivity of 83% with IS6110 gene, 87.7% with MPB64 gene and 90% when either of the two was taken as positive [17].

(c) Commercial Assays.

GeneXpert MTB/RIF assay is a commercial semi-automated machine working on the real-time PCR chemistry that allows for simultaneous detection of tubercle bacilli as well as resistance to rifampicin. It is a cartridge-based test wherein the sample is to be inoculated without much processing, thereby decreasing the risk of contamination and requiring minimum expertise. With a turn-around time of 1–2 hours, it gives results for both the presence of tubercle bacilli and rifampicin resistance. It, however, cannot rule out tuberculosis. Different studies have evaluated GeneXpert for STB. In a study by Tang et al., [18] the sensitivity of GeneXpert was 97% in comparison to culture and pus was the most useful sample for diagnosis followed by granulation tissue, with caseous necrotic tissue being the least useful sample. In another study, GeneXpert had a sensitivity of 87% in comparison to histopathology and 63% in comparison to composite reference standard [19]. Patel et al. [20] reported a sensitivity and specificity of 86% and 85%, respectively, in comparison to culture for diagnosing STB and a sensitivity and specificity of 76% and 96%, respectively, as compared to phenotypic drug susceptibility testing for determining rifampicin resistance. However, there were four false rifampicin resistance and eleven false rifampicin-susceptible cases reported.

GeneXpert MTB/RIF ULTRA is the next generation of GeneXpert. Ultra has increased sensitivity of detection and lower limit of detection that GeneXpert (16 colony forming units (CFU)/ml vs. 131 CFU/ml). It involves usage of high-resolution melt curve analysis along with the incorporation of two gene targets (IS6110 and IS1081) that allows for better detection of tubercle bacilli as well as rifampicin resistance [21]. Ultra has been proposed as the first-line test for diagnosing tuberculosis in place of GeneXpert, and WHO has released the guidelines for the same [22]. Currently, there are no studies evaluating Ultra for STB.

Another commercial format is Truenat MTB, MTB Plus and RIF that also allows detection of both tuberculosis and rifampicin resistance, albeit sequentially and not simultaneously. Truenat is also microchip-based real-time PCR developed in India. It works on a battery-operated device, making it suitable for outreach settings that are devoid of continuous electricity supply. Truenat has been recommended as a first-line test for diagnosing pulmonary tuberculosis in the year 2020, [23] though its extrapolation to extrapulmonary samples is not yet made pending evaluation studies.

(d) Line Probe Assay.

As the name suggests, line probe assay consists of a strip on which probes are already integrated. On addition of the amplified product to this strip, the hybridization occurs between the corresponding genes and a band is formed in case of positive amplification. These probes are specific for detection of *M. tuberculosis* as well as detection of various mutations associated with rifampicin and isoniazid resistance. The patterns of hybridization on the strip help to interpret whether *M. tuberculosis* was present or not and whether there was any mutation representing resistance to either rifampicin or isoniazid or both. Line probe assay has a definite advantage of simultaneous detection of multi-drug resistant tuberculosis. However, it needs a specifically trained staff, ample laboratory area for carrying out all the three steps separately and is costly. While GeneXpert costs around \$22/test, Truenat with and without rifampicin resistance costs \$20 and \$12, line probe assay costs around \$25/test. No study has yet evaluated line probe assay for the diagnosis of STB.

(e) Sequencing of Gene/Genome.

Whole genome sequencing is the ultimate blueprint of any organism, and specific genes from the genome can also be targeted for a fool-proof identification. Gene sequencing involves amplification of specific pathogen genes, purifying the amplified product, processing and decoding the product in terms of nucleotides and then matching of the nucleotide pattern with publicly-available databases available online. The best match given the unambiguous identity of the organism.

Whole genome sequencing has also been applied on various extrapulmonary specimens to map the genetic diversity of isolates and reveal clinically relevant mutations conferring drug resistance [24].

Further, gene sequencing forms the molecular gold standard for determining drug resistance. Cases reported rifampicin resistant by other methods like GeneXpert and line probe assay may be confirmed by sequencing of the concerned gene. The technique of gene sequencing is highly specialized, requiring scientific equipment, software and fully-trained staff.

5. Drug Susceptibility Testing.

   Drug susceptibility testing for commonly used drugs against *M. tuberculosis* should be performed using phenotypic and genotypic methods. Among phenotypic methods, susceptibility testing on solid medium can be performed using 1% proportion method, absolute concentration method and the resistant ratio method. The 1% proportion method is the most commonly employed, however, the absolute concentration method is technically more simpler to perform and read [25].

   Susceptibility testing using liquid culture method greatly shortens the turnaround time and can be performed in MGIT. Commercially-available or in-house prepared microtiter plates can also be used for determining not only the susceptibility but also the minimum inhibitory concentration of different drugs to different strains of *M. tuberculosis*.

   Among the genotypic methods, susceptibility can be ascertained either using commercial platforms like GeneXpert, Truenat or line probe assay; or performing sequencing of specific genes to ascertain mutations conferring resistance.

   There are several reports of emerging drug resistance is STB [3, 26] and the need of the hour is universal testing for drug resistance and individualized therapy on the basis of drug susceptibility profile and penetration into the bony tissues.

References

1. Jain A, Rajsekaran S, Jaggi R, Myneedu V. Tuberculosis of the spine. J Bone Jt Surg. 2020;102A(7):617–28.
2. Jain AK. Tuberculosis of the spine: a fresh look at an old disease. J Bone Jt Surg - Ser B. 2010;92(7):905–13.
3. Arockiaraj J, Karthik R, Michael JS, Amritanand R, David KS, Krishnan V, et al. "Need of the hour": Early diagnosis and management of multidrug resistant tuberculosis of the spine: an analysis of 30 patients from a 'high multidrug resistant tuberculosis burden' country. Asian Spine J. 2019;13(2):265–71.
4. Merino P, Candel FJ, Gestoso I, Baos E, Picazo J. Microbiological diagnosis of spinal tuberculosis. Int Orthop. 2012;36(2):233–8.
5. Das R, Chandrasekar S, Purohit G, Satapathy AK, John J, Mohapatra S, et al. "There is more than what meets the eye"–Extensive spinal tuberculosis presenting as ocular tuberculosis. Indian J Tuberc. 2020;67(3):404–6. https://doi.org/10.1016/j.ijtb.2019.11.017.
6. Kim CJ, Kang SJ, Choe PG, Park WB, Jang HC, Jung SI, et al. Which tissues are best for microbiological diagnosis in patients with pyogenic vertebral osteomyelitis undergoing needle biopsy? Clin Microbiol Infect. 2015;21(10):931–5.
7. Rahyussalim AJ, Kurniawati T, Rukmana A. Mycobacterium tuberculosis contaminant risk on bone marrow aspiration material from iliac bone patients with active tuberculous spondylitis. Biomed Res Int. 2016;2016
8. Francis IM, Das DK, Luthra UK, Sheikh Z, Sheikh M, Bashir M. Value of radiologically guided fine needle aspiration cytology (FNAC) in the diagnosis of spinal tuberculosis: a study of 29 cases. Cytopathology. 1999;10(6):390–401.

9. Diffre C, Jousset C, Roux AL, Duran C, Noussair L, Rottman M, et al. Predictive factors for positive disco-vertebral biopsy culture in pyogenic vertebral osteomyelitis, and impact of fluoroscopic versus scanographic guidance. BMC Infect Dis. 2020;20(1):1–9.
10. Morgan MA, Horstmeier CD, DEYoung DRRGD. Comparison of a radiometric method (BACTEC) and conventional culture media for recovery of mycobacteria from smear-negative specimens. J Clin Microbiol. 1983;18(2):384–8.
11. Shang X, Wang L, Liu Y, Liu X, Lv J, Zhou X, et al. Diagnostic value of CXCR3 and its ligands in spinal tuberculosis. Exp Ther Med. 2020;21(1):1–8.
12. Chen X, Jia X, Lei H, Wen X, Hao Y, Ma Y, et al. Screening and identification of serum biomarkers of osteoarticular tuberculosis based on mass spectrometry. J Clin Lab Anal. 2020;34(7):1–10.
13. Hajdu T, Fóthi E, Kovári I, Merczi M, Molnár A, Maász G, et al. Bone tuberculosis in Roman Period Pannonia (western Hungary). Mem Inst Oswaldo Cruz. 2012;107(8):1048–53.
14. Wang G, Dong W, Lan T, Fan J, Tang K, Li Y, et al. Diagnostic accuracy evaluation of the conventional and molecular tests for Spinal Tuberculosis in a cohort, head-to-head study. Emerg Microbes Infect [Internet]. 2018;7(1):1–8. https://doi.org/10.1038/s41426-018-0114-1.
15. Sharma K, Meena RK, Aggarwal A, Chhabra R. Multiplex PCR as a novel method in the diagnosis of spinal tuberculosis–a pilot study. Acta Neurochir (Wien) [Internet]. 2017;159(3):503–7. https://doi.org/10.1007/s00701-016-3065-0.
16. Notomi T, Mori Y, Tomita N, Kanda H. Loop-mediated isothermal amplification (LAMP): principle, features, and future prospects. J Microbiol. 2015;53(1):1–5.
17. Sharma K, Sharma M, Batra N, Sharma A, Dhillon MS. Diagnostic potential of multi-targeted LAMP (loop-mediated isothermal amplification) for osteoarticular tuberculosis. J Orthop Res. 2016;32(2):361–5.
18. Tang L, Feng S, Gao R, Han C, Sun X, Bao Y, et al. A comparative study on the role of xpert MTB/RIF in testing different types of spinal tuberculosis tissue specimens. Genet Test Mol Biomarkers. 2017;21(12):722–6.
19. Yu Y, Kong Y, Ye J, Wang A. Performance of conventional histopathology and GeneXpert MTB/RIF in the diagnosis of spinal tuberculosis from bone specimens: A prospective clinical study. Clin Biochem [Internet]. 2020;85(July):33–7. https://doi.org/10.1016/j.clinbiochem.2020.08.010.
20. Patel J, Upadhyay M, Kundnani V, Merchant Z, Jain S, Kire N. Diagnostic efficacy, sensitivity, and specificity of xpert MTB/RIF assay for spinal tuberculosis and rifampicin resistance. Spine (Phila Pa 1976). 2020;45(3):163–9.
21. Chakravorty S, Simmons AM, Rowneki M, Parmar H, Cao Y, Ryan J, et al. The new Xpert MTB/RIF ultra: improving detection of Mycobacterium tuberculosis and resistance to Rifampin in an assay suitable for point-of-care testing. MBio. 2017;8(4):1–12.
22. World Health Organization. Meeting Report of a Technical Expert Consultation: Non-inferiority analysis of Xpert MTB/RIF Ultra compared to Xpert MTB/RIF. World Heal Organ. 2017; https://apps.who.int/iris/handle/10665/254792. Lic.
23. WHO consolidated guidelines on tuberculosis Module 3: diagnosis; rapid diagnostics for tuberculosis detection. Geneva: world health organization. 2020. Licence: CC BY-NC-SA 3.0 IGO.
24. Sharma K, Verma R, Advani J, Chatterjee O, Solanki HS, Sharma A, et al. Whole Genome Sequencing of Mycobacterium tuberculosis Isolates from Extrapulmonary Sites. Omi A J Integr Biol. 2017;21(7):413–25.
25. Kim SJ. Drug-susceptibility testing in tuberculosis: methods and reliability of results. Eur Respir J. 2005;25(3):564–9.
26. Upadhyay M, Patel J, Kundnani V, Ruparel S, Patel A. Drug sensitivity patterns in Xpert-positive spinal tuberculosis: an observational study of 252 patients. Eur Spine J [Internet]. 2020;29(7):1476–82. https://doi.org/10.1007/s00586-020-06305-x.

Chapter 8
Radiology in TB Spine (X-rays, Ultrasound, CT, MRI)

Anindita Sinha, Stanzin Spalkit, Anuj Prabhakar, and Mahesh Prakash

Abstract Spine is the most common site of skeletal involvement by tuberculosis (TB). Imaging plays an important role in its diagnosis, deciding management strategies, detects and predicts complications and monitors response to therapy. Out of the different modalities available,

The paradiscal, central, anterior subligamentous and neural arch are the common patterns of vertebral involvement. Thoracolumbar junction is the most common site of involvement. Plain radiographs are usually the initial investigation in spinal TB. A minimum of 30% bone mineral loss is required for the lesion to be conspicuous on a plain radiograph. Computed tomographic scanning provides better bony detail and delineation of the pattern of bone destruction, especially in areas that are inaccessible to evaluation by plain X-ray. Its major role lies in the detection of subtle calcification in the paraspinal collection as well as in providing guidance for targeted aspiration or biopsy. Magnetic resonance imaging (MRI) is the modality of choice for Pott's spine and is more sensitive as well as specific than other modalities. MRI demonstrates involvement of all the components of the spine, including vertebral body, intervertebral disc, the posterior elements, epidural extension of disease and the spinal cord involvement. The exact extent of paraspinal granulation tissue and collection is demarcated well on MRI. It also has a crucial role in post-treatment response assessment besides detection of complications.

Keywords Tuberculosis · Spine · MRI · Radiograph · Vertebra · Central · Paradiscal · Subligamentous · Neural

India accounts for 23% of the worldwide TB burden [1]. Around 10% of the extrapulmonary TB are contributed by skeletal TB, with spinal TB being the most common site of involvement [2].

A. Sinha (✉) · S. Spalkit · A. Prabhakar · M. Prakash
Department of Radiodiagnosis, Post Graduate Institute of Medical Education & Research, Chandigarh, India
e-mail: Official-sinha.anindita@pgimer.edu.in

S. S. Dhatt, V. Kumar (eds.), *Tuberculosis of the Spine*,
https://doi.org/10.1007/978-981-16-9495-0_8

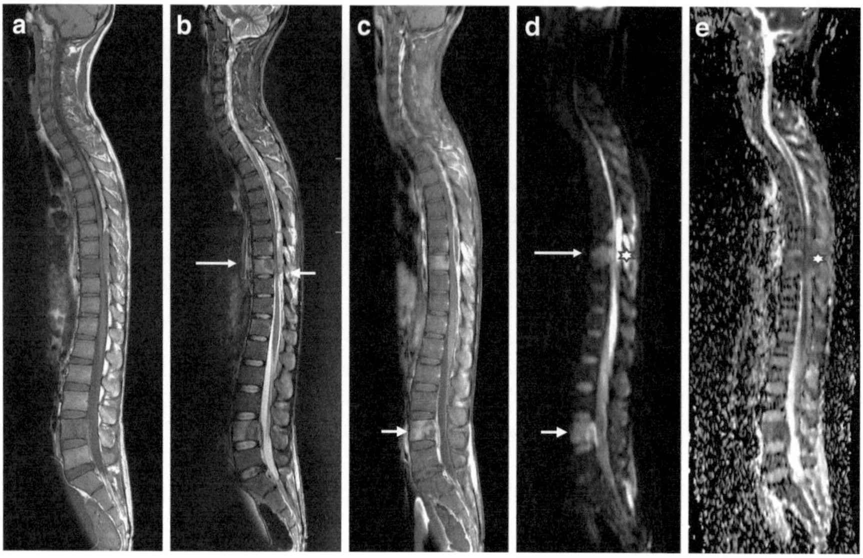

Fig. 8.1 Sagittal T1 (**a**), T2 (**b**), T1 post-contrast (**c**), DWI (**d**) and (**e**) ADC images of the whole spine in a case of multifocal caries spine reveal T1 hypointensity, T2 hyperintensity, post-contrast enhancement and diffusion restriction involving D8, D9 vertebral body (arrow) with an epidural peripherally enhancing collection (empty arrow) and posterior spinous process involvement from D7 to D9 level (asterix). Similar vertebral involvement also seen at L4 level (small arrow). A small epidural component is also seen at this level

Plain radiographs may be normal in early disease. A 30% mineral loss must occur before the lesions become conspicuous radiographically. An average of 3.4 to 3.8 vertebral involvement has been reported by various authors over the years [3, 4]. Extensive vertebral involvement may be seen in immunocompromised state, diabetics and hemoglobinopathies.

'Skipped lesion' where two non-contiguous vertebrae are involved without the involvement of intervening vertebral bodies and intervertebral discs are seen in 7% of the cases; the spread of infection along the Batson's perivertebral plexus of veins is proposed to be the mechanism (Fig. 8.1) [5].

Most common site of involvement is dorsal spine followed by the lumbar region. The vertebral body is more frequently affected than the posterior arch.

Four distinct radiological types of vertebral involvement have been described: paradiscal (most common), anterior, central, neural arch or appendiceal (pedicles, laminae, spinous process or transverse processes) [6].

8.1 Paradiscal Type

It is the most common pattern of vertebral involvement where simultaneous involvement of two contiguous vertebrae adjacent to the disc space is seen. This suggests a common blood supply to this region. On radiographs, it is manifested as reduction

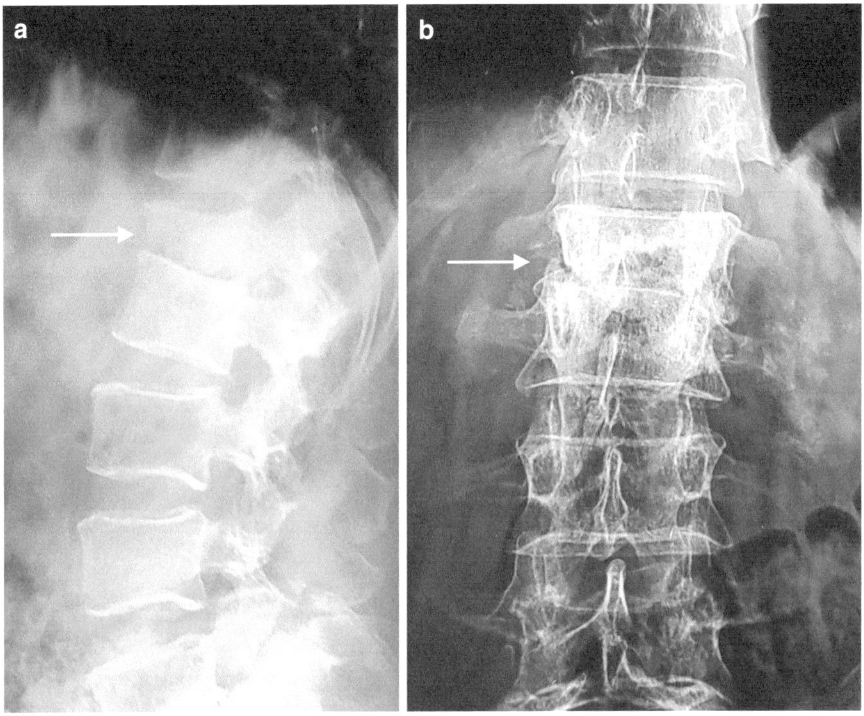

Fig. 8.2 Radiograph lateral (**a**) and AP (**b**) view reveal loss of intervertebral disc space associated with destruction of the anteroinferior aspect of L1 vertebral body (arrow)—*marginal variety of caries*

in intervertebral disc space associated with irregularity of endplates in the adjacent vertebrae (Figs. 8.2 and 8.3) [7].

Paravertebral shadow: Tuberculous granulation tissue as well as abscess formation in the paravertebral region is seen on plain radiographs in the form of soft tissue shadows adjacent to the spine. In the cervical region, it is best seen on a lateral radiograph as increased prevertebral soft tissue shadow [8]. The normal space between the vertebral bodies and pharyngeal/tracheal shadow measures approximately 5 mm above the cricoid cartilage level and 15 mm below this level. Anteroposterior diameter of the prevertebral soft tissue shadow should not exceed that of the adjacent vertebral bodies [9].

In the upper dorsal spine region (from the C7 to D4 region), it may manifest on an AP view as widening of the superior mediastinum. A good quality X-ray may help in early diagnosis in this region. In the lateral view, the contour of the posterior tracheal wall should be looked for, which normally appear concave anteriorly [7]. Any change in the normal contour (anterior convexity of the tracheal shadow) and/or a distance >8 mm from the vertebrae should prompt a search for vertebral disease from C7 to D4 level. Abscesses below the D4 vertebral level produce typical fusiform-shape (bird nest appearance), a larger sized abscess may produce a broad

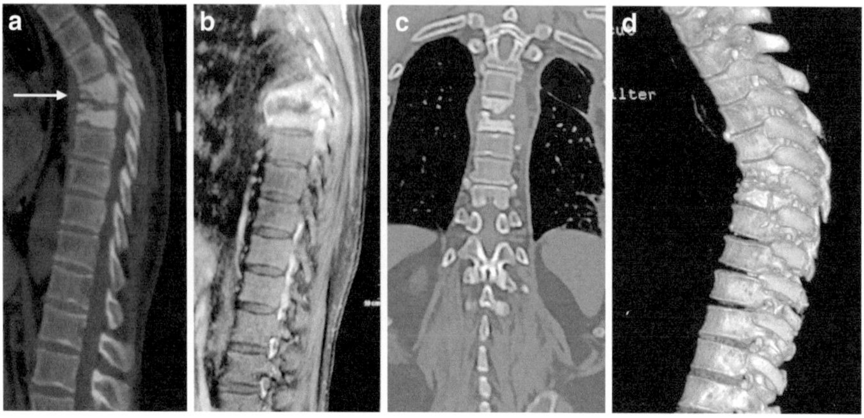

Fig. 8.3 CT spine sagittal (**a**), coronal CT (**c**) and virtual reconstructed 3D image (**d**) reveals loss of D4/5 intervertebral disc space with simultaneous destruction of the adjacent contiguous vertebrae (D4 and D5) causing a focal kyphotic deformity (arrow). T1 weighted post-contrast sagittal image (**b**) showing the paradiscal involvement of the D4 and D5 vertebrae with intervening disc involvement

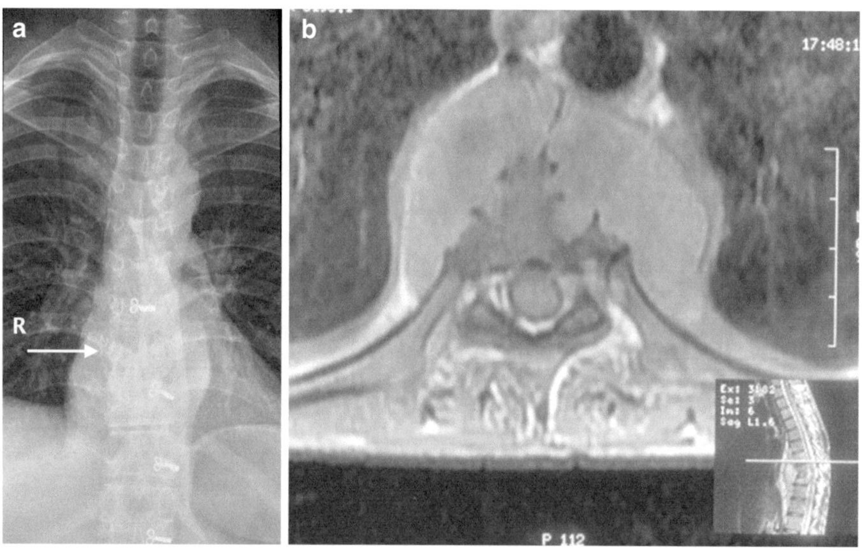

Fig. 8.4 Chest X-ray PA view (**a**) of a patient with tuberculosis D8–10 vertebrae seen as a retrocardiac shadow.(arrow) Axial T1 weighted MRI (**b**) of the same patient reveals a pre and paravertebral abscess at D8 level

posterior mediastinal shadow. (Fig. 8.4) An abscess under tension may give rise to a globular-shaped shadow. In the lumbar region, abscess tracking along the psoas muscle appear as widening of the psoas shadow.

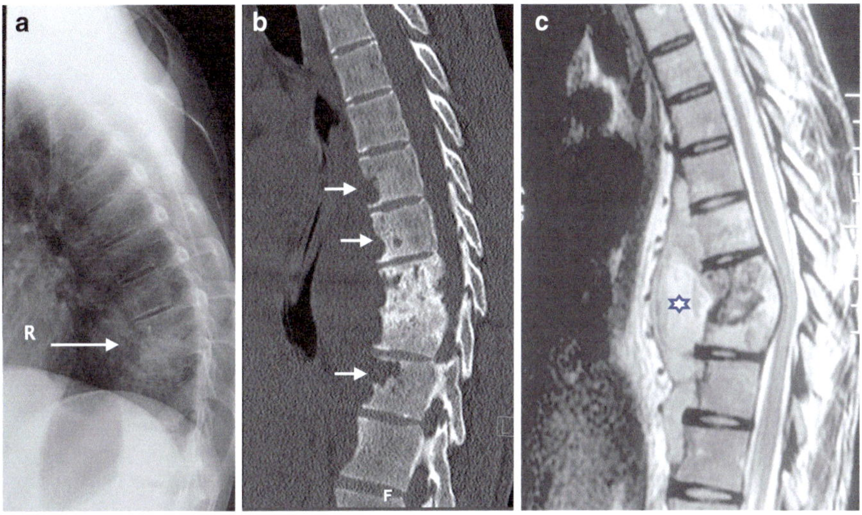

Fig. 8.5 X-ray lateral view DL spine (**a**) showing loss of D9/10 disc space with adjacent vertebral destruction with focal kyphosis (arrow), NCCT spine sagittal view (**b**) additionally shows destruction along the anterior aspect of D7,D8 and D11 (short arrow) with relative preservation of the disc spaces at these levels giving the 'saw tooth appearance' along with large prevertebral soft tissue. T2 weighted MRI sagittal view (**c**) reveals the large subperiosteal collection deep to Anterior Longitudinal Ligament (ALL) (asterix) with destruction of adjacent anterior vertebral cortices besides the paradiscal destruction at D9/10 level

An absence of osseous disease in the presence of a large paraspinal abscess may be identified rarely at radiography. CT may help demonstrate a small focus of vertebral involvement. Small perivertebral abscess may not be visible on radiography [10].

An 'aneurysmal phenomenon' is described where a paravertebral abscess remains under tension for a long time and causes erosion along the anterior margin of the vertebral bodies with sparing of the intervertebral discs because of its elasticity giving rise to the 'saw tooth' appearance [11] (Fig. 8.5).

Calcification within an abscess is pathognomonic of spinal tuberculosis. It is proposed to occur due to lack of proteolytic enzymes in *Mycobacterium tuberculosis*. Plain X-rays are superior to MRI for the evaluation of calcification [12] (Fig. 8.6).

Deformity: In long-standing cases, contiguous paradiscal vertebral bodies are destroyed, and one or both bodies show wedge collapse and angulation of spine with convexity posteriorly. Involvement of the dorsal vertebrae leads to a kyphotic deformity which is the most common spinal deformity (Fig. 8.3). Involvement of multiple adjacent vertebrae may result in a severe kyphotic deformity [13].

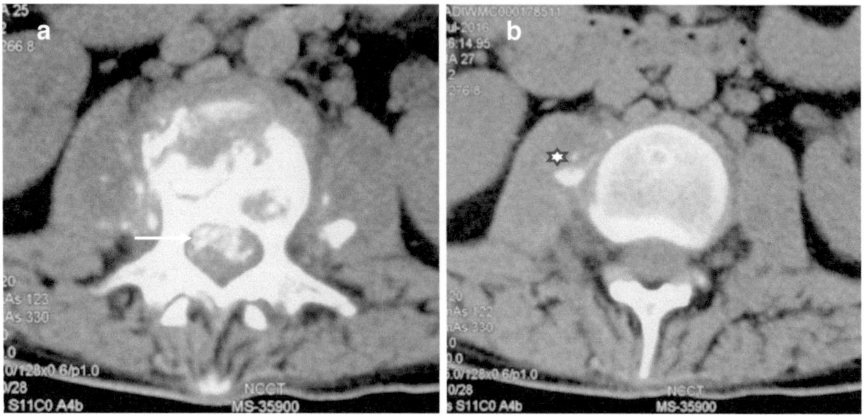

Fig. 8.6 NCCT Axial section (**a**) through the lumbar region reveals fragmentary vertebral destruction with associated paravertebral collection showing calcification within. Destroyed bone fragments are also seen in the epidural space (arrow). Axial CT section at a lower level (**b**) showing a right psoas abscess with few specks of calcification (asterix)

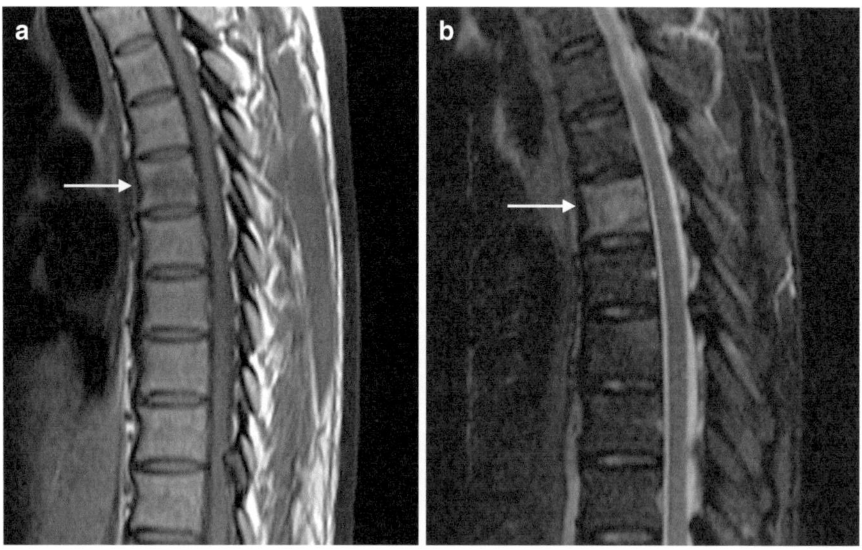

Fig. 8.7 Sagittal T1 (**a**) and fat-suppressed T2 weighted (**b**), post-contrast images showing altered signal intensity within the vertebral body (arrow) (T1 hypointensity and T2 hyperintensity) with preserved cortices and discs

8.2 Central Type

This pattern of involvement arises when the infection starts from the centre of the vertebral body when the bacteria inseminates through Batson's venous plexus or via the posterior vertebral artery branches (Fig. 8.7). Later, due to loss of trabeculae

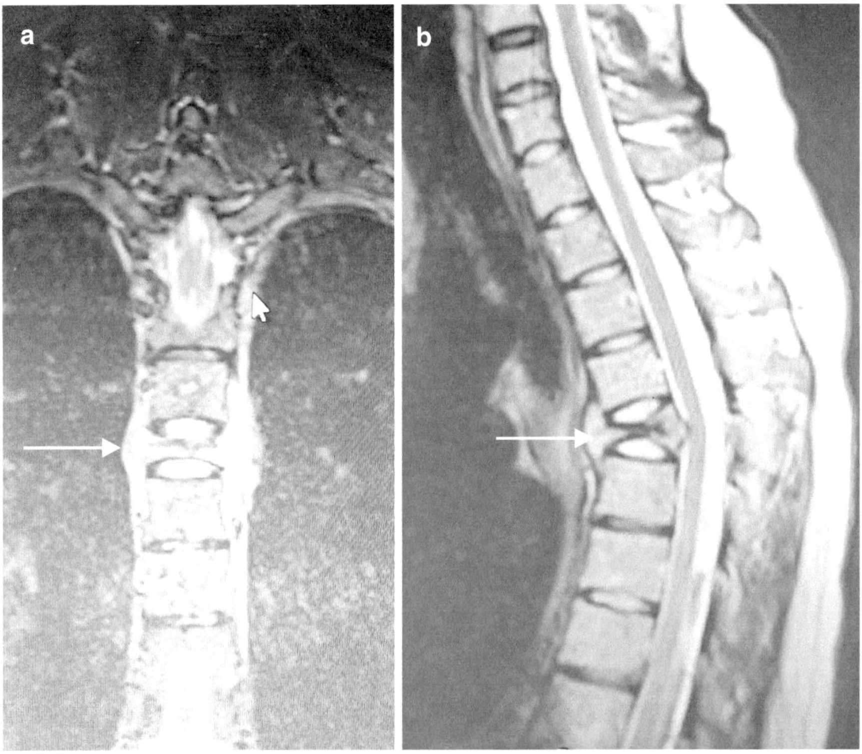

Fig. 8.8 T2 weighted coronal (**a**) and sagittal (**b**) images showing D5 complete collapse (arrow) with a small pre and paravertebral collection. Note the sparing of the contiguous discs

there is collapse of the diseased vertebral body on axial loading [5]. In contrast to the paradiscal type, loss of disc space and paravertebral shadow is minimal, hence, it is often confused with neoplastic aetiology (Fig. 8.8). However with longer follow up, diminution of adjacent disc space may be observed [14].

8.3 Anterior Type

This pattern is seen when disease process begins just deep to the anterior longitudinal ligament and periosteum (Fig. 8.5). This causes erosions of the anterior aspect of vertebral body, which is seen on lateral radiographs as irregular cortical margins. With extension of the disease underneath the anterior or posterior longitudinal ligaments, there may be involvement of multiple contiguous vertebrae. Vertebral body collapse with diminution of adjacent disc space is usually minimal and is seen at a later stage [5].

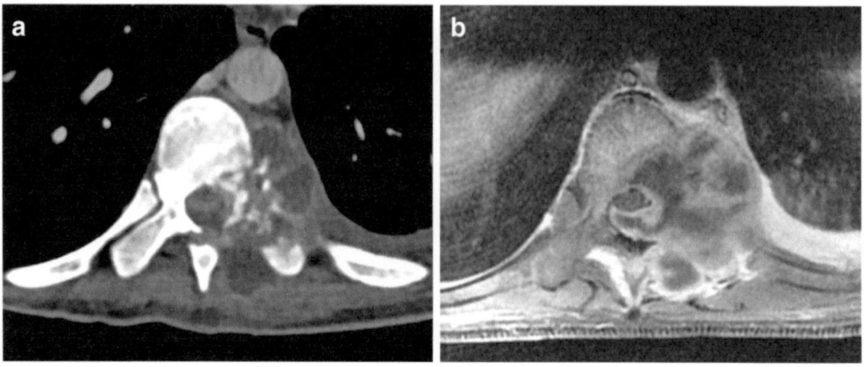

Fig. 8.9 Axial CT (**a**) sections soft tissue window showing lytic lesions involving the left pedicle, adjacent lamina and posterior body of dorsal vertebra. On axial T1 post-contrast study (**b**: associated soft tissue extending into the spinal canal is also seen—Neural arch tuberculosis

8.4 Appendiceal Type

This includes involvement of the neural arch (pedicles and laminae), transverse processes and spinous process either in isolation or combined (Fig. 8.9). Radiographically, these lesions may be suspected when indirect signs of involvement are seen, such as paravertebral shadows or erosive changes with an intact disc [15]. The involvement of posterior spinal joints is difficult to appreciate on routine radiography [16]. Posterior spinal articulations may also be involved and give rise to a rare deformity called lateral translation in addition to the more common paradiscal lesions [17].

The main disadvantage of radiographs is its low sensitivity in the early stages of the disease. Vertebral sites that are difficult to assess on X-ray include craniovertebral and cervicodorsal junction [18]. Assessment of spinal cord changes, involvement of soft tissue, exact site and extent of abscesses is difficult to decipher on plain X-rays. Hence, visualization of any of the radiographic signs may indirectly mean that the disease process has reached a relatively advanced stage [19, 20].

Simultaneous presence of pulmonary tuberculosis is common in patients with spinal tuberculosis. A primary focus in the lung or a history of pulmonary tuberculosis can be obtained in 67% of patients spinal tuberculosis [21].

Ultrasound can help diagnose the presence of tubercular abscesses, assess the nature (solid or fluid) of iliopsoas mass and quantify the drainable content especially in lumbar vertebral disease.

8.5 Computed Tomography

Findings are conspicuous much earlier on CT than plain radiography as it demonstrates better detail of bony irregularity/disruption, sclerosis and disc collapse. Various patterns of bone destruction have been described; fragmentary (Figs. 8.10,

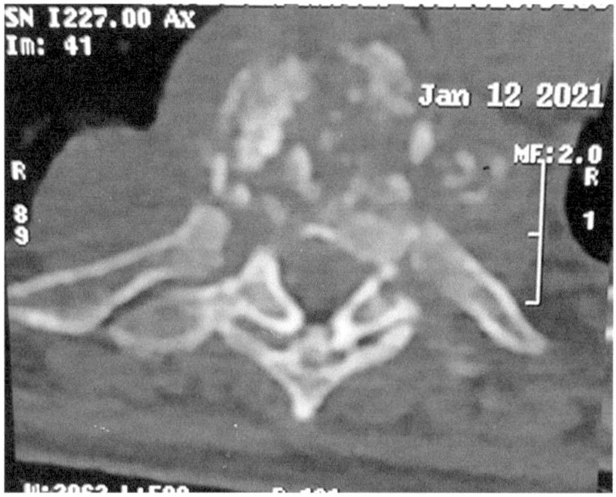

Fig. 8.10 Axial NCCT section through the dorsal vertebral body showing gross destruction of bone with numerous residual small bone fragments

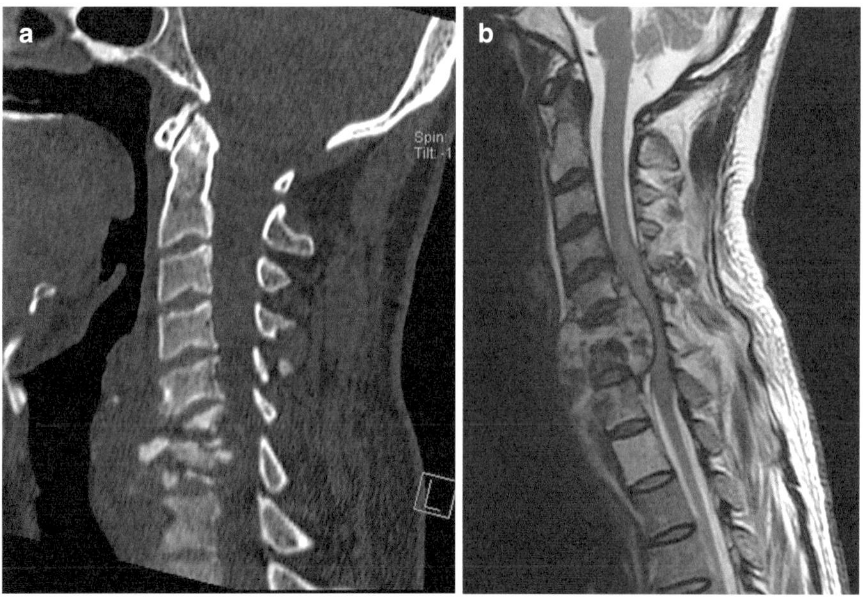

Fig. 8.11 Sagittal NCCT (**a**) and T2W images (**b**) cervical spine MR scans of a patient with tuberculosis of C5–7 show fragmentary destruction and collapse of C6 and C7 vertebral body with the destruction of the intervening disk space. A prevertebral abscess lifting up the anterior longitudinal ligament and a small ventral epidural collection are also seen

and 8.11), osteolytic, sclerotic and subperiosteal (Fig. 8.5). Besides bony detail, paraspinal abscesses are also better evaluated than plain radiography. It has a crucial role in demonstration of calcification within an abscess or bone fragments within epidural lesions (Fig. 8.6). It is of great value in providing guidance for percutaneous diagnostic sampling, especially in inaccessible sites. The major disadvantage is in evaluation of effect of the disease on neural structures for which MRI scores over CT.

Radiological evidence of healing lags behind the clinical and laboratory findings in spinal tuberculosis. X-rays or MRI done after few months after the start of multi-drug therapy may not show any signs of improvement in many patients and should not be labelled as treatment failure. However, if the images do not show improvement when repeated more than 6 months after the onset of treatment, one should consider the possibility of an alternative pathology or a therapeutically refractory disease. Once the disease has healed, the bony architecture is restored. Rarely the healing is accompanied by fat replacement of the healed area.

8.6 MRI

MRI scores over other imaging modalities with its superior soft tissue contrast and its ability to detect and delineate changes in the marrow, the intervertebral disc and the spinal cord [6].

MRI is the modality of choice for the overall evaluation of tuberculous spine. It has a special role in the evaluation of disease in difficult sites like craniovertebral junction (Fig. 8.12), cervicodorsal junction, neural arch elements and vertebral appendages, the sacroiliac joint region (Fig. 8.13), sacrum and coccyx.

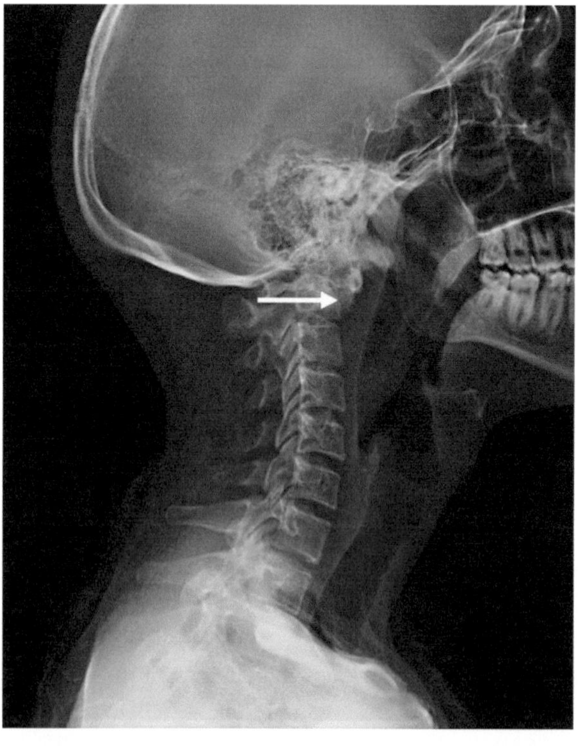

Fig. 8.12 Lateral view cervical spine show increased atlanto-dental interval and indistinct cortical margins of the odontoid process, subtle amorphous calcification is seen anterior to the D2 body (arrow)

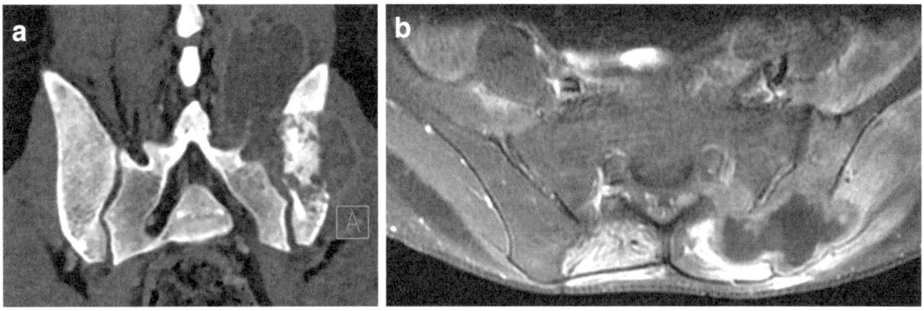

Fig. 8.13 (**a**). CT through the sacroiliac (SI) joint reveal left iliac bone destruction with periarticular fluid collection (**b**) Axial T1 weighted post-contrast image MRI image of the same patient showing abnormal enhancement and destruction of the left iliac bone with peripherally enhancing collection in posterior aspect of the left SI joint

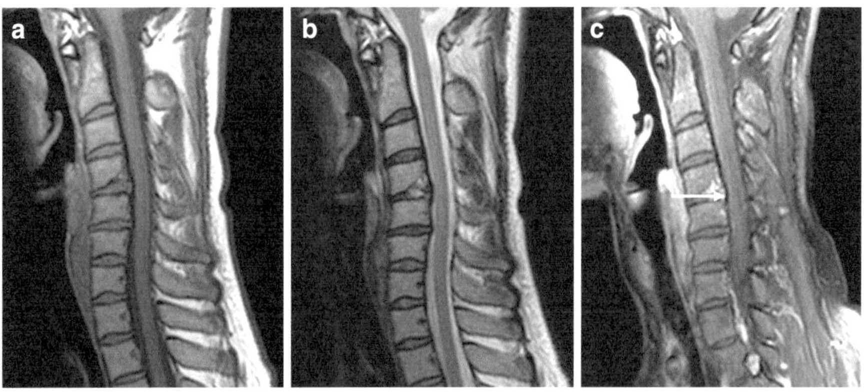

Fig. 8.14 Sagittal T1(**a**), T2(**b**) weighted and post-contrast T1 (**c**) weighted images showing altered signal within C4/5 intervertebral disc which appears T2 hyperintense and show post-contrast enhancement in the posterior aspect s/o discitis (arrow). There is endplate irregularity with enhancement of inferior sub endplate region of C4 vertebral body -spondylodiscitis

Usual MRI protocol includes non-contrast T1-weighted (T1W), T2-weighted (T2W) and short tau inversion recovery (STIR) sequences in axial, sagittal and coronal planes along with contrast-enhanced T1W fat-suppressed sequences after gadolinium contrast injection.

MRI appearances can be described according to the phase or activity of the disease process.

In the Active Stage: The vertebral body involvement is seen as abnormal marrow signal intensity, which appears hypointense on T1W and hyperintense on T2W sequences showing heterogeneous enhancement associated with loss of cortical definition [16, 22] (Fig. 8.14). Contiguous vertebral body disease with disc destruction (osteitis and discitis) is common. Disc involvement manifests as loss of normal internuclear cleft with increased signal on T2-weighted images and post-contrast enhancement. Due to the lack of proteolytic enzymes in mycobacterium, disc involvement occurs relatively late compared to pyogenic spondylitis. The 'floating disc sign' may appear rarely if there is significant vertebral destruction with sparing of the disc. In paediatric cases, the disc is well hydrated and is more prone for infection [23].

Abscess formation in and around the vertebral lesion is a characteristic feature of spinal tuberculosis, with occurrence of prevertebral, paravertebral and epidural masses seen in approximately 71% of the cases on MRI [23] (Fig. 8.15). MRI is highly accurate in distinguishing granulation tissue from abscess. Both granulation tissue and abscess appear hypointense on T1 and hyperintense on T2; however, on post-contrast study an abscess reveals thick rim enhancement while a granulation tissue or phlegmon reveals more uniform enhancement [16, 22, 23] (Figs. 8.15 and 8.16). In thoracic

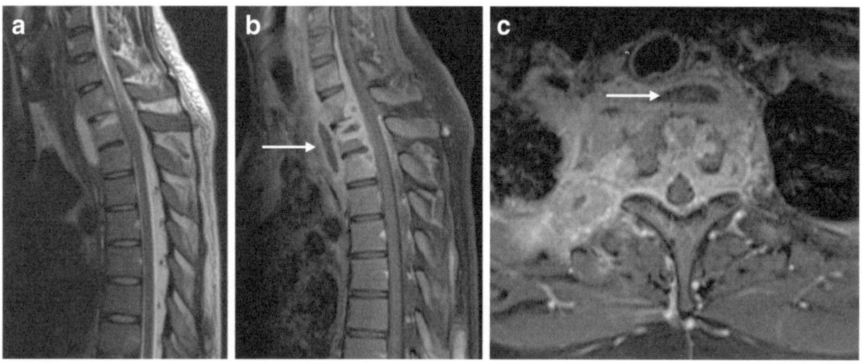

Fig. 8.15 Sagittal T2 weighted (**a**), T1 post-contrast sagittal (**b**) and axial (**c**) images show altered signal with enhancement of multiple contiguous upper dorsal vertebrae with associated prevertebral collection with thick peripheral enhancement (arrow) suggestive of abscess with homogenously enhancing paravertebral granulation tissue in right paravertebral area. Extradural extension of the granulation tissue circumferentially around the spinal cord is seen

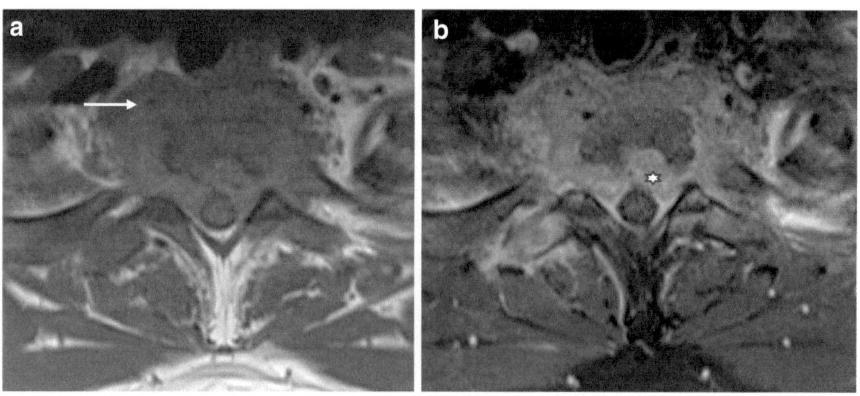

Fig. 8.16 Axial T1 non-contrast (**a**) and T1 post-contrast (**b**) scan of the same patient as in Fig. 8.15 show T1 isointense and homogenous post-contrast enhancement within the pre and paravertebral tissue (arrow). A ventral epidural extension is also seen (asterix)

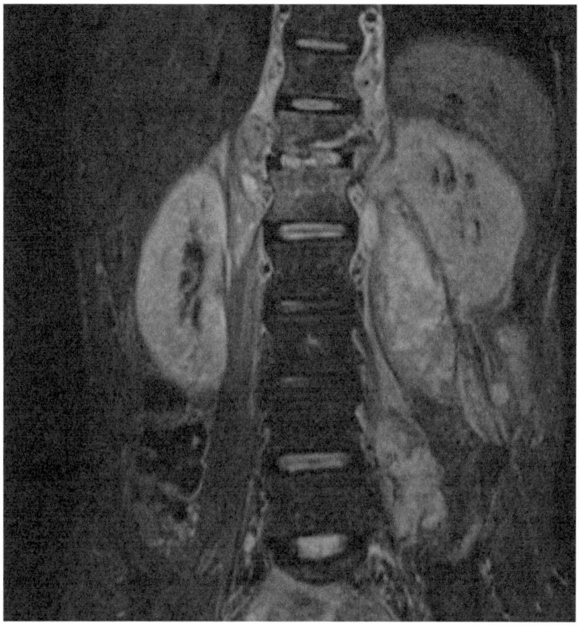

Fig. 8.17 T1 post-contrast coronal scan in a patient with dorso-lumbar TB spine depicts partial collapse of D12 and enhancement of D12 and L1 vertebrae. There is a disproportionately large psoas abscess on the left side posterosuperiorly displacing the left kidney

region, the paraspinal collection can extend along the intercostal space or track into the mediastinum or pleural cavity, or rarley encase the intercostal arteries as they barely penetrate the anterior longitudinal ligament [24]. In the lumbar region, in case of psoas muscle involvement, there is loss of normal muscle morphology, increase muscle bulk with uniform signal intensity on T1W images. On T2W images, the psoas abscess is seen as high signal fluid with thick peripheral post-contrast enhancement (Fig. 8.17).

The following MRI features show high sensitivity and specificity for spinal tuberculosis: end plate disruption, 100 and 81.4%, respectively, paravertebral soft tissue shadow (96.8%, 85.3%) and an increased T2 signal intensity of intervertebral disk (80.6%, 82.4%) [25].

Posterior element involvement is rare in tuberculosis, however, it is more common than in pyogenic infection. Involvement by the disease manifests as abnormal signal and inhomogeneous enhancement of the affected site. The posterior elements may be affected in isolation (Fig. 8.18), however, more commonly they are seen in combination with the anterior element lesions. Combined involvement of the posterior and anterior elements is referred to as 'composite lesions or pan vertebral lesion' [26]. There may be associated granulomatous lesions within the spinal canal either with involvement of epidural/subdural space or that of spinal cord. Epidural extension is detected by MRI in about 61% of involved vertebrae [23]. Compressive myelopathy may result due to compression of the spinal cord from posterior aspect [27–29] or from anterior aspect [30] (Fig. 8.11).

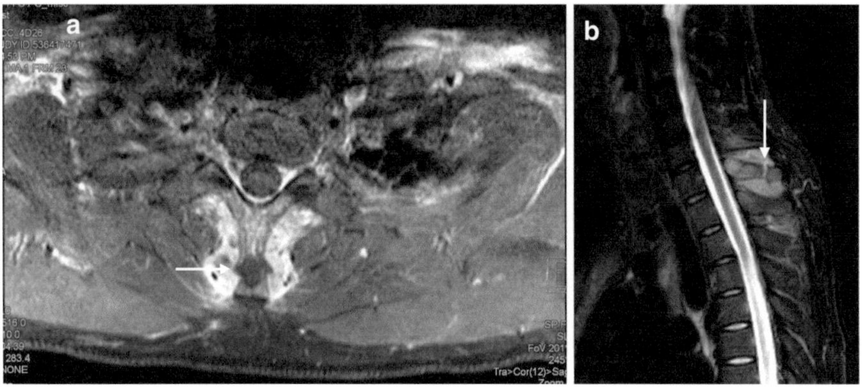

Fig. 8.18 Post-contrast T1W axial MR (**a**) and sagittalT2 weighted image (**b**) of a patient with TB spine showing T2 hyperintensity and abnormal enhancement of the spinous process of C6 vertebra with an undisplaced fracture line through it (arrow in **b**). There is surrounding homogenous enhancement

8.7 Cord Changes

Neurological deficit due to involvement of posterior element by tuberculosis is not uncommon [1, 17]. Common causes include extrinsic mechanical compression on the cord by abscesses, granulation tissue or debris, internal gibbus and subluxation. It is rarely due to direct involvement of the cord by the disease process as the cord can withstand slowly developing pressure exerted over a long period of time due to relatively high physiologic reserve, such that even a significant reduction in cord diameter is compatible with good cord function. Most patients present with compression paraplegia rather than sensory deficit, this is because motor fibres are more susceptible to pressure effect, while sensory fibres are relatively more susceptible to ischemia, collateral formation prevents ischemia for quite some time [31].

Direct involvement of the cord may result in inflammatory oedema (myelitis) and rarely it may lead to granuloma formation within the cord [32]. Oedema is seen as hyperintense signal on T2W images with minimal signal alteration on T1W images (Fig. 8.19). Myelitis with a relatively preserved cord associated with fluid collection in the epidural space shows good response to conservative treatment, provided neurological deficit is predominantly due to mechanical compression. However, myelitis associated with granulation tissue with little fluid component as a cause for neurological deficit calls for surgical decompression [33].

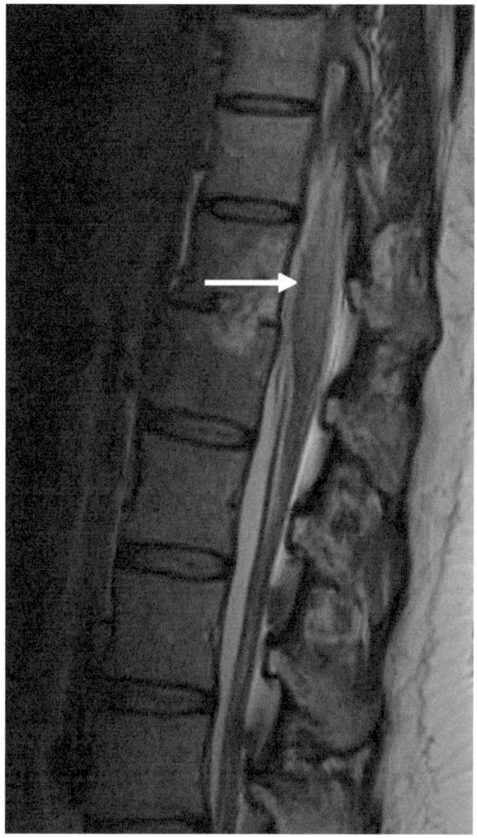

Fig. 8.19 Sagittal T2W MR scan shows altered signal in the marrow and intervening disk of lumbar vertebrae. The cord is mildly expanded at this level with T2 hyperintense signal due to cord edema (arrow) –myelitis

8.8 Cord Changes in Chronic Disease

Include myelomalacia, cord atrophy and syringomyelia. Myelomalacia is seen as hyperintense signal on T2w images with a T1 hypointense signal (higher than that of CSF) and may be associated with thinning of the cord. A syrinx is a well-defined tubular, fluid-filled region (showing CSF signal characteristics) within the spinal cord which is usually tapered to one or both ends and can be septated (Fig. 8.20). It is associated with poor neurological outcomes, [32, 34] however, mild atrophy of the cord can still be compatible with successful neurological outcomes.

Paraplegia may occur even with healed disease due to a residual severe deformity, even after many years. It is produced either due to stretching of the spinal cord over internal bony deformity, with resultant gliosis, or due to dural scarring causing constriction of cord [33].

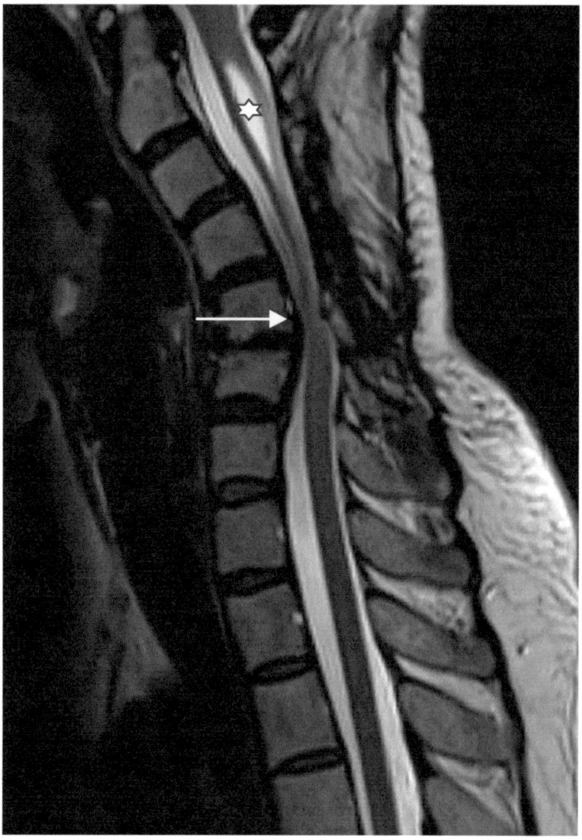

Fig. 8.20 Sagittal T2 weighted MRI scan in an old TB spine at C5/6 level post decompression shows residual deformity in the form of reversal of normal cervical lordosis and thinning of the cord at the same level (arrow). An elongated tubular structure showing CSF like signal within the spinal cord from C2 to C3 level (asterix)–syrinx formation

8.9 Atypical Spinal Tuberculosis: [5, 35]

The common paradiscal lesion is readily diagnosed and treated. Atypical spinal tuberculosis can be defined as compressive myelopathy with no visible spinal deformity with the absence of the radiological appearance of a typical vertebral lesion. Such lesions are rare, however, it is crucial that they are not missed as late diagnosis may lead to more chances of complications. Atypical lesions include: single vertebral disease (Fig. 8.8), ivory vertebra, isolated involvement of the neural arch (Fig. 8.18), circumferential vertebral involvement, multifocal vertebral disease, skipped lesion (Fig. 8.1).

Patients with tubercular granulomas in the intradural, epidural or intramedullary spaces may have symptoms of compressive myelopathy, radiculopathy or both, without any obvious spinal deformity or radiological signs, which is also described

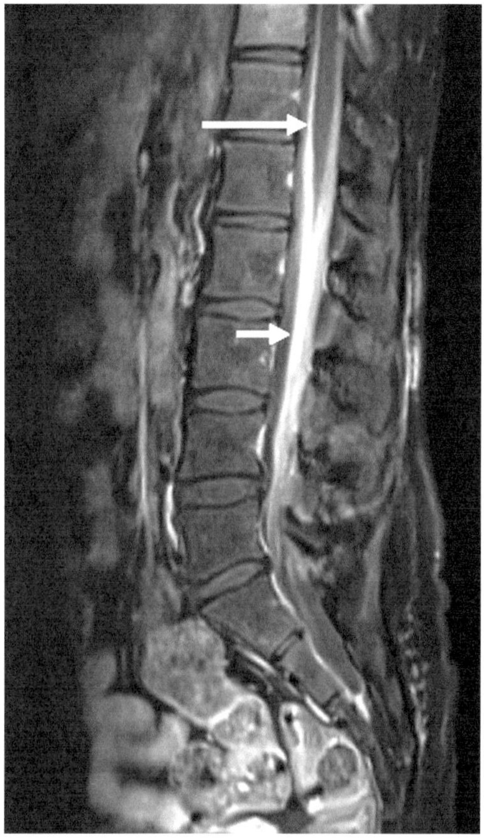

Fig. 8.21 Sagittal T1 weighted post contrast through the lumbosacral region reveals thick dural around the distal visualized cord (arrow) and enhancement around the adherent roots(short arrow)-arachnoiditis

as 'spinal tumor syndrome'. Final diagnosis in such conditions is usually made at surgery or histopathological evaluation.

Extraosseous extradural granuloma is when an extradural granulomatous lesion is seen in the absence of bone involvement. Hematogenous dissemination is the likely cause. This manifestation is more common in the dorsal epidural space and in the thoracic segment of spine. Clinically patients present with compressive radiculomyelopathy. On pathologic examination, a granulomatous reaction is found encircling and causing compression of the spinal cord or cauda equina. These findings are well evident on MRI as T1 isointense (relative to the cord) and T2 mixed signal intensity lesions showing homogenous enhancement [36]. Extradural abscess may occur either as primary lesions or may be seen associated with myelitis, arachnoiditis (Fig. 8.21), intramedullary tuberculoma etc. [37]

8.10 Post-Treatment Follow Up

8.10.1 Conventional Radiograph

When the disease is diagnosed at an early stage and treated promptly, healing process may result in complete resolution of radiological findings except for a decreased disc space. Radiological evidence of healing lags behind the clinical features of healing by about 3 months [38].

Moreover, bone destruction or loss of vertebral height and soft tissue paravertebral masses may progress for months while on treatment, however, this should not necessarily be considered as a sign of failed treatment [39].

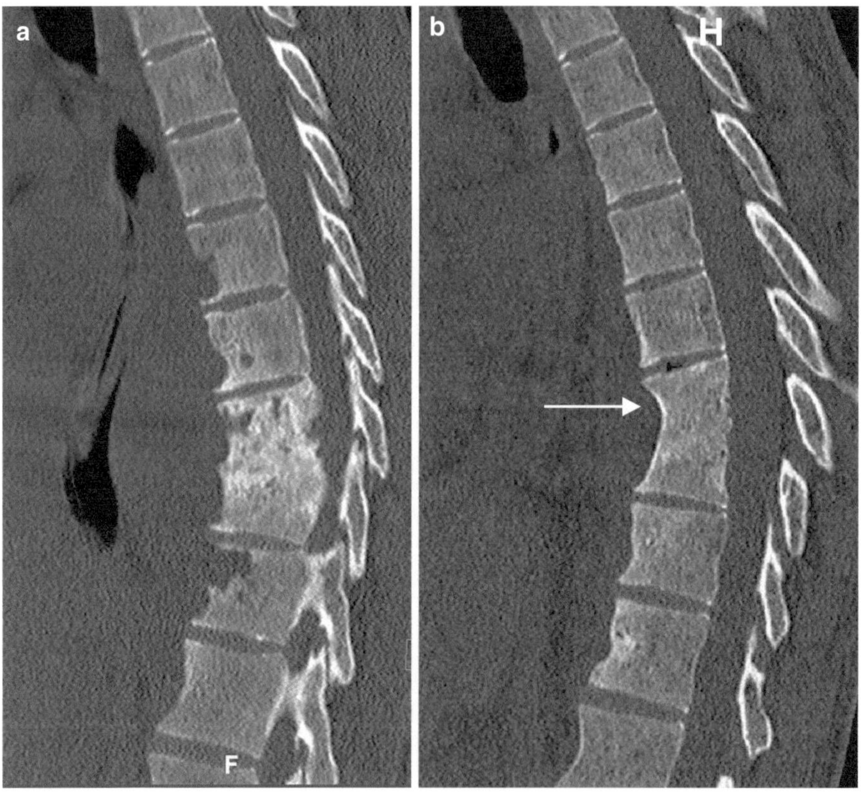

Fig. 8.22 Sagittal CT dorsolumbar spine of a patient with Potts spine before and after treatment. (**a**) Multiple contiguous vertebral destruction with a large prevertebral abscess (**b**) post treatment there is reduction in the prevertebral abscess with bony ankylosis(arrow) of D9 and D10 vertebral bodies, there is regeneration of the D7,8 and D11 vertebral bodies with mild sclerotic reaction.

Early signs of healing on radiology include sharpening of the irregular endplate margins, reappearance and mineralization of the trabeculae which were absorbed earlier. In the early stage of healing, a sclerotic reaction to the diseased bone may give rise to an 'ivory vertebra' i.e. diffuse increase in density of vertebral body [5]. Modern antitubercular drugs result in significant regeneration of the destroyed vertebrae as seen on radiology. Healing by fibrous ankylosis usually occurs when several vertebrae are destroyed with a large gap. Uncommonly, if the disc is completely destroyed with obliteration of the disc space due to collapse and apposition of the vertebrae, healing may take place by bony ankylosis or bone-block formation [1] (Fig. 8.22).

8.11 MRI

Decrease in the size of paraspinal soft issue involvement is the earliest sign of healing. It must be noted, however, that persistence of bone destruction with an altered signal intensity on MRI does not necessarily indicate failed treatment. T1 non-fat saturated images are crucial in follow up, a high T1 signal at the rim of the osseous lesion is an MRI sign of healing. This sequential increase in T1 signal can be followed up in post-treatment imaging as it is found to correlate with clinical healing as well. Besides the non-contrast T1 non-fat suppressed images, T1 fat-suppressed post-contrast images may also reveal reduction in enhancement with healing. Again, the persistence or mild increase in enhancement does not necessarily indicate a failed treatment. MRI also has a role in detection of reactivation of old healed tubercular disease, it is seen as appearance of high signal on T2 images in areas that had turned hypointense during healing. Rarely reactivation may be in the form of an isolated paraspinal collection without osseous involvement. It must be stressed, however, that MRI alone cannot determine disease healing and termination of treatment must be considered only after correlation with clinical and laboratory findings [40].

8.12 Differential Diagnosis

1. Degenerative Spondylosis:

   T2 signal and contrast study can help differentiate the two. The degenerated disc appears T2 hypointense and shows occasional faint enhancement, while the infected disc appears T2 hyperintense and shows strong enhancement [41].
2. Pyogenic Infection: It is often difficult to differentiate the two, however, certain features that favour the diagnosis of tubercular aetiology rather than pyogenic are; Osteoporotic changes with lack of reactive sclerosis on X-ray, late involvement of the intervertebral disc, presence of multiple contiguous vertebral disease

with subligamentous spread, disproportionately large paraspinal abscess showing calcification, neural arch involvement and skip lesions [41, 42].
3. Brucellosis: Intradiscal gas, minimal paraspinal soft tissue involvement with lower lumbar predilection are ommon.
4. Sarcoidosis: It is the great masquerader; hence it may occasionally be identical to tuberculous involvement of multiple vertebrae [42].
5. Others: In case of single vertebral involvement due to metastatic disease or eosinophilic granuloma, differentiation from tubercular disease could be done by observing the disc involvement and paraspinal soft tissue with/without calcification. Other differential diagnosis that an involve consecutive vertebral bodies involvement include lymphoma, multiple myeloma, chordoma. [22, 42, 43].

References

1. Kumar K. Spinal tuberculosis, natural history of disease, classifications and principles of management with historical perspective. Eur J Orthop Surg Traumatol Orthop Traumatol. 2016 Aug;26(6):551–8.
2. Rajasekaran S, Soundararajan DCR, Shetty AP, Kanna RM. Spinal Tuberculosis: Current Concepts. Glob Spine J. 2018 Dec;8(4 Suppl):96S–108S.
3. Hodgson AR, Stock FE, Fang HSY, Ong GB. Anterior spinal fusion the operative approach and pathological findings in 412 patients with pott's disease of the spine. Br J Surg. 1960 Sep;48(208):172–8.
4. Agrawal V, Patgaonkar P, Nagariya S. Tuberculosis of spine. J Craniovertebral Junction Spine. 2010;1(2):74.
5. Pande KC, Babhulkar SS. Atypical Spinal Tuberculosis. Clin Orthop. 2002 May;398:67–74.
6. Ansari S, Amanullah MF, Rauniyar R, Ahmad K. Pott′s spine: Diagnostic imaging modalities and technology advancements. North. Am J Med Sci. 2013;5(7):404.
7. Garg RK, Somvanshi DS. Spinal tuberculosis: A review. J Spinal Cord Med. 2011 Sep;34(5):440–54.
8. V A, Pr P, Sp N. Tuberculosis of spine [Internet]. Vol. 1, Journal of craniovertebral junction & spine. J Craniovertebr Junction Spine; 2010 [cited 2020 Dec 3]. Available from: https://pubmed.ncbi.nlm.nih.gov/21572628/
9. Bhargava SK, Gupta S. Large retropharyngeal cold abscess in an adult with respiratory distress. J Laryngol Otol. 1990 Feb;104(2):157–8.
10. Boachie-Adjei O, Squillante RG. Tuberculosis of the spine. Orthop Clin North Am. 1996 Jan;27(1):95–103.
11. Rivas-Garcia A, Sarria-Estrada S, Torrents-Odin C, Casas-Gomila L, Franquet E. Imaging findings of Pott's disease. Eur Spine J. 2013 Jun;22(Suppl 4):567–78.
12. Kukreja R, Mital M, Gupta PK. Evaluation of Spinal Tuberculosis by Plain X-Rays and Magnetic Resonance Imaging in a Tertiary Care Hospital in Northern India. A Prospective Study. 2018;5(2):6.
13. Jain AK. Tuberculosis of the skeletal system. Indian J Orthop. 2016;50(3):337.
14. Sagane SS, Patil VS, Bartakke GD, Kale KY. Assessment of Clinical and Radiological Parameters in Spinal Tuberculosis: Comparison between Human Immunodeficiency Virus-Positive and Human Immunodeficiency Virus-Negative Patients. Asian Spine J. 2020 Dec 31;14(6):857–63.

15. Kumar K. Posterior Spinal Tuberculosis: A Review. Mycobact Dis [Internet]. 2017; [cited 2020 Dec 27];07(02). Available from: https://www.omicsonline.org/open-access/posterior-spinal-tuberculosis-a-review-2161-1068-1000243.php?aid=90703
16. Abdelwahab IF, Camins MB, Hermann G, Klein MJ. Vertebral arch or posterior spinal tuberculosis. Skelet Radiol. 1997 Dec 9;26(12):737–40.
17. Kumar K. A clinical study and classification of posterior spinal tuberculosis. Int Orthop. 1985 Nov;9(3):147–52.
18. Department of Radiology, Nagpur NKPSIMS, Patil DS. Assessment of imaging finding in Spinal tuberculosis. J Med Sci Clin Res [Internet]. 2019; Jan 20 [cited 2020 Dec 31];7(1). Available from: http://jmscr.igmpublication.org/v7-i1/93%20jmscr.pdf
19. Moon M-S. Tuberculosis of Spine: Current Views in Diagnosis and Management. Asian Spine J. 2014;8(1):97.
20. Rasouli MR, Mirkoohi M, Vaccaro AR, Yarandi KK, Rahimi-Movaghar V. Spinal Tuberculosis: Diagnosis and Management. Asian Spine J. 2012 Dec;6(4):294–308.
21. Harisinghani MG, McLoud TC, Shepard J-AO, Ko JP, Shroff MM, Mueller PR. Tuberculosis from Head to Toe. Radiographics. 2000 Mar 1;20(2):449–70.
22. Sharif HS, Morgan JL, al Shahed MS, al Thagafi MY. Role of CT and MR imaging in the management of tuberculous spondylitis. Radiol Clin N Am. 1995 Jul;33(4):787–804.
23. Gouliamos AD, Kehagias DT, Lahanis S, Athanassopoulou AA, Moulopoulou ES, Kalovidouris AA, et al. MR imaging of tuberculous vertebral osteomyelitis: pictorial review. Eur Radiol. 2001;11(4):575–9.
24. Hong SH, Choi J-Y, Lee JW, Kim NR, Choi J-A, Kang HS. MR Imaging Assessment of the Spine: Infection or an Imitation? Radiographics. 2009 Mar 1;29(2):599–612.
25. Danchaivijitr N, Temram S, Thepmongkhol K, Chiewvit P. Diagnostic accuracy of MR imaging in tuberculous spondylitis. J Med Assoc Thail Chotmaihet Thangphaet. 2007 Aug;90(8):1581–9.
26. Corea JR, Tamimi TM. Tuberculosis of the Arch of the Atlas: Case Report. Spine. 1987 Aug;12(6):608–11.
27. Rao BD, Rao KS, Subrhamanian MV, Reddy MV. Granulomatous lesions of the spinal epidural space. Neurol India. 1965 Sep;13(3):89–92.
28. Kocen RS, Parsons M. NEUROLOGICAL COMPLICATIONS OF TUBERCULOSIS: SOME UNUSUAL MANIFESTATIONS. QJM Int J Med. 1970 Jan 1;39(1):17–30.
29. Kak VK, Pani KC, Chopra JS. Epidural spinal tuberculoma presenting as 'spinal tumour syndrome'. Tubercle. 1972 Jun 1;53(2):139–42.
30. Solomon A, Sacks AJ, Goldschmidt RP. Neural arch tuberculosis: a morbid disease. Radiographic and computed tomographic findings. Int Orthop. 1995;19(2):110–5.
31. Bosworth DM, Della Pietra A, Rahilly G. PARAPLEGIA RESULTING FROM TUBERCULOSIS OF THE SPINE. JBJS. 1953 Jul;35(3):735–40.
32. Kumar R. Spinal tuberculosis: with reference to the children of northern India. Childs Nerv Syst ChNS Off J Int Soc Pediatr Neurosurg. 2005 Jan;21(1):19–26.
33. Negi SS, Khan SFB, Gupta S, Pasha ST, Khare S, Lal S. Comparison of the conventional diagnostic modalities, bactec culture and polymerase chain reaction test for diagnosis of tuberculosis. Indian J Med Microbiol. 2005 Jan;23(1):29–33.
34. Andronikou S, Bindapersad M, Govender N, Waner JI, Segwe A, Palliam S, et al. Musculoskeletal tuberculosis - imaging using low-end and advanced modalities for developing and developed countries. Acta Radiol Stockh Swed 1987. 2011 May 1;52(4):430–41.
35. JaypeeDigital | Tuberculosis of the Spine [Internet]. [cited 2021 Jan 12]. Available from: https://www.jaypeedigital.com/book/9789350258835/chapter/ch7
36. Hsu LC, Leong JC. Tuberculosis of the lower cervical spine (C2 to C7). A report on 40 cases. J Bone Joint Surg Br. 1984 Jan;66(1):1–5.
37. Trivedi R, Saksena S, Gupta RK. Magnetic resonance imaging in central nervous system tuberculosis. Indian J Radiol Imaging. 2009 Jan 10;19(4):256.

38. Jaypee Brothers: Book Details [Internet]. [cited 2020 Dec 27]. Available from: https://www.jaypeebrothers.com/pgDetails.aspx?cat=s&book_id=9788194709022
39. Boxer DI, Pratt C, Hine AL, McNicol M. Radiological features during and following treatment of spinal tuberculosis. Br J Radiol. 1992 Jun 1;65(774):476–9.
40. Le Page L, Feydy A, Rillardon L, Dufour V, Le Hénanff A, Tubach F, et al. Spinal tuberculosis: a longitudinal study with clinical, laboratory, and imaging outcomes. Semin Arthritis Rheum. 2006 Oct;36(2):124–9.
41. Sharif HS, Aideyan OA, Clark DC, Madkour MM, Aabed MY, Mattsson TA, et al. Brucellar and tuberculous spondylitis: comparative imaging features. Radiology. 1989 May;171(2):419–25.
42. Yao DC, Sartoris DJ. Musculoskeletal tuberculosis. Radiol Clin N Am. 1995 Jul;33(4):679–89.
43. Moore SL, Rafii M. Imaging of musculoskeletal and spinal tuberculosis. Radiol Clin N Am. 2001 Mar;39(2):329–42.

Chapter 9
Role of Nuclear Medicine in TB Spine

Rajender Kumar, Apurva Sood, and Anish Bhattacharya

Abstract Spinal tuberculosis (TB), also known as Pott's spine, is one of the most debilitating and common forms of extrapulmonary TB. Clinical presentation of spinal TB depends on the stage and site of the disease. The symptoms are usually insidious and progress slowly, leading to delayed presentation and delayed diagnosis. Early diagnosis and rapid intervention can significantly reduce morbidity and mortality. The clinician relies on serological, hematological, and radiological imaging for diagnosis and management of spinal TB. Nuclear Medicine imaging is molecular imaging modality that uses various SPECT and PET radiotracers to evaluate oncological and non-oncological conditions. The past decade has seen a surge in radiotracers, particularly PET tracers, to manage infections like TB. Radiotracers used in nuclear medicine can be utilized in spinal TB for early diagnosis, identifying the most appropriate biopsy site, evaluating disease extent, detecting drug resistance, and monitoring treatment response. The following chapter aims at understanding the various features of nuclear medicine molecular imaging that can be used in the management of spinal TB.

Keywords Tuberculosis · Spinal · Imaging: positron emission tomography/computed tomography

Rajender Kumar and Apurva Sood contributed equally with all other contributors.

R. Kumar (✉) · A. Sood · A. Bhattacharya
Department of Nuclear Medicine and PET/CT, Post Graduate Institute of Medical Education and Research, Chandigarh, India

S. S. Dhatt, V. Kumar (eds.), *Tuberculosis of the Spine*,
https://doi.org/10.1007/978-981-16-9495-0_9

Abbreviations

ATT	anti-tubercular therapy
CT	computed tomography
EPTB	Extrapulmonary tuberculosis
FDG PET/CT	^{18}F-fluoro-2-deoxy-D-glucose (FDG) positron emission tomography/computed tomography
MDR	Multi-drug resistance
MRI	magnetic resonance imaging
SUV	standardized uptake value
TB	tuberculosis

9.1 Introduction

Tuberculosis (TB) continues to be the top leading cause of death from a single infectious disease, ranking above HIV/AIDs according to the World Health Organization (WHO) report 2020. An estimated 10.0 million people fell ill with TB, and 1.2 million TB deaths occurred among HIV-negative people. The problem continues to increase, with a growing incidence of multi-drug resistance and HIV co-infection despite various programs and efforts by governments to curtail the disease [1].

Although pulmonary TB is the most frequent presentation, amounting to 80% of the cases, TB can essentially involve any tissue or organ by the hematogenous or lymphatic spread. Around 20% of the cases are of extrapulmonary TB (EPTB) and can involve lymph nodes (LNs), musculo-skeleton, gastrointestinal tract, pleura, genitourinary system, and central nervous system [2, 3]. Spinal tuberculosis, popularly known as Potts' disease (named after Percival Pott, who first described the classic presentation in 1779) is one of the most debilitating and common forms of EPTB [4]. Approximately 10% of EPTB cases have skeletal involvement, with the spine being the most commonly affected site, followed by hip and knee joints [5]. Spinal TB is the result of hematogenous spread of the *Mycobacterium tuberculosis* bacilli into the vasculature of the vertebral bodies and is usually secondary to lung or abdominal involvement. The clinical presentation of spinal TB depends on the stage and site of the disease. Furthermore, the symptoms are typically insidious and progress slowly, leading to delayed presentation and late diagnosis (ranging from weeks to years), resulting in substantial morbidity and mortality. This presents a particular challenge to the clinician, as he has to rely on serological, microbiological, and radiological tests for the diagnosis of spinal TB [6, 7].

Nuclear medicine imaging is based on the compounds labeled with single-photon emitting isotopes or positron-emitting isotopes. These radiopharmaceuticals can identify pathophysiological reactions preceding morphological changes and can play a useful role in the early diagnosis of spine TB. Various SPECT and PET tracers are available to diagnose infectious bone disease. Still, with the advantage of high sensitivity and better resolution at acceptable radiation dose, PET/CT with F18-fluoro-2-deoxy-D-glucose (FDG) has been extensively used and studied in the management of TB spine.

9.2 Spect Imaging

9.2.1 Skeletal Scintigraphy

Bone scan with 99mTc-diphosphonates is highly sensitive in detecting bone remodeling, resulting in various pathological processes like infection, fracture, or neoplastic involvement [8]. Increased uptake in all three phases of triple-phase scintigraphy is suggestive of infection, and additionally, SPECT/CT improves anatomical localization and specificity. Advantages of skeletal scintigraphy include high sensitivity (80–95%), low cost, easy availability, and scanning of the entire skeleton in a single setting [9]. Consequently, a normal bone scan can very reliably rule out bone infection/inflammation. But in spondylodiscitis, false-negative are not uncommon, and an inadequate blood supply or osteolytic lesion with loss of osteal tissue can lead to photopenic defects. The specificity of bone scan further decreases in the setting of previous vertebral surgeries or injuries [10].

9.2.2 Gallium-67-Citrate Scintigraphy

Ga-67 shows a high concentration in infectious foci. Increased vascular membrane permeability, binding to transferrin and lactoferrins, direct uptake by bacteria through siderophores are a plausible mechanism of uptake of Ga67 in the tuberculous lesion. Ga-67 accurately identifies chronic infection of the spine. Combined with a bone scan, it can efficiently detect both osseous and soft tissue infection with a sensitivity of 90% and specificity of 78%, and uptake on Ga67 higher than the bone scan suggests an infectious origin [11]. Ga67 is less affected by bone remodeling and can monitor treatment response and identify residual disease [12]. The drawback of Ga67 includes poor image quality, high radiation burden and time-consuming acquisition (48–72 hours) [10, 13].

9.2.3 Scintigraphy with Autologous Radiolabeled Leukocytes

Leukocytes significantly accumulate in the site of infection to fight with the microbial agent. Labeling of the leukocyte with tracers like Tc99m, In111, and PET tracer (FDG) can help in diagnosing infection. But most of the labeled cells are neutrophils and therefore are more useful in identifying neutrophil mediated inflammatory processes, unlike TB, where the cellular response is predominantly lymphocytes. It lowers the sensitivity of labeled leukocytes for the identification of Pott's spine [14]. Physiological uptake of leukocytes by haematopoietically active bone marrow further reduces sensitivity to identify SD. Photopenic lesions at scintigraphy with labeled leukocytes were seen in about 50% of patients affected by SP, probably due to encapsulation of the infected site and therefore reduced migration of leukocytes [10, 15, 16].

9.3 PET Imaging

Molecular imaging using PET/CT with F18-FDG, a glucose analog, has been extensively used to detect high metabolism cells. It is now regularly used for diagnosis, staging, and treatment response assessment of oncologic diseases [17]. FDG also gets accumulated in infection and inflammatory conditions besides cancer cells. Increased glycolysis seen in activated macrophages, lymphocytes, and granulocytes in the granuloma of an active tuberculous lesion cause increased FDG accumulation, which can be employed for metabolic assessment of the disease [18]. Thus, the molecular and anatomical information provided by PET/CT can prove beneficial for the management of spinal TB.

9.3.1 PET/CT in Diagnosis

Early diagnosis and timely treatment of spinal TB is of paramount importance to prevent neurological deficit and spinal deformities. Low incidence and slow development of clinical features are probable causes for its late identification and pose a challenge to the clinician. Spinal TB is a *great mimicker* due to its ability to mimic other diseases like pyogenic spondylitis, brucellar spondylitis, sarcoidosis, metastases, multiple myeloma, and lymphoma, especially in HIV infected patients [19]. Consequently, once an abnormality is detected, it becomes essential for the physician to differentiate spinal TB from these diseases.

Growth of *Mycobacterium* obtained from infected tissue is considered the gold standard for diagnosis of spinal TB but has a lower sensitivity. Demonstration of a classical granuloma on histopathology examination and acid-fast bacilli is considered the reference standard for all diagnostic modalities. Apart from these, hematological and serological tests and radiological imaging are also essential to clinch the diagnosis. Plain radiographs, Computed Tomography (CT), and Magnetic Resonance Imaging are commonly used to diagnose and identify the disease extent [6, 7].

Although not typically used to determine the presence of spinal TB, FDG PET/CT-based molecular imaging shows promising results in recent literature. PET

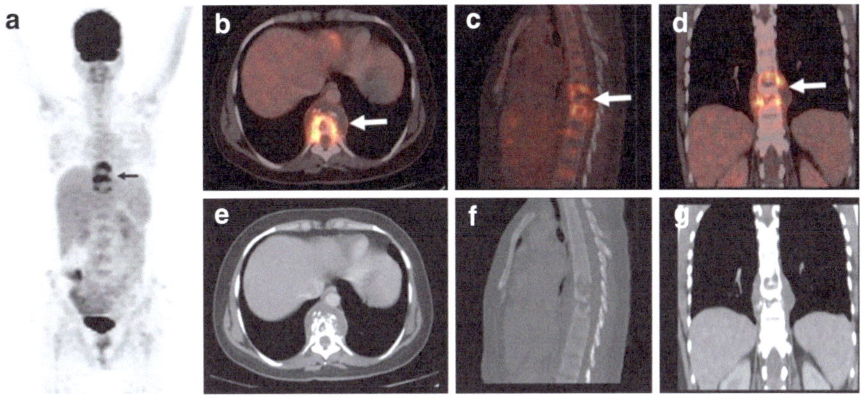

Fig. 9.1 Forty-five years old female presented with pain in the lower back and loss of weight. CT scan of the region showed a lytic lesion with abscess involving D8-D10 vertebrae. A sample from the lesion tested positive for acid-fast bacilli suggestive of TB. The patient underwent 18F-FDG PET/CT to look for the activity and pattern of the disease. Maximum Projection Image (MIP) (**a**), PET/CT fused (**b**, **c**, **d**), and CT only (**e**, **f**, **g**) images show FDG uptake in a lytic destructive lesion with soft tissue component (abscess) involving D8-D10 vertebrae (white arrow, **b**, **c**, and **d**). FDG uptake higher than the healthier vertebra is suggestive of FDG positive disease (Black arrow, **a**). No abnormal FDG uptake was seen elsewhere in the visualized organs

highlights glucose utilization, which may be evident before anatomical changes. A PET/CT is considered positive when FDG uptake is higher than that seen in healthy vertebral bone (Fig. 9.1) [20].

Schmitz et al., in 16 patients with suspected spinal TB found that all 12 patients with histopathological diagnosis of spinal TB had increased FDG uptake in PET/CT with SUVmax of 7.5 ± 3.8 and showed 100% sensitivity. Additionally, PET/CT also helped to identify paraspinal abscesses [21]. Gulhmann et al. found that FDG showed 96% sensitivity in diagnosing osteomyelitis of the central skeleton [22]. Compared to bone scan and Ga67 scintigraphy to diagnose spondylodiscitis (SD), F18-FDG PET/CT reported the best diagnostic accuracy with 89% sensitivity, 88% specificity, 89% negative predictive value, 89% positive predictive value, and 88% accuracy [23].

Magnetic resonance imaging (MRI) is the preferred imaging technique for evaluating spinal TB. It can detect infection in its early stages and provide excellent anatomic information of the epidural space, soft tissue involvement, the spread of abscess, spinal cord and neural compression [7, 24]. The high sensitivity of FDG to detect spinal TB is advantageous, especially in conditions where patients cannot undergo MRI due to metallic implants in situ or recent surgery. Gratz et al. found that FDG hybrid PET was superior to MRI and bone scan in patients with a history of surgery and those with low-grade spondylitis or discitis. Additionally, osteo-degenerative changes showed low FDG uptake compared to infective changes [25].

A joint European Association of Nuclear Medicine (EANM), European Society of Neuroradiology (ESNR), and European Society of Clinical Microbiology and InfectiousDiseases(ESCMID)endorsedconsensusdocumentfordiagnosisofSDstatesthat:-

1. MRI is the first diagnostic imaging modality in the absence of contraindications.
2. When MRI is contraindicated, the imaging modality of choice is FDG PET/CT.
3. In post-surgical SD, with or without spinal hardware, PET/CT can detect both spine infection and soft tissue infection.
4. In patients with suspected spine infection and elevated Erythrocyte sedimentation rate (ESR) and/or c-reactive protein (CRP) and doubtful MRI, PET/CT should be performed.
5. In the case of negative MRI or negative PET/CT, the diagnosis of SD should be excluded [20].

PET/CT can be used as a complimentary imaging modality to MRI for distinguishing between tuberculous and pyogenic spondylitis [26]. A retrospective case-control study with FDG PET/CT found that tuberculous SD was seen more frequently in younger patients with multiple vertebral involvements. Higher FDG uptake was noticed in TB compared to pyogenic SD (SUVmax 12.4 vs. 7.3) with a higher specificity [27]. Another study documented that FDG uptake in the spleen was significantly higher in pyogenic spondylitis as compared to TB spondylitis. SUVmax of spleen >1.49, spleen to marrow ration >0.957 and spleen to liver ratio > 0.889 favored pyogenic spondylitis [28]. Conversely, a dual time point FDG PET/CT performed in 23 patients to differentiate TB spondylitis from pyogenic spondylitis showed no significant difference in SUVmax or change in SUVmax between the two entities [29].

Patients with known malignancy and HIV are immunocompromised and have a higher risk of acquiring TB or reactivation of latent TB [30, 31]. Patients with malignancy undergoing PET/CT might show increased uptake in the spine with or without paravertebral soft tissue component suggestive of TB (Fig. 9.2). But neither dual time point imaging nor semiquantitative analysis can differentiate between TB from other malignant lesions, and only histopathological/microbiological examination is a prerequisite for definitive diagnosis. Another indication where FDG PET/CT is advocated due to its high sensitivity is pyrexia of unknown origin (PUO), aiming to rule out infection, inflammation, and malignancy. In developing nations like India, TB is the most common cause of infection, and PET/CT might help to identify spinal TB, especially where the radiological features are subtle [32–34].

One of the most promising and forthcoming roles of PET/CT in both oncological and non-oncological conditions is its ability to guide sampling of the most metabolically active lesions, described as PET-guided biopsy [35, 36]. Metabolic and anatomical information provided by combined PET/CT is ideal for guiding a percutaneous needle to sample the most appropriate site, particularly in lesions with necrotic components and relatively inaccessible locations. Another benefit of PET-guided biopsy is that metabolic changes occur before anatomical changes, which, when sampled, can help in the early diagnosis of spinal TB [37, 38].

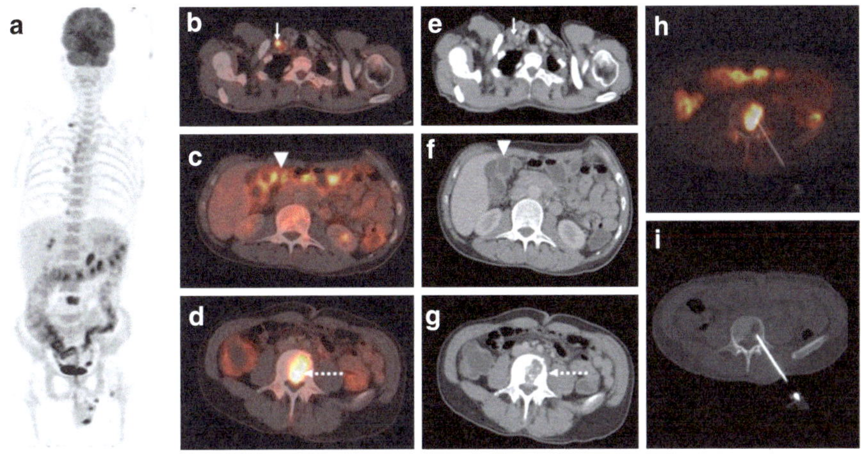

Fig. 9.2 A forty-one-year-old male diagnosed with ulcerative colitis for the past one year on treatment (immunosuppressive drugs) presented with persistent fever for one month. The patient underwent 18F-FDG PET/CT to look for disease activity and identify any other abnormal focus of FDG uptake. MIP (**a**), PET/CT fused (**b**, **c**, **d**, **h**), and CT only (**e**, **f**, **g**, **i**) images show FDG avid subcentimetric right supraclavicular (Arrow **b**, **e**) and mediastinal (not shown) lymph nodes. FDG uptake in diffuse mucosal thickening involving the large bowel (Arrowhead, **c**, **f**) and FDG uptake in lytic lesion involving the L4 vertebral body. He underwent a PET/CT guided biopsy (**h**, **i**) from the L4 vertebral lesion, which on histopathology was suggestive of TB. The patient was started on ATT, and his fever subsided

Hence, FDG PET/CT is a one-stop-shop imaging modality for whole-body evaluation with high negative predictive value, short acquisition time, high-quality imaging, its ability to detect disease at an early stage and guiding the biopsy from an appropriate site. The disadvantages include relatively limited availability (compared to CT/MRI), higher cost, low specificity and inability to differentiate infection from neoplastic lesions reliably.

9.3.2 *PET/CT for Staging*

A PET/CT usually includes images from head to mid-thigh, which allows a physician to assess all the organs in a single sitting and identify sites of disease involvement. Spinal TB is usually secondary to lung or abdominal involvement, and 60–70% of spinal TB cases have active primary lung focus or have a history of pulmonary TB. Moreover, detection of pulmonary TB becomes essential to reduce the risk of transmission [39, 40]. Usually, it involves two to three continuous vertebrae, but several vertebrae may be affected with skip lesions seen in 4–10% of cases. Lower thoracolumbar vertebrae are the most common site of involvement, followed by middle thoracic and cervical vertebrae [6, 41].

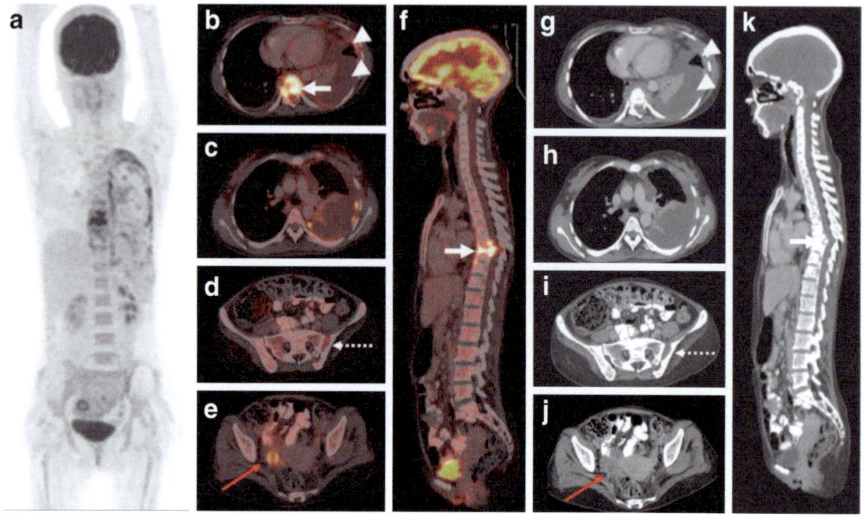

Fig. 9.3 Thirty years old female presented with paraplegia of bilateral lower limbs for one month. MRI spine revealed the collapse of the D7-D9 vertebra with paravertebral soft tissue mass. FNAC from paravertebral soft tissue mass—s/o Tuberculosis. The patient underwent 18F-FDG PET/CT to look at the disease extent. Maximum Projection Image (MIP) (**a**), PET/CT fused (**b**, **c**, **d**, **e**, **f**) and CT only (**g**, **h**, **i**, **j**, **k**) images show FDG uptake in FDG lytic lesion with soft tissue component D7–D9 vertebrae with the collapse of the D8 vertebra (arrow **b**, **f**, and **k**). FDG avid left-sided pleural thickening and pleural effusion (**b**, **g**, arrowhead). FDG avid lesion with soft tissue component involving the left sacroiliac joint (**d**, **i** dashed arrow). Physiological FDG uptake in the right ovary (**e**, **j**, red arrow)

A study detected occult non-contiguous lesions in 63% of the patients (Fig. 9.3). It attributed this significantly high number to either increased sensitivity of FDG PET for detecting lesions with subtle or no morphological change on CT, evaluation of the whole spine in contrast to regional X-ray/CT or MRI images, or an overestimation due to small sample size ($n = 33$) [34]. Zinn et al. investigated the use of FDG PET/CT in treatment-naïve cases of spinal TB. They found that PET/CT detected active pulmonary disease in 6/16 (38%) patients and 75% of the subjects had two or more spinal lesions. PET/CT also detected 60 of 60 (100%) clinically observed extra-spinal sites, including pulmonary TB, nodal disease and other musculoskeletal sites, vs. the 43 of 60 (71%) on CT imaging. PET/CT was superior to CT alone in detecting nodal involvement [37]. Furthermore, studies have demonstrated that the involvement of five or more nodal basins had more chances of treatment resistance [42].

Early identification of spinal involvement in pulmonary and non-skeletal extra-pulmonary TB cases is essential. It warrants a longer duration of anti-tubercular treatment (ATT) and helps the physician take appropriate steps to prevent complications. A study including 87 patients of TB found that FDG PET/CT detected skeletal involvement in 7/27 (26%) cases of pulmonary TB and detected extra-skeletal sites in 17/27 (63%) cases of skeletal TB [43]. Thus, FDG PET/CT in a single setting can help in documenting the disease extent, metabolic activity, and extra-skeletal sites in spinal TB.

9.3.3 Response assessment

Response to ATT can be assessed by the following parameters like,

1. Symptomatic improvement.
2. Reduction in inflammatory markers [ESR, CRP, Total leukocyte count (TLC)] and.
3. Radiological improvement.

While assessing response to treatment, a substantial variability of radiological changes has been reported on CT imaging that might occur despite clinical response to ATT. Sclerosis in an initial osteolytic lesion suggests healing. But in an initial sclerotic lesion, CT imaging provided little information about improvement. Recovery of vertebral height is seen after 15 months, and ankylosis, which occurs in over 50% of cases, is considered the surest sign of healing. Change in soft tissue masses with the progression of calcifying debris is also valuable [44].

Signs of MRI response are decreased edema and loss of contrast enhancement starting a few weeks to months after the ATT. It may persist in successfully treated cases, and enhancement might not necessarily mean treatment failure [38]. PET/CT for response assessment is a quintessential application of this modality that might prove beneficial in the individualization of therapy and shorten ATT duration, varying from 9–18 months in spinal TB cases.

In a prospective study, Martinez et al. monitored the response to ATT in 21 HIV-negative TB patients. They found that a lower SUVmax at 1 month after treatment initiation is a marker for a favorable response. They found a higher SUVmax suggests a lack of adherence to treatment, drug resistance or misdiagnosis [45].

In a study cohort of 28 patients with multi-drug resistant (MDR) -TB, Chen et al. demonstrated that F18-FDG PET/CT performed at 2 months had a sensitivity of 96% for predicting treatment success and a specificity of 79% for predicting treatment failure (Figs. 9.4 and 9.5). CT scans also achieved similar results but after 6 months of treatment initiation [46].

Implying that metabolic change often occurs before the morphological response is evident. In a cohort of 33 cases of spinal TB, Dureja et al. demonstrated a decrease in SUVmax on FDG PET/CT done at 6, 12, and 18 months of ATT initiation. The reduction in SUVmax at 6 and 12 months significantly correlated with the patient's clinical improvement assessed with Visual analog Score and showed no correlation with ESR change [34]. ESR is used for follow-up of treatment response, but it has been reported in the literature that ~10% of TB cases might have normal ESR or total WBC at the start of therapy. In a series, scan findings of the appearance of new lesions or an increase in SUVmax in PET/CT done at 3–4 months showed that these patients had a higher risk of mortality, drug resistance and longer ATT intake duration [43].

Kim et al. evaluated the prognostic effectiveness of follow-up imaging with FDG PET/CT in 30 patients with spinal infection (11 TB spine cases) after therapy. They found that FDG PET/ CT is useful for evaluating residual infection after treatment.

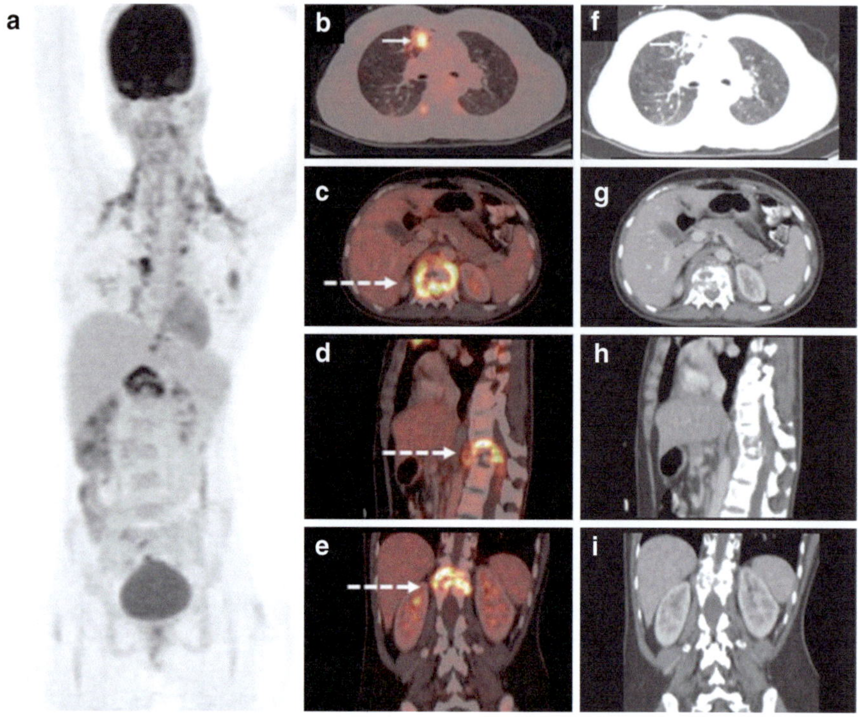

Fig. 9.4 Twenty-eight-year-old woman with a history of treated pulmonary TB 5 years back now presented with back pain for two months. MRI of the thoracolumbar spine revealed the pathological collapse of the D12 vertebra. The patient underwent 18F-FDG PET/CT to look for the activity and pattern of the disease. Maximum Projection Image (MIP) (**a**), PET/CT fused (**b**, **c**, **d**, **e**), and CT only (**f**, **g**, **h**, **i**) images show FDG uptake in a fibro-consolidatory change in the anterior segment of the RUL and parenchymal nodules (**b**, **f**, arrow). Intense FDG uptake is noted in the collapsed body of the D12 vertebra with contiguous involvement of the adjacent D11 and L1 vertebral discs with pre and paravertebral collection—cold abscess (**c**, **d**, **e**, dashed arrow)

In the patient-based analysis, a change in SUVmax of <46.14% had 100% sensitivity and 79.9% specificity in differentiating residual from the non-residual disease [47]. In a recent study, Davis et al. investigated the difference in participant characteristics between positive and negative PET/CT activity at the spinal TB site following 12 months of appropriate ATT. A total of 18 patients were included in the study, and five were PET-positive. PET-positive patients were of a younger age group and had multiple infected vertebrae. Among these five patients, smear microscopy was negative in all. The Gene Xpert was positive in four patients. Among them, one patient showed typical TB histopathology. They concluded that PET/CT can be over-sensitive and show metabolic activity in sterile inflammation areas and requires further studies [48].

This implies that PET/CT might show activity in recovered patients due to the continued reactive process. The FDG uptake at the end of treatment PET should be

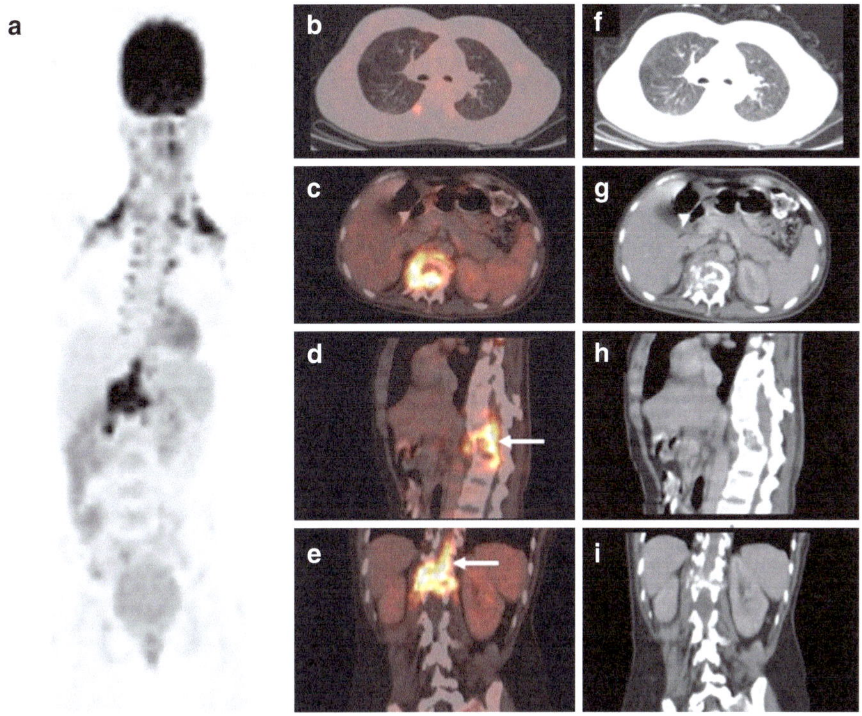

Fig. 9.5 The patient underwent 18F-FDG PET/CT 4 months after initiation of ATT. Maximum Projection Image (MIP) (**a**), PET/CT fused (**b**, **c**, **d**, **e**), and CT only (**f**, **g**, **h**, **i**) images show resolution of lung lesions. D11-L1 vertebral lesion shows the persistence of tracer activity with an increase in the extent of the associated soft tissue component (**d**, **e**, white-arrows), suggestive of disease progression. A repeat biopsy from the skeletal lesion revealed drug resistance to rifampicin and isoniazid (MDR-TB)

interpreted keeping clinical and biochemical data in mind. Khandelwal et al. evaluated the role of FDG PET/CT to detect infection in post-operative cases of spinal TB. Out of the ten subjects recruited in the study, nine patients showed FDG positivity after 6 months and continued ATT. At 1 year, FDG activity resolved in all cases except two, where a biopsy of the lesions revealed MDR-TB [49]. Therefore, an interim PET/CT can facilitate the evaluation of the efficacy of the treatment regimen and help decide the treatment protocol. End of treatment PET/CT should be aimed at seeking residual disease, which may require further treatment. Vanino E et al. proposed the use of FDG PET/CT for treatment response in cases of spinal TB in the following circumstances:

1. If bacteriological confirmation of TB is not obtained.
2. Poor clinical/MRI response, mainly in clinically diagnosed TB and.
3. MDR-TB cases [24].

9.3.4 PET/MRI in Spinal Tuberculosis

PET/MRI is a technology that combines the advantages of MRI like increased soft tissue contrast and lack of ionizing radiation exposure with metabolic/physiological information provided by PET. Although PET/MRI is promising, its higher cost, limited availability and technical difficulties make it less appealing. MRI is the imaging of choice for spinal lesions and it is logical that PET/MRI might offer an advantage over PET/CT in the diagnosis and characterization of spinal TB [50]. Data on the use of PET/MRI in spinal TB is minimal. Jeon et al. assessed therapeutic response using FDG PET/MRI in three cases of spinal TB. They found that high FDG uptake in the spinal lesion at 12 months, even in the presence of signs of healing on MRI, warrants the continuation of ATT. However, this requires validation in a large prospective study [51].

9.4 Conclusion and Future Perspectives

Metabolic and anatomical information provided by SPECT and PET imaging modalities are useful clinical tools for the clinical management of spinal TB. They are non-invasive imaging biomarker and can help diagnose spinal TB in its early stages. PET/CT or Ga67 scintigraphy is useful in diagnosing spinal TB in patients who are immunocompromised or with PUO. Patients who cannot undergo MRI or have undergone recent surgery of the spine can be evaluated using PET/CT. PET/CT can also help in identifying the most metabolically active and accurate site for biopsy. Baseline PET/CT can provide information about the extent of disease and other organs involved with sensitivity higher than CT alone. Real-time metabolic information provided by PET/CT can be used for treatment response assessment, prognostication and help identify the residual disease and even resistance to ATT. Finally, PET/CT can direct treatment duration and individualize therapy instead of using empirical treatment in all cases.

One of the inherent challenges of these radiotracers, especially FDG is its low specificity. To overcome this challenge, the development of new tracers that are specific for the tubercular process is required. Besides, new radiotracer development to better understand the disease process and anti-tubercular drugs may play a pivotal role in TB management and warrants further research.

Further large prospective studies are required to evaluate the optimal time between baseline scan and response evaluation scan, identify quantitative parameters that can detect responders from non-responders and individualize therapy based on PET findings.

FDG PET/CT is costly, not readily available and involves radiation exposure. Its use in all cases of TB is not justified. Even though its role in managing TB management is likely to evolve as new data becomes available, guidelines for the use of FDG PET/CT in spinal TB clinical management need to be formulated.

Acknowledgments none.

Conflicts of Interest No conflict of interest.

References

1. Licence: CC BY-NC-SA 3.0 IGO. In: Global tuberculosis report 2020. Geneva: World Health Organization; 2020.
2. Ankrah AO, Glaudemans AWJM, Maes A, et al. Tuberculosis. Semin Nucl Med. 2018;48:108–30.
3. Golden MP, Vikram HR. Extrapulmonary tuberculosis: an overview. Am Fam Physician. 2005;72:1761–8.
4. Chauhan A, Gupta BB. Spinal tuberculosis. Indian Acad. Clin Med. 2007;8:110–3.
5. Davies PD, Humphries MJ, Byfield SP, et al. Bone and joint tuberculosis. A survey of notifications in England and Wales. J Bone Joint Surg Br. 1984;66:326–30.
6. Ansari S, Amanullah MF, Ahmad K, et al. Pott's Spine: Diagnostic Imaging Modalities and Technology Advancements. N Am J Med Sci. 2013;5:404–11.
7. Rajasekaran S, Soundararajan DCR, Shetty AP, et al. Spinal Tuberculosis: Current Concepts. Glob spine J. 2018;8:96S–108S.
8. De Rossi G, Focacci C, Maini CL, et al. The particular usefulness of radioisotope methods in some benign bone diseases. Eur J Nucl Med. 1979;
9. Pandit HG, Sonsale PD, Shikare SS, et al. Bone scintigraphy in tuberculous spondylodiscitis. Eur Spine J. 1999;8:205–9.
10. Treglia G, Focacci C, Caldarella C, et al. The role of nuclear medicine in the diagnosis of spondylodiscitis. Eur Rev Med Pharmacol Sci. 2012;16(Suppl 2):20–5.
11. Lin WY, Wang SJ, Cheng KY, et al. Diagnostic value of bone and Ga-67 imaging in skeletal tuberculosis. Clin Nucl Med. 1998;23:743–6.
12. Tyrrell PN, Cassar-Pullicino VN, McCall IW. Spinal infection. Eur Radiol. 1999;9:1066–77.
13. Leitha T. Nuclear medicine diagnosis of osteomyelitis. Radiologe. 1996;36:813–22.
14. Palestro CJ, Torres MA. Radionuclide imaging of nonosseous infection. Q J Nucl Med. 1999;43:46–60.
15. Gratz S, Braun HG, Behr TM, et al. Photopenia in chronic vertebral osteomyelitis with technetium-99m-antigranulocyte antibody (BW 250/183). J Nucl Med. 1997;38:211–6.
16. Palestro CJ, Kim CK, Swyer AJ, et al. Radionuclide diagnosis of vertebral osteomyelitis: indium-111-leukocyte and technetium-99m-methylene diphosphonate bone scintigraphy. J Nucl Med. 1991;32:1861–5.
17. El-Haddad G, Zhuang H, Gupta N, et al. Evolving role of positron emission tomography in the management of patients with inflammatory and other benign disorders. Semin Nucl Med. 2004;34:313–29.
18. Kubota R, Kubota K, Yamada S, et al. Microautoradiographic study for the differentiation of intratumoral macrophages, granulation tissues and cancer cells by the dynamics of fluorine-18-fluorodeoxyglucose uptake. J Nucl Med. 1994;35:104–12.
19. Garg RK, Somvanshi DS. Spinal tuberculosis: a review. J Spinal Cord Med. 2011;34:440–54.
20. Lazzeri E, Bozzao A, Cataldo MA, et al. Joint EANM/ESNR and ESCMID-endorsed consensus document for the diagnosis of spine infection (spondylodiscitis) in adults. Eur J Nucl Med Mol Imaging. 2019;46:2464–87.
21. Schmitz A, Risse JH, Grünwald F, et al. Fluorine-18 fluorodeoxyglucose positron emission tomography findings in spondylodiscitis: preliminary results. Eur Spine J. 2001;10:534–9.
22. Guhlmann A, Brecht-Krauss D, Suger G, et al. Chronic osteomyelitis: detection with FDG PET and correlation with histopathologic findings. Radiology. 1998;206:749–54.

23. Fuster D, Solà O, Soriano A, et al. A prospective study comparing whole-body FDG PET/CT to combined planar bone scan with 67Ga SPECT/ct in the diagnosis of spondylodiskitis. Clin Nucl Med. 2012;37:827–32.
24. Vanino E, Tadolini M, Evangelisti G, et al. Spinal tuberculosis: proposed spinal infection multidisciplinary management project (SIMP) flow chart revision. Eur Rev Med Pharmacol Sci. 2020;24:1428–34.
25. Gratz S, Dörner J, Fischer U, et al. 18F-FDG hybrid PET in patients with suspected spondylitis. Eur J Nucl Med Mol Imaging. 2002;29:516–24.
26. Lee IS, Lee JS, Kim S-J, et al. Fluorine-18-fluorodeoxyglucose positron emission tomography/computed tomography imaging in pyogenic and tuberculous spondylitis: preliminary study. J Comput Assist Tomogr. 2009;33:587–92.
27. Bassetti M, Merelli M, Di Gregorio F, et al. Higher fluorine-18 fluorodeoxyglucose positron emission tomography (FDG-PET) uptake in tuberculous compared to bacterial spondylodiscitis. Skelet Radiol. 2017;46:777–83.
28. Kim K, Kim S-J, Kim IJ, et al. Diffuse increased splenic F-18 fluorodeoxyglucose uptake may be an indirect sign of acute pyogenic cause rather than tuberculous in patients with infectious spondylitis. Nucl Med Commun. 2011;32:1155–61.
29. Lee JS, Kim S-J, Suh KT, et al. Differentiation of Tuberculous and Pyogenic Spondylitis Using Double Phase F-18 FDG PET. Open Med Imaging J. 2008;2:1–6.
30. Kamboj M, Sepkowitz KA. The Risk of Tuberculosis in Patients with Cancer. Clin Infect Dis. 2006;42:1592–5.
31. Simonsen DF, Farkas DK, Horsburgh CR, et al. Increased risk of active tuberculosis after cancer diagnosis. J Infect. 2017;74:590–8.
32. Meller J, Sahlmann C-O, Scheel AK. 18F-FDG PET and PET/CT in fever of unknown origin. J Nucl Med. 2007;48:35–45.
33. Kouijzer IJE, Mulders-Manders CM, Bleeker-Rovers CP, et al. Fever of Unknown Origin: the Value of FDG-PET/CT. Semin Nucl Med. 2018;48:100–7.
34. Dureja S, Sen IB, Acharya S. Potential role of F18 FDG PET-CT as an imaging biomarker for the noninvasive evaluation in uncomplicated skeletal tuberculosis: a prospective clinical observational study. Eur Spine J. 2014;23:2449–54.
35. Kumar R, Mittal BR, Bhattacharya A, et al. 18F-FDG PET/CT-Guided Real-Time Automated Robotic Arm–Assisted Needle Navigation for Percutaneous Biopsy of Hypermetabolic Bone Lesions: Diagnostic Performance and Clinical Impact. Am J Roentgenol. 2018;212:W10–8.
36. Radhakrishnan RK, Mittal BR, Gorla AKR, et al. Real-time intraprocedural (18)F-FDG PET/CT-guided biopsy using automated robopsy arm (ARA) in the diagnostic evaluation of thoracic lesions with prior inconclusive biopsy results: initial experience from a tertiary health care centre. Br J Radiol. 2017;90:20170258.
37. Zinn C, Vorster M, Sathekge MM. Spinal tuberculosis evaluated by means of 18F-FDG PET/CT: Pilot study. Open Nucl Med J. 2014;6:6–11.
38. Rivas-Garcia A, Sarria-Estrada S, Torrents-Odin C, et al. Imaging findings of Pott's disease. Eur Spine J. 2013;22(Suppl 4):567–78.
39. Dharmalingam M. Tuberculosis of the spine-the Sabah experience. Epidemiology, treatment and results. Tuberculosis. 2004;84:24–8.
40. Schirmer P, Renault CA, Holodniy M. Is spinal tuberculosis contagious? Int J Infect Dis. 2010;14:e659–66.
41. Kaila R, Malhi AM, Mahmood B, et al. The incidence of multiple level noncontiguous vertebral tuberculosis detected using whole spine MRI. J Spinal Disord Tech. 2007;20:78–81.
42. Sathekge M, Maes A, Kgomo M, et al. Impact of FDG PET on the management of TBC treatment. A pilot study Nuklearmedizin. 2010;49:35–40.
43. Sood A, Mittal BR, Modi M, et al. 18F-FDG PET/CT in Tuberculosis: Can Interim PET/CT Predict the Clinical Outcome of the Patients? Clin Nucl Med. 2020;45:276–82.
44. Boxer DI, Pratt C, Hine AL, et al. Radiological features during and following treatment of spinal tuberculosis. Br J Radiol. 1992;65:476–9.

45. Martinez V, Castilla-Lievre MA, Guillet-Caruba C, et al. (18)F-FDG PET/CT in tuberculosis: an early non-invasive marker of therapeutic response. Int J Tuberc Lung Dis. 2012;16:1180–5.
46. Chen RY, Dodd LE, Lee M, et al. PET/CT imaging correlates with treatment outcome in patients with multidrug-resistant tuberculosis. Sci Transl Med 2014;6:265ra166.
47. Kim S-J, Kim I-J, Suh KT, et al. Prediction of residual disease of spine infection using F-18 FDG PET/CT. Spine. 2009;34:2424–30.
48. JH D, MC B, Pienaar G, et al. 18F-FDG PET/CT as a modality for the evaluation of persisting raised infective markers in patients with spinal tuberculosis. SA Orthop J 2020;19:23–27.
49. Khandelwal RCS, Nathan S, Deo T, et al. Role of Fluorodeoxyglucose - Positron Emission Tomography Scan in Detection of Residual Pus Pocket Post-Operatively in Tuberculosis of Spine and Juxta Articular Tuberculosis. J Spine. 2018;7:424.
50. Jadvar H, Colletti PM. Competitive advantage of PET/MRI. Eur J Radiol. 2014;83:84–94.
51. Jeon I, Kong E, Kim SW. Simultaneous 18F-FDG PET/MRI in tuberculous spondylitis: an independent method for assessing therapeutic response - case series. BMC Infect Dis. 2019;19:845.

Chapter 10
FNAC and Biopsy Techniques in TB Spine

Chirag Kamal Ahuja and Bharat Hosur

Abstract The image-guided fine needle aspiration (FNA) and biopsy are of utmost importance in the effective management of spinal tuberculosis (TB), providing a definitive diagnosis. The spinal TB mimics like brucellosis, pyogenic infections, post-traumatic spinal degeneration, lymphoma, metastases, etc. may bear a close resemblance in clinico-radiological profile. Meticulous planning with a detailed pre-procedural clinical assessment, contrast-enhanced MRI, and attention to serial imaging and clinical course of the disease is crucial. Screening the patients for coagulopathies, neurological deficits requiring urgent surgical treatment in synchronization with the treating team averts complications. Thorough knowledge of the regional anatomy in the target area of biopsy bundled with a judicial choice of hardware and modality of imaging for guidance ensures precise access as well as the optimal yield of the tissue sample. The transpedicular coaxial approach is the commonest method used for the dorsolumbar spine, through the "bull's eye view of pedicle" if fluoroscopic guidance is used. Ultrasound or MRI guidance can be used in apt locations in pregnant or pediatric patients. Optimal patient comfort using local anesthesia, sedation and apt positioning, observing radiation safety measures and post-procedural care is sine-qua-non for patient safety and satisfaction as well as an efficient workflow.

Keywords Aspiration · Biopsy · CT guided · Spinal · Tuberculosis

---

C. K. Ahuja (✉)
Division of Neuroradiology, Department of Radiodiagnosis, PGIMER, Chandigarh, India

B. Hosur
Department of Radiodiagnosis, Command Hospital, Panchkula, Haryana, India

S. S. Dhatt, V. Kumar (eds.), *Tuberculosis of the Spine*,
https://doi.org/10.1007/978-981-16-9495-0_10

10.1 Introduction

The spinal FNAC or biopsy can be an effective adjunct to the clinical management of spinal tuberculosis when strategically planned with meticulous pre-procedural imaging, technical details of the procedure and post-procedural care. The coordinated team efforts between the operator and the referring clinician without communication gaps is a sin-a-qua-non for the meaningful outcome of the procedure as well as the patient safety. The attendants of the patient need to be kept informed at all the stages of the procedure apart from the initial detailed informed consent, to enhance patient satisfaction.

Identity of the patient, side and location of the affliction, correlation with the most recent imaging prior to the procedure and referring to the timely clinical notes bear immense medico-legal importance as well as save everyone from the unnecessary mismatch between the expected and performed procedures. Strict protocols regarding the vertebral numbering and labeling the levels craniocaudally on the pre-procedural imaging films can help to prevent inappropriate needle placement. The GATA classification (GATA = Gulhane Askeri Tip Akademisi) from the Gulhane Military Medical Academy provides relatively simplistic guidance for the surgical or interventional management approach of spinal tuberculosis [1]. A clinically stable patient without any neurological deficit, with the involvement of a single vertebra or single disc with no collapse and no abscess, is classified as Type 1A and is the right candidate for FNAC/Biopsy followed by medical management. The presence of abscess and/or involvement of two vertebral levels, which is Type 1B, mandates abscess drainage with debridement. Also, the presence of a stable spinal deformity is labeled Type-2 and treated with a surgical fusion of the vertebrae, while the unstable deformity, especially with neurological deficits, is urgently managed with surgical decompression.

The needle biopsy/microbiological confirmation is of utmost importance even in presence of obvious imaging features suggestive of spinal tuberculosis, especially in the endemic regions, due to the close resemblance of the clinico-radiological profile of the mimics [2]. Brucellosis, pyogenic infections, rheumatoid arthritis, post-traumatic spinal degeneration, lymphoma, metastases, and rarely, Rosai-Dorfman disease form the close differential diagnosis for spinal TB. The imaging phenotypes may be further distorted with immunocompromised status, coexisting infection with malignancy, and multifocal disease. Also, the locoregional and temporal variations in the presentations and natural history of the spondylodiscitis similar to the spinal TB mandate the definitive evidence before starting the non-tubercular drug therapy [3]. In a recent study, the MRI was shown to have a sensitivity of 85.71% and a specificity of 86.48% for the diagnosis of spinal tuberculosis. The initial biopsy had a sensitivity of 71.42% and specificity of 100% for the diagnosis of infection [4]. The image-guided needle-based microbiological diagnosis is shown to provide reliable, timely, and clear management decisions, avoiding unnecessary diagnostic dilemmas, delays, and failures in the treatment [5].

10.2 Anatomical Factors

The soft tissue spaces around the spine from skull base to coccyx can be accessed for aspiration cytology or biopsy safely adhering to the locoregional peculiarities at various spinal segments. The cervical spine has relatively smaller vertebral bodies with broader posterior elements that lie nearly in the same plane. Both anterolateral as well as posterolateral approaches are feasible in the cervical spine provided the needle path avoids the carotid space. The cervical exiting nerves traverse anteriorly nearly in the same plane of the respective discs, unlike the obliquity seen in the subsequent caudal levels. Also, the vertebral arteries, veins, and sympathetic nerves traverse the transverse foramina of the cervical vertebrae.

The dorsal spine, a relatively common site for tubercular involvement, has lungs and mediastinal vital structures in the immediate vicinity of the prevertebral space. The descending aorta on the left side is usually closely abutting the vertebral bodies and the discs upto the D10 level. The adjacent pleura overlying the lungs are pain-sensitive structures and can accumulate dangerous pneumothorax if breached inadvertently. The left atrium is the cardiac chamber closest to the spine and can be injured with unsafe needle access.

The lumbar spine, by far the technically least difficult location for needle access is also the commonest site for aspiration or biopsy. Owing to the larger size of the vertebrae and abundance of paraspinal muscle and subcutaneous fat, the delineation of the tissue planes and the needle access path is relatively simpler [6]. However, the presence of abnormal curvature due to kyphoscoliosis may render the target tissue inaccessible for safe passage of the needle. The lumbar curvature can be manipulated by placing the pillows under the hip or chest in addition to the CT gantry tilt to achieve a feasible cross-sectional plane for the optimal needle visualization. Inadvertent injury to the obliquely traversing lumbar nerve plexus and the closely hugging sympathetic chain can be carefully avoided by choosing the apt paramedian distance from the midline at the skin entry. The sacral lesions being in close proximity to the recto-sigmoid parts of the large bowel are amenable for external and endorectal access options. There is also a risk of gut perforation and contamination of the sample. The peculiarities of the regional anatomy need focused heed on a case-to-case basis before the invasive procedure.

10.3 Pre-Procedural Evaluation

The clinical inputs regarding the spinal localization, timeline, and severity of the illness should be elicited in detail. Comorbidities, immune status, and bleeding/clotting disorders should be meticulously recorded. The serial imaging, including the spinal radiographs, CT and contrast-enhanced MRI images, should be reviewed along with the chest and abdominal imaging if available. Only the most recent MRI (performed within two weeks before the procedure) is to be relied upon for planning the needle access. Pre-procedural contrast-enhanced MRI with axial and coronal reformats, preferably done in the same center performing the procedure, are to be stressed upon; since the canulation of the pathological site may distort the imaging appearance.

The patterns of vertebral involvement in spinal TB can be paradiscal (via spinal arteries), central (along the venous plexus of a single vertebra), anterior marginal (subligamentous spread along anterior longitudinal ligament and adjacent periosteum), posterior-involving only the posterior elements (via external venous plexus or direct contiguous spread), synovial (usually around the craniovertebral junction (CVJ), spread via the synovial arteries) and multilevel or skipped lesions along the Batson's venous plexus [7, 8]. The commonest imaging features typical for spinal TB are subligamentous spread to more than two spinal levels, enhancing paraspinal components of the spondylodiscitis with or without sparing the intervertebral disc [9]. Identification of the sinister imaging patterns that need urgent surgical management without the prior FNAC and locating the site of best possible diagnostic yield are the main advantages of the contrast-enhanced MRI, without the risks of radiation hazards.

Pre-procedural PET/PET-CT in the presence of multilevel and multifocal disease is essential, especially when the imaging features are not conclusive of spinal tuberculosis or a previous image-guided needle biopsy has been inconclusive. The whole-body PET adds the non-spinal target sites for a guided biopsy which is vital when the spinal target access is difficult. The conundrum of PET-CT in hypermetabolic inflammation like spinal TB is about the wide range of uptake values that can also have temporal variations. The cutoff maximum Standardized Uptake Value (SUVmax) in spinal TB has been reported to be as low as 2 and as high as 21 in tuberculosis [10]. No definite single cutoff value discriminating the spinal TB from the mimics has been established. Thus, despite being a very sensitive modality, the lack of its specificity in a hypermetabolic spinal lesion on PET makes the needle biopsy a sine-qua-non for effective treatment.

The spinal needle biopsy or aspiration is an invasive procedure and it should not be planned in isolation but in consultation with the managing team consisting of a Neurosurgeon, Neurologist, Interventional Radiologist & Pathologist. The contraindications (Table 10.1) and risk factors (Table 10.2) associated with the procedure

Table 10.1 Contraindications to image-guided percutaneous biopsy

Absolute
Uncorrected bleeding diathesis
Platelet count <50,000/mm3
Acute cord compression
Relative
Lesions closely abutting or encasing aorta / major vessels
Coexistent vascular malformations
Small dimension (<5 mm in diameter)
Lesions in other locations that are safer to biopsy
Noncooperative patient
Clinically unstable patient when not fit for general anesthesia

Table 10.2 Complications and Risks associated with Spinal Needle Aspiration/Biopsy

Complications
Pneumothorax
Spinal cord/Cauda equina injury
Vascular injury Carotid/Vertebral/Aortic/intercostal artery dissection Pseudoaneurysm formation Uncontrolled bleed Distal thromboembolism
Severe pain due to pleural/peritoneal injury
Inappropriate needle placement Hematomyelia Spinal extradural or intradural hematoma Injury to exiting nerve roots (Neuropraxia) Injury to the sympathetic chain
Technical failure Sampling wrong level / side / person Inadequate tissue sampling Biopsy system failure
Anesthesia-related Respiratory depression Aspiration Airway compromise Anaphylactic reactions

should be discussed along with the risk-benefit analysis. The emergency systems to effectively handle the sudden cardiac arrest and the anaphylactic shock should be ensured to be intact. Urgent blood availability should also be preemptively ensured in case of uncontrolled hemorrhage requiring blood transfusions. The neurosurgery team should be kept informed for the backup of emergency laminectomy in case of hematoma within the spinal canal or hematomyelia.

10.4 Procedural Details

The accuracy of the image-guided percutaneous biopsy for providing the definitive diagnosis ranges from 74–92% depending upon the variations in the imaging modality used for guidance, hardware, and technical protocols [11]. The Biopsy scores over FNAC in the tissue sample yield available for analysis hence avoiding unnecessary repetitions, at the cost of the procedural safety, due to the more invasive nature of the involved hardware and techniques. Availability of trained manpower and advanced laboratory facilities, including the GeneXpert polymerase chain reaction test (sensitivity of 95.6% and specificity of 96.2% for spinal TB), are necessary for a seamless workflow and outcome [12].

10.5 Instrumentation

A variety of needles are available for the safe and accurate practice of spinal FNAC and Biopsy.

FNA Needles Commonly, 20 to 22 gauge needles are used with variable bevel angles (spinal—30°; Chiba—25°; Meditech, Boston Scientific, Natick, MA; Turner-45°, Cook, Bloomington, IN). The beveled edges provide a sharp cutting end for tissue penetration and increase the cross-sectional area for aspiration. Greene (Cook, Bloomington, IN), E-2-Em (E-2-EM, Westbury, NY), Crown (Meditech, Boston Scientific, Natick, MA), and Franseen (Meditech) are the aspiration cutting needles that increase the yield of the tissue with variable tip configurations [13]. They can also act as adjuvant access for coaxial biopsy systems in addition to providing extra material for microbiological analysis. Comparatively, smaller dimensions of the needles scores over the biopsy hardware in terms of safety, ease of access and patient compliance throughout the procedure and thereafter.

Biopsy Needles Automated cutting needles: ASAP, Meditech, Boston Scientific, Natick, NY; MaxCore, CR Bard, Covington, GA Trephine needle system: Craig (10-gauge, Becton Dickinson, Rutherford, NJ) and the Ackerman (12-gauge, Cook, Bloomington, IN) trephine needles.

Trephine needle systems have a large outer cannula with a fitted obturator, which is advanced to the bone surface. Trephine needle devices for subsequent FNA and cutting needle biopsies may be used as a coaxial device. FNA and cutting needles will be progressed through the outer cannula into the medullary cavity through the bone biopsy defect until the trephine needle has crossed the cortex during a core biopsy. Serial FNA and biopsies for cutting may be done. The Elson (Cook, Bloomington, IN) and Geremia (Cook, Bloomington, IN) coaxial systems use a 22-gauge needle with a removable stylet and hub to serve as a coaxial guiding the biopsy needle subsequently.

Combination Needles These have an outer hollow cutting needle and an inner trocar-boring needle. (Jamshidi, Manan Medical Products, Northbrook, IL; Ostycut, CR Bard, Covington, GA; Osteosite Cook, Bloomington, IN), thus combining the advantages of both the cutting needle & the trephine.

10.5.1 MRI-Compatible Needles

MRI-compatible FNA (18- to 22-gauge, E2-EM, Westbury, NY) and core (Comatex, Berlin, Germany Biogun, E-2-EM, Westbury, NY; Daum, Schwerin, Germany) biopsy systems can be used under MR-imaging guidance without radiation risks.

Pregnant and pediatric patients and the previously failed procedures with small lesions can be benefitted from superior soft tissue resolution and lesion delineation [14].

10.5.2 Robotically Driven FNAC/Biopsy

The newer, robotically driven artificial intelligence-based hardware advances for the CT-guided FNAC can enhance precision and safety without the radiation hazards to the operator [15]. However, the loss of tactile feedback, especially with a suboptimally cooperative patient, sophisticated infrastructure and higher cost-related setbacks are shortcomings of the robotic systems.

10.6 Aseptic and Safety Precautions

Diligent and proper hand wash with copious soap and disinfection before the procedure has no replacement. Use of disposable gown, cap and masks and sterile gloves without contaminating any of the useful surfaces as a planned step-by-step protocol, preferably in front of an observer is the best way to avoid chances of contamination (Fig. 10.1). Centrifugal dermal painting around the skin entry site with betadine and draping the surrounding unsterile parts, taking care of the smooth table movements in CT or fluoroscopy are important.

Preemptive intubation in the earmarked area as per the extant institutional infectious disease (e.g., Covid-19) protocols in a dyspneic patient to avoid emergency intubation and related aerosolization risk is the best approach. Non-intubated patients in the author's institute are made to wear a double mask with inner N-95

Fig. 10.1 Strict aseptic precautions with full protection need to be followed while performing the aspiration/ biopsy procedure

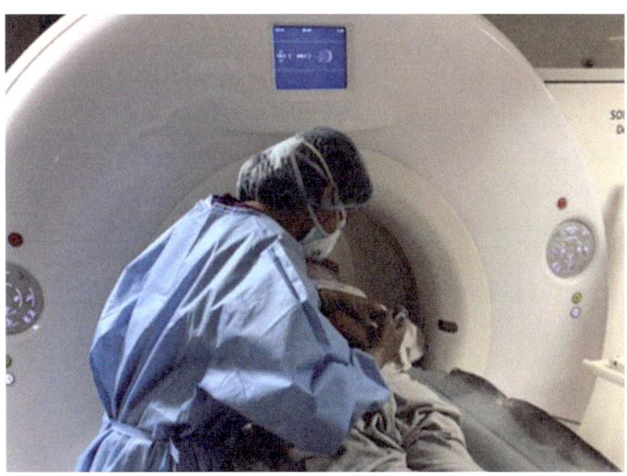

type and an outer surgical mask. If MRI-guided procedures are being performed, metallic content masks are avoided to prevent focal burns around the nose. Donning and doffing with strict personal protection equipment (PPE) protocols are to be followed, especially in patients harboring highly infectious disease (e.g., Covid positive).

10.7 Positioning and Needle Access

The cervical spine lesions can be accessed in both prone and supine positions depending on the location. A trans-oral approach with a secured open-mouth for the CVJ lesions and transpharyngeal access to upper cervical segments are also described. For the thoracic spine lesions, the patient is usually in a prone position with a pillow under the neck and arms by the side or above the head to suit the comfort of the patient for a posterolateral, transpedicular, or transcostovertebral approach. Many a time, letting the patients hold the cranial edge of the table with flexed elbows allows them to be comfortable motionless [16]. Lumbo-sacral lesions are usually targeted from posterior aspects after adjusting for the curvature of deformities if any, with pillows making it perpendicular to the expected needle path. Sometimes, the patient may also be in a lateral or oblique decubitus position to cater to the painful spinal deformities and obtain a motionless setup and maximum patient comfort [17]. The sacral lesions can be targeted by a posterior, perineal, or endorectal approach based on the lesion [18].

In the dorsal spine, the transcostovertebral approach offers safer, faster, and more reliable access due to easy visualization of the costovertebral joint on the axial CT images and stable positioning of the access hardware for coaxial passes [19]. The coaxial system consisting of initial access with a thinner needle and using it as a guide for insertion of the actual thicker trocar over the initial needle makes it safer and reliable for an effective yield of the tissue sample [20]. A tram-track technique of CT-guided biopsy has also been described, which involves placing a thin 23-25G spinal needle transcutaneously until the periosteum for initial marking of the access route [21]. The bone biopsy needle is subsequently introduced parallel to the spinal needle just by its side and further introduced into the bone. Choice of skin penetration site, depth, and angle of needle advancement should be decided once the patient assumes a comfortable position. Marking the skin entry after pin-pointing with laser pointers of CT gantry (Fig. 10.2), adhering to the careful progress of the needle tip with meticulous image guidance at every step is crucial. Maintaining the precise angle and depth of the needle during aspiration and biopsy maneuvers are also equally important. The patient should be adequately counseled about the importance of avoiding inadvertent body movements at all the steps.

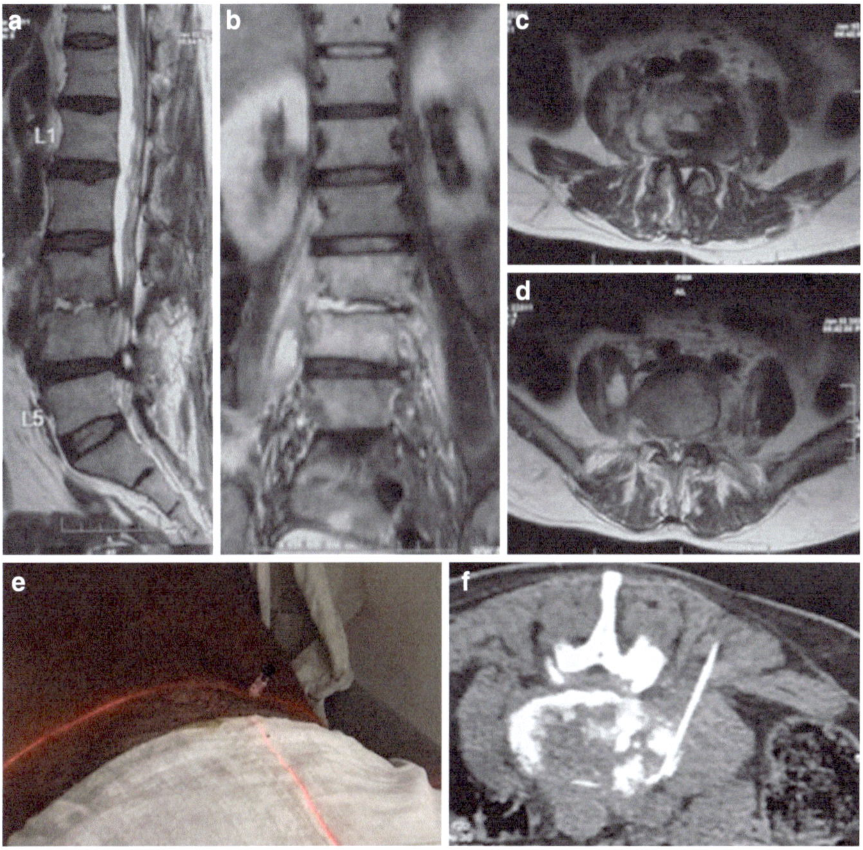

Fig. 10.2 Sagittal T2 (**a**), coronal T2 fat saturated (**b**) and axial T2 (**c**, **d**) weighted MR images demonstrating spondylodiscitis involving the L3 and L4 vertebral bodies with associated right psoas abscess. Patient lying prone on CT table with needle in situ (**e**) precisely guided and confirmed by the red laser pointers. Needle in situ evident on the CT image (**f**)

10.8 Methods of Image Guidance

Although an intact cortex of the bone restricts penetration of the ultrasound waves, the destructive lesions of spinal tuberculosis, especially in the cervicodorsal segments, readily allow the usage of sonographic guidance for needle biopsies (Fig. 10.3). Apart from the thinner subcutaneous tissue planes in these regions, continuous real-time visualization of the needle penetration up to the target tissue offers more advantages for a seamless procedure [22]. CT-guided procedures are usually the commonest amongst the FNAC/Biopsy. Most of the procedures are performed in the prone position (Figs. 10.2, 10.3, 10.4, 10.5 and 10.6). However, different

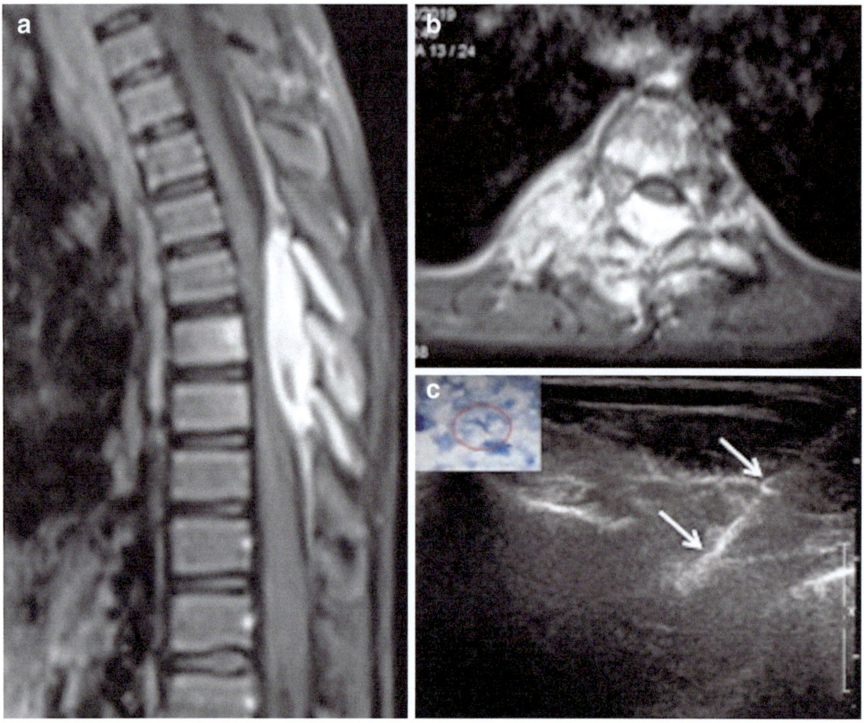

Fig. 10.3 Ultrasound-guided fine needle aspiration of tuberculous inflammatory lesion centered at the posterior arch elements of the dorsal vertebrae with contiguous involvement at three spinal levels with associated paravertebral and intraspinal extradural soft tissue component evident on sagittal (**a**) and axial (**b**) post-contrast T1 weighted MR images. Needle in situ (arrows) targeting the lesion. Acid fast bacilli evident on the aspirate slide in Fig. C (inset)

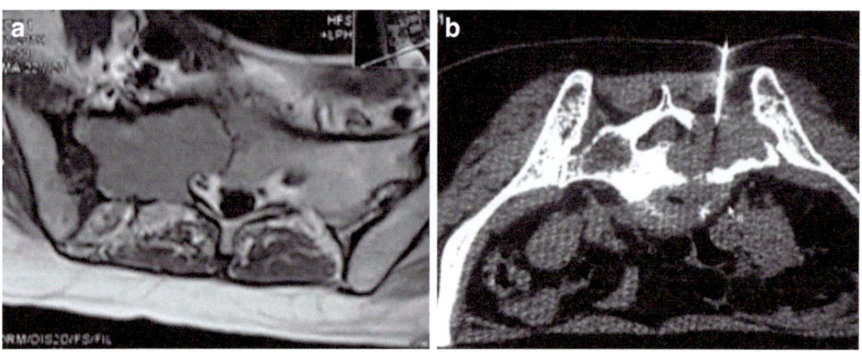

Fig. 10.4 Axial T1 weighted MRI (**a**) reveals a bone lesion in the right sacral ala. CT-guided fine needle aspiration (**b**) with the patient in prone position. The needle easily punctures the thin residual enveloping bone along the posterior aspect

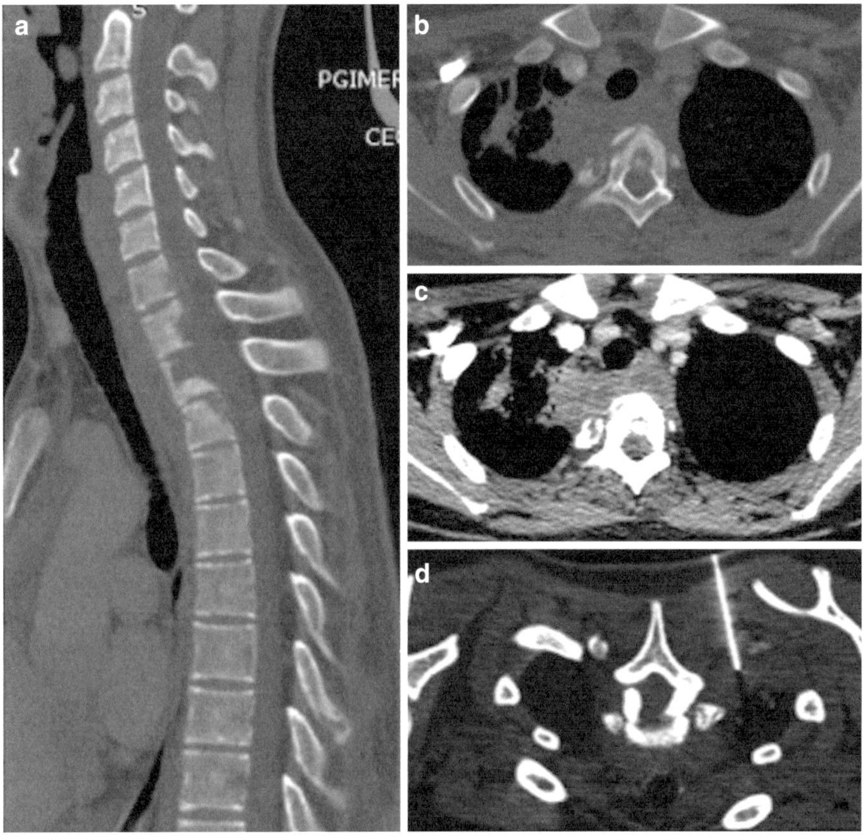

Fig. 10.5 Sagittal (**a**) and axial (**b**) CT bone window images showing lytic destructive lesion involving the vertebral bodies at D1 to D3 levels. Extensive associated soft tissue is seen on axial CT (**c**) mediastinal window section. Presence of soft tissue makes aspiration of the lesion (**d**) safe as the needle need not be directed to the vertebral body and surrounding neurovascular structures. Cytopathology revealed granulomatous lesion

convenient positions may be chosen depending on which area of the vertebra needs to be targeted. The laser pointer helps in accurately targeting the skin surface and helps to significantly reduce the navigation errors (Fig. 10.2). The following approaches are described [23] for various vertebral biopsy sites:

1. Transpedicular approach—It can be employed at any spinal level, however is most suitable for lumbar vertebral biopsy (Fig. 10.6).
2. Posterolateral extrapedicular approach—It is preferred for lumbar vertebrae where when the transpedicular approach is not feasible.
3. Superior costotransverse approach—It is the technique of choice, if feasible, for mid and lower thoracic vertebrae. The vertebral lesion is approached through superior costotransverse joint space.

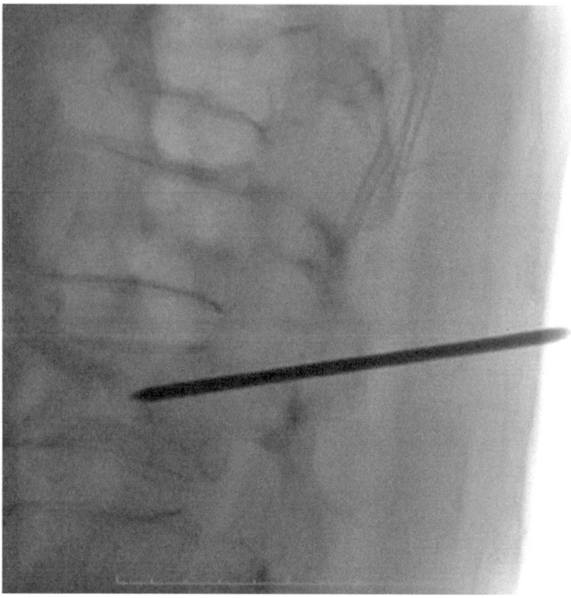

Fig. 10.6 Fluoroscopically guided transpedicular approach for a lumbar vertebral body lesion

4. Inferior costotransverse approach—This is employed in upper thoracic vertebral biopsy in which the needle is introduced through the inferior costotransverse joint space.
5. Pedicular biopsy—It is done for lesions of the pedicle when the vertebral body is collapsed.
6. Anterolateral or lateral approach—It is chosen for cervical vertebra biopsy with the patient in supine position. The operator has to be careful about the key neurovascular structures in these approaches.

Presence of soft tissue helps in reducing complications as the needle may be directed away from the central spinal and neurovascular structures (Fig. 10.5). Lesions with significant bony destruction may actually be easily targeted. The thin intact cortex can be easily breached with some pressure applied on the fine needle during its introduction at the directed target (Fig. 10.4). Choosing the low dose protocols (like the manual reduction of the kV to around 80–90) or use of dedicated-based biopsy protocols helps to avoid artifacts as well as reduce radiation exposure. Covering only the limited area of interest and providing radiation protection to the patient (like lead goggles, lead shields around the genitals) can also reduce inadvertent exposure. MRI guidance for the needle biopsy should be done with an entirely MRI-compatible kit after the screening of the patient as per the MRI-safety protocols as well as Gadolinium-based contrast safety requirements. Preferably, a lower gradient strength magnet (1.5 Tesla or lower) should be chosen, and faster gradient T1-based sequences are used for tissue localization.

Fluoroscopic guidance is also commonly used for dorsolumbar lesions (Fig. 10.6) by attaining "bull's eye view of the pedicle" from the anteroposterior plane providing direct transpedicular access [11]. CT-fluoroscopy can also be used in case the lesion is closer to the aorta or major vessels, and appropriate confirmation of the needle tip position can be done with selective angiograms. Fusion imaging guidance with CT-fluoroscopy and matched sections of the contrast-enhanced MRI becomes helpful in cases with difficult access with unsuccessful prior attempts.

10.9 Radiation Exposure and Prevention

The risk of radiation hazards in the CT/fluoroscopically guided needle biopsy is negligible owing to the short procedure time. However, the repetitive procedures with difficult access and lack of operator experience may add to the radiation time and dose. The operator must observe strict radiation protection for the self and the entire team. Lead aprons, thyroid shield, lead goggles, if possible, lead gloves should be used while performing CT/fluoroscopic guidance. Portable lead shields and separators are also effective in warding off the scattered radiation. Iterative reconstruction and the newer artificial intelligence-based advances in post-processing of the CT images can be applied for the reduction of needle artifacts.

10.10 Conclusion

FNAC/Biopsy in spinal TB is an important part of the management, providing timely definitive diagnostic decisions and avoiding inadvertent delay and failure of therapy. Image-guided needle aspiration or biopsy is best practiced as a team effort with no communication gaps, consisting of radiologist, spine surgeon, neurologist, and pathologist. Detailed pre-procedural assessment of clinical and imaging features with clear delineation of target tissue with contrast-enhanced MRI and apt planning of the required hardware and image guidance modality are a sine-qua-non. Ensuring optimal patient positioning, adequate anesthesia, pain management with strict radiation safety protocols and post-procedural care are important adjuvants of the procedure. CT forms the dominant image-guided modality to secure access for spinal aspirations. Ultrasound and MRI guidance can be alternative options in pregnant and pediatric patients with radiation hazard-related concerns. Fusion imaging with advanced robotic systems can be useful aids in apt set up for safe and precise needle access without radiation to the operator.

References

1. Oguz E, Sehirlioglu A, Altinmakas M, Ozturk C, Komurcu M, Solakoglu C, Vaccaro AR. A new classification and guide for surgical treatment of spinal tuberculosis. Int Orthop. 2008;32:127–33.
2. Kumaran S, Thippeswamy P, Reddy B, Neelakantan S, Viswamitra S. An institutional review of tuberculosis spine mimics on MR imaging: Cases of mistaken identity. Neurol India. 2019;67:1408.
3. Aithala JP, Attar A, Imthiaz AKA, Rai M. Is there a change in trend towards pyogenous spondylodiscitis compared to tubercular spondylodiscitis in India-A study of percutaneous biopsy evaluation in spondylodiscitis. Indian J Tuberc. 2020;67:509–14.
4. Aithala JP. Role of percutaneous image guided biopsy in spinal lesions: adequacy and correlation with MRI findings. J Clin Diagn Res. 2016;10:RC11–155.
5. Francis IM, Das DK, Luthra UK, Sheikh Z, Sheikh M, Bashir M. Value of radiologically guided fine needle aspiration cytology (FNAC) in the diagnosis of spinal tuberculosis: a study of 29 cases. Cytopathology. 1999;10:390–401.
6. Ortiz AO. Image-Guided Percutaneous Spine Biopsy. Springer; 2017. p. 125–62.
7. Garg RK, Somvanshi DS. Spinal tuberculosis: a review. J Spinal Cord Med. 2011;34:440–54.
8. Diehn FE. Imaging of spine infection. Radiol Clin N Am. 2012;50:777–98.
9. Torres C, Riascos R, Figueroa R, Gupta RK. Central nervous system tuberculosis. Top Magn Reson Imaging. 2014;23:173–89.
10. Meena R, Aggarwal A, Bhattacharya A, Gupta V, Dhandapani S, Chhabra R. Non traumatic vertebral lesions: incremental utility of PET-CT over MRI and FNAC in a suggested diagnostic algorithm. Br J Neurosurg. 2019;33:25–9.
11. Sahoo MM, Mahapatra SK, Sethi GC, Sahoo A, Kar BK. Role of percutaneous transpedicular biopsy in diagnosis of spinal tuberculosis and its correlation with the clinico-radiological features. Indian J Tuberc. 2019;66:388–93.
12. Held M, Laubscher M, Zar HJ, Dunn RN. GeneXpert polymerase chain reaction for spinal tuberculosis: an accurate and rapid diagnostic test. Bone Joint J. 2014;96-B:1366–9.
13. Davis TM. Spinal Biopsy Techniques. In: McGraw JK, editor. Interventional Radiology of the Spine. Totowa, NJ: Humana Press; 2004. p. 181–96.
14. Liu M, Sequeiros RB, Xu Y, He X, Zhu T, Li L, Lü Y, Huang J, Li C. MRI-guided percutaneous transpedicular biopsy of thoracic and lumbar spine using a 0.23t scanner with optical instrument tracking: Biopsy of Thoracic and Lumbar Spine. J Magn Reson Imaging. 2015;42:1740–6.
15. Hiraki T, Kamegawa T, Matsuno T, et al. Robotically Driven CT-guided Needle Insertion: Preliminary Results in Phantom and Animal Experiments. Radiology. 2017;285:454–61.
16. Bayley E, Clamp J, Boszczyk BM. Percutaneous approach to the upper thoracic spine: optimal patient positioning. Eur Spine J. 2009;18:1986–8.
17. Peh W. CT-guided percutaneous biopsy of spinal lesions. Biomed Imaging Interv J. 2006; https://doi.org/10.2349/biij.2.3.e25.
18. Tehranzadeh J, Tao C, Browning CA. Percutaneous Needle Biopsy of the Spine. Acta Radiol. 2007;48:860–8.
19. Brugieres P, Gaston A, Heran F, Voisin MC, Marsault C. Percutaneous biopsies of the thoracic spine under CT guidance: transcostovertebral approach. J Comput Assist Tomogr. 1990;14:446–8.
20. Yaffe D, Greenberg G, Leitner J, Gipstein R, Shapiro M, Bachar GN. CT-guided percutaneous biopsy of thoracic and lumbar spine: A new coaxial technique. AJNR Am J Neuroradiol. 2003;24:2111–3.
21. Singh DK, Sharma A, Boruah T, Kumar N, Suman S, Jaiswal B. Computed Tomography-Guided Vertebral Biopsy in Suspected Tuberculous Spondylodiscitis: Comparing a New Navigational Tram-Track Technique versus Conventional Method. J Clinic Interv Radiol ISVIR. 2020;4(03):159–66.

22. Gupta S, Takhtani D, Gulati M, Khandelwal N, Gupta D, Rajwanshi A, Gupta S, Suri S. Sonographically guided fine-needle aspiration biopsy of lytic lesions of the spine: technique and indications. J Clin Ultrasound. 1999;27:123–9.
23. Singh DK, Kumar N, Nayak BK, Jaiswal B, Tomar S, Mittal MK, Bajaj SK. Approach-based techniques of CT-guided percutaneous vertebral biopsy. Diagn Interv Radiol. 2020;26(2):143–6.

Chapter 11
Differential Diagnosis of Spinal Infections

Jayesh Trivedi and Rishi Trivedi

Abstract Spinal infections encompass a wide group of clinical conditions affecting all age groups with a variety of causative pathogens. These include pyogenic (bacterial), granulomatous infections (prototype being tuberculosis) and parasitic. The clinical presentation of spinal infections may range from subtle symptoms mimicking mechanical back pain to the florid with abscess formation and neurological deficits. The plethora of pathogens, the wide age group affected, and a constellation of symptoms make diagnosis of spinal infection difficult, resulting in delay in treatment often with deleterious consequences. Furthermore, the radiological features of spinal infections maybe similar to other non-infectious clinical entities. Degenerative disease of spine, metastatic disease, osteoporotic fractures, myeloma, and Charcot joints of the spine form the differential diagnosis of spinal infections. Multiple diagnostic tools maybe needed to establish accurate diagnosis. Magnetic Resonance Imaging (MRI) is the imaging modality of choice in diagnosing spinal infections.

Keywords Spinal infections · Vertebral osteomyelitis · Tuberculosis · Diagnosis

11.1 Diagnosis of Spinal Infections

The spine is a frequent site of affection by both pyogenic and tubercular infections. It accounts for 2–7% of pyogenic infections [1, 2], and spinal TB is the most common form of osteoarticular TB accounting for 50% of cases [3]. A wide variety of

J. Trivedi (✉)
Robert Jones and Agnes Hunt Orthopaedic Hospital, Oswestry, UK

Alder Hey Children's Hospital, East Prescot Road, Liverpool, UK

R. Trivedi
East Sussex healthcare NHS trust, Eastbourne, UK
e-mail: Rishi.trivedi2@nhs.net

S. S. Dhatt, V. Kumar (eds.), *Tuberculosis of the Spine*,
https://doi.org/10.1007/978-981-16-9495-0_11

pathogens are responsible for spinal infections. Pyogenic infections are predominantly caused by *Staphylococcus aureus* although *Staphylococcus epidermidis*, *Escherichia coli*, *Pseudomonas*, *Propionibacterium acnes*, and *Enterococcus* are some of the other bacteria responsible for pyogenic vertebral osteomyelitis [1, 2, 4–8]. *Mycobacterium tuberculosis* is the most common granulomatous disease of the spine [3, 5]. Vertebral osteomyelitis accounts for 1% of patients affected by tuberculosis and 50% of osteoarticular TB [3]. 150,000 new cases of TB develop annually [3]. Brucellosis is more prevalent in the Mediterranean areas along with countries where TB is also prevalent and accounts for 6–12% of cases of spinal osteomyelitis [7]. Worldwide there is an increase in the incidence of spinal infections, attributed to a rising ageing population, increased incidence of diabetes mellitus, immune-suppression, intravenous drug abuse, and an increase in HIV infections [1, 5, 9, 10].

Delayed diagnosis and misdiagnosis is one of the main issues in the assessment of spinal infections [1, 5]. In one series of 101 patients, misdiagnosis occurred in 33.7%, and the average delay from the onset of clinical manifestations to diagnosis was 2.6 months [8]. Colmenero et al. in a review of 219 cases of spinal infections found that the mean duration of symptoms was 14 weeks when there was no preceding surgical procedure and 2.4 weeks if there had been a surgical procedure leading to the infection [7]. Pyogenic spondylitis had a mean delay in diagnosis of 7.1 weeks, brucellosis 14.3 weeks, and TB spondylitis 22.9 weeks in their series [7]. Butler et al. in a review of 48 pyogenic spinal infections over a 12-year period noted a delay in presentation from 2 weeks to 6 months [11]. In addition, patients with immune deficiency may have a subtle clinical picture lacking outward symptoms and signs, compromising early diagnosis and appropriate care.

When the physician suspects a spinal infection, a careful review of the patient's history and a detailed physical examination is required, followed by a thorough laboratory testing and immediate imaging evaluation.

Symptoms of back pain, fever, and worryingly neurological deficit may be associated with spinal infections, but there is a wide variation in this presentation. Pain is often the presenting complaint [1, 4, 6], but 15% of patients may be pain-free [1]. Localized back pain aggravated by percussion was present in 90% of patients with vertebral osteomyelitis according to Kapeller et al. [12]. Contrary to this, Priest et al. reported this feature in less than a fifth of their patients [13]. Fever however is not a constant feature in adults. Pyrexia may be present in only 35–60% of cases [6]. In children the infection may commence as discitis. The mean age of children with discitis is approximately 2.8 years [14]. Although any level of the spine can be affected, the infection is localized in the lumbar or lumbosacral region in approximately 75% of patients [14, 15]. Presenting symptoms in children who are under 2 years of age may include a refusal to walk and standing with a tendency to support their hands on their thighs, whereas older children often complain of back or abdominal pain [5, 14].

Laboratory analysis almost always shows an elevation in the level of C-reactive protein, an elevated erythrocyte sedimentation rate, and an increase in the white blood-cell count, but cultures are necessary to determine the specific pathogen.

Determination of the white blood cell (WBC) count, C-reactive protein (CRP) levels, and erythrocyte sedimentation rate (ESR) measurements are part of the initial evaluation for all patients with spinal infections [1, 4, 9]. In a series of 101 patients, laboratory studies such as leukocyte count and ESR were not found to be sensitive tests in the diagnosis of spondylodiscitis as they were elevated in 42.6% and 81.3% of the patients, respectively [8]. Elevation of WBC has been reported in 13% to 60% of series [8, 16–18]. In Hadjipavlou's [8] series these tests were more sensitive in the presence of epidural abscess (leukocyte count in 89.6%; ESR in 100%).

The CRP level may be more specific and sensitive than the ESR or WBC count [5]. The CRP value and the ESR can be used to assess response to treatment or to detect postoperative disc space infection, especially in situations where there is persistence of pain after surgery [19]. A gradual decline of both values correlates well with normal postoperative course, whereas a failure to normalize raises the suspicion of a postoperative infection [19].

There is conflicting evidence about the sensitivity of cultures obtained from blood samples, aspirate, and biopsy. Hadjipavlou et al. in their series of 101 patients with pyogenic vertebral osteomyelitis found a positive tissue culture in 76 patients. In their series a single pathogen was isolated in 52 patients, whereas 2 or more pathogens were noted in a total of 24 of 101 patients [8]. In 41 children, Wenger et al. reported that 6 of 9 biopsy samples and 9 of 22 blood specimens that were cultured were positive for growth of *Staphylococcus aureus* [15]. In another series of 36 children with discitis, Fernandez et al. obtained biopsies from a series of 8 patients with discitis, none of which showed bacterial growth. From the blood specimens cultured for 32 children in the same series, 4 (13%) were positive for bacterial growth: *Staphylococcus* was isolated from 2 specimens, *Streptococcus* from 1, and gram-positive rods (not further identified) from another. When an organism is identified, it is most often *Staphylococcus aureus*, which is present in 50% to 67% of cultures [20].

11.2 Imaging

Radiological imaging may form the mainstay of the diagnostic work up in spinal infections. Modalities of plain radiographs, computerized tomography (CT) scans, Magnetic Resonance Imaging (MRI) scan, and positron emission tomography (PET) (Figs. 11.1, 11.2 and 11.3) may all be utilized for the evaluation of spinal infections.

11.2.1 Plain Radiographs

In the very early stages of an infective process, plain radiographs may be essentially normal. Features suggestive of infection may take 2–8 weeks to appear on plain radiographs [2]. Pyogenic spondylitis often commences in the antero-superior

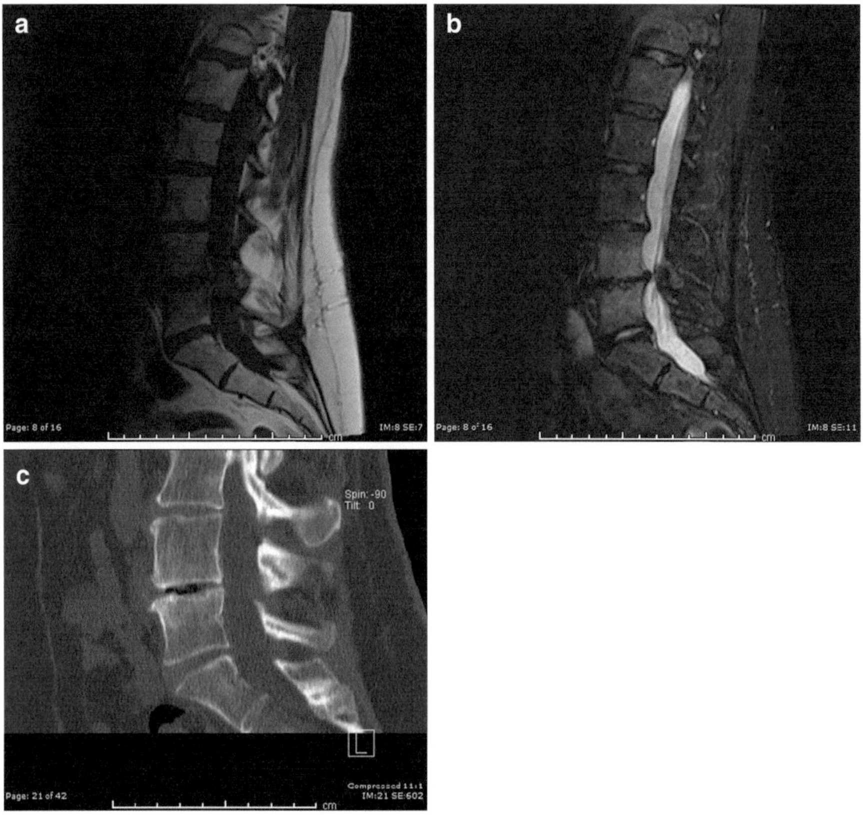

Fig. 11.1 (**a**) T1 weighted sagittal MRI scan of the lumbar spine of a 35-year-old with low back pain. MRI revealing Modic type 1 change at L4/5 with reduction of disc space. The features may mimic an infective process, but the disc appears unaffected which is more in keeping with a degenerative process. (**b**) T2 weighted sequence of the same patient showing increased signal adjacent to the disc space in keeping with Type 1 Modic change of degenerative disc disease. Note the reduction in the disc space height and the low signal intensity of the disc in keeping with degeneration within the disc. In infectious discitis the disc would exhibit a high signal. (**c**) CT scan of the patient revealing gas in the disc space more suggestive of a degenerative pathology rather than infection. Also note osteophytic spurring in keeping with a degenerative pathology

corner of the vertebral body. Loss of disc height may ensue. These changes are visualized best on the lateral view but may mimic degenerative disc disease (DDD). One of the differentiating features between infectious spondylitis and DDD is the presence of gas in the disc space in DDD, which is absent in infections [2, 21] (Fig. 11.1c). Sclerosis of the end plates appears usually at the 8–12 week stage (Fig. 11.2d). In advanced stages vertebral body destruction and kyphosis occur, whereas the end stage of a healed infective process maybe an ankylosis across the disc space (Fig. 11.2e).

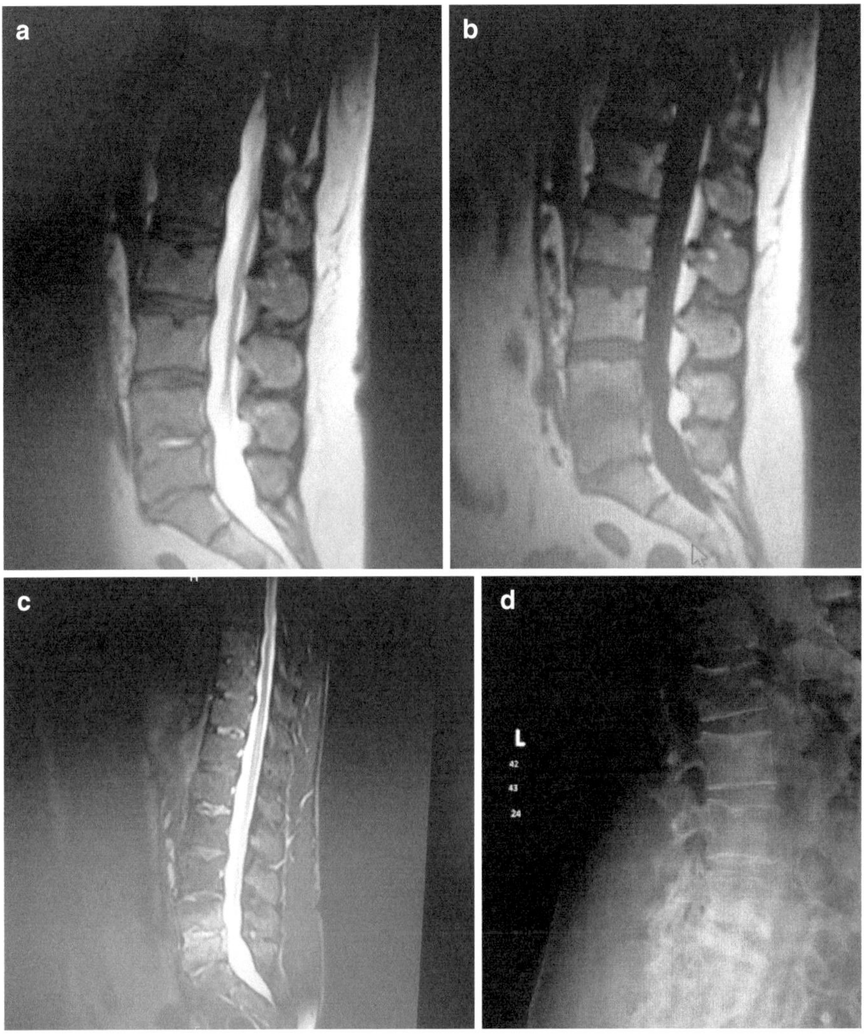

Fig. 11.2 (**a**) T2 weighted sagittal MRI scan of the lumbar spine of a 53-year-old lady with rheumatoid arthritis and a non-healing ulcer on her foot. She presented with low back pain, and MRI scan reveals discitis at L4/5. Note the high signal within the disc space. (**b**, **c**) T1 weighted MRI scan of the above patient along with (**c**) a fat suppressed STIR sequence revealing the marrow changes in the adjacent vertebrae secondary to the infection. (**d**) Lateral X-ray of the same patient showing sclerosis of the end plates with loss of definition of the end plate secondary to the discitis. The plain X-ray may take some time to show changes of infection. (**e**) Healed discitis showing ankylosis of the L4/5 disc in the same patient

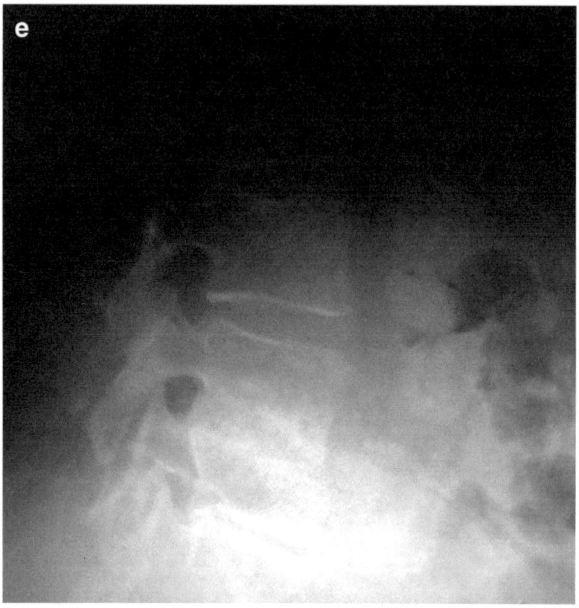

Fig. 11.2 (continued)

Three major sites of involvement of the vertebral body in TB include the peri-discal, central, and anterior areas. The most common form is the peridiscal type. It occurs adjacent to the vertebral end plate with the infection spreading around a motion segment. Extension to the adjacent vertebra occurs as the abscess tracks beneath the anterior longitudinal ligament (Fig. 11.3a and b). Central involvement affecting the vertebral body may be mistaken for a tumor. Anterior disease causes scalloping of the vertebral body. The thoracic spine is more commonly affected in TB, whereas brucellosis and pyogenic spondylitis have a greater predilection for the lumbar area. Multilevel affection is more commonly seen in brucellosis and TB [7] (Fig. 11.3a and b). Calcification of the wall of a large abscess cavity is a very typical feature of tuberculous involvement. Thoracic vertebral involvement with lesions affecting the posterior portion of the vertebral body and the presence of a paravertebral soft tissue mass point towards a tuberculous pathology [7].

11.2.2 Scintigraphy

With the widespread availability of MRI scans, the use of scintigraphy has become less prevalent. Scintigraphy has a high degree of sensitivity (90%) but lower specificity (78%) [4]. Also scintigraphy does not provide anatomic detail of the affected area, and there is a lag between scintigraphy results and healed infections. 3-phase

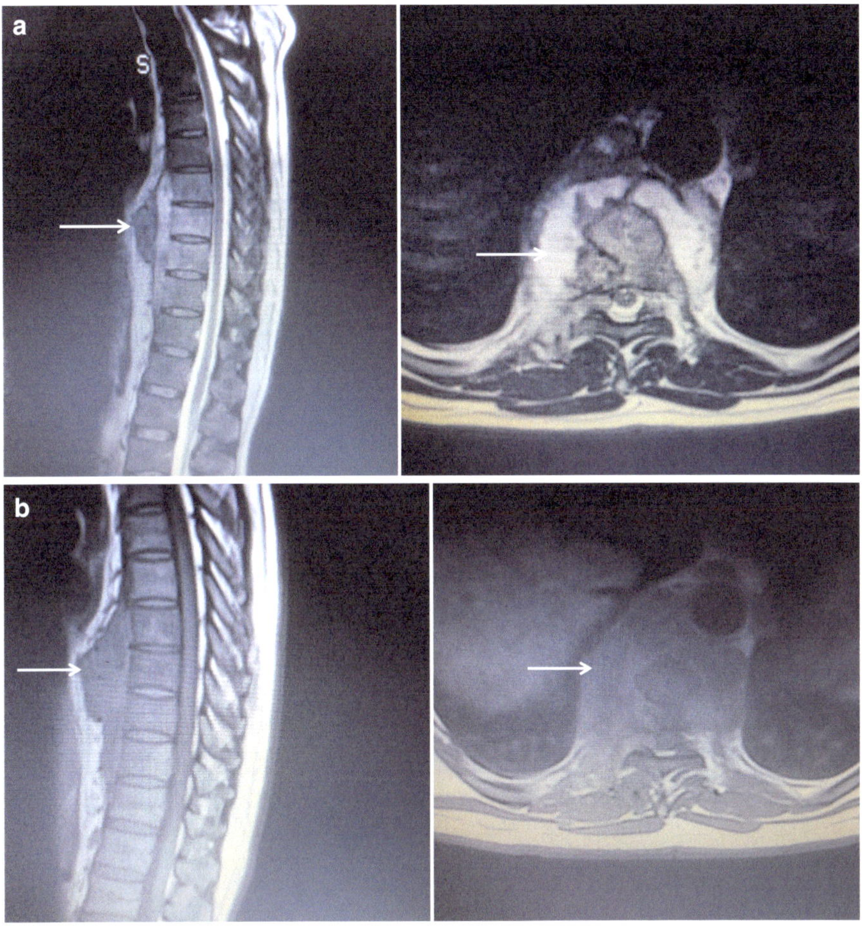

Fig. 11.3 (**a**) T2 sagittal and axial MRI scan images of a 65-year-old with spinal tuberculosis of the paradiscal variety. Note the large anterior cold abscess (solid white arrow). (**b**) T1 sagittal and axial MRI scans of patient with tuberculosis. Note the relative sparing of the discs in the initial stages. Large anterior abscess (solid arrow)

technetium-99 m, gallium-67 citrate, and indium 111-labelled leucocyte scans have been utilized in the diagnosis of spinal infections [4].

11.2.3 Computer Tomography (CT)

CT scan is useful in defining osseous involvement particularly when the focus of infection may be within the posterior elements. Biopsies of affected areas are best undertaken under CT guidance [2].

11.2.4 Magnetic Resonance Imaging

MRI remains the gold standard in the diagnosis of spinal infections [2, 4, 22]. It has 96%, 92%, and 94% sensitivity, specificity, and accuracy in the diagnosis [4]. The characteristic changes in MRI include hypointense signal within the vertebral body and disc on T1 weighted sequence and a hyperintense signal of these structures on T2 sequences (Fig. 11.2a, b, and c). Contrast enhancement using gadolinium particularly of the disc, vertebral body, and soft tissues aids in further diagnosis and differentiation from tumors and degeneration [21]. Skip lesions involving non-contiguous discovertebral levels are rare in pyogenic infection, but constitute a not so uncommon feature in spinal tuberculosis. In TB large paravertebral soft tissue masses may indicate cold abscess formation [22] (Fig. 11.3a and b).

11.2.5 Positron Emission Tomography (PET) Scan

Smids et al. undertook a study comparing the efficacy of ^{18}F-FDG-PET/CT and MRI scans in diagnosing spondylodiscitis [23]. They evaluated 68 patients of whom 49 were diagnosed with spondylodiscitis. In their series, in the first 2 weeks of onset of symptoms, ^{18}F-FDG-PET/CT showed a sensitivity of 96% and a specificity of 95%, with no relation to the interval between the scan and the start of symptoms. On the other hand, MRI scan had a diagnostic accuracy of 58% in the first 2 weeks improving to 82%, when performed more than 2 weeks after onset of symptoms.

A PET scan has other advantages. It is particularly useful in the presence of metal implants that may create metal artefacts on MRI scans. It is also particularly useful where an MRI may be contra-indicated, e.g., in patients with non-MRI compatible pacemakers or in those patients who are severely claustrophobic and cannot tolerate an MRI scan.

A limitation of ^{18}F-FDG-PET/CT scans is its low specificity in differentiating spinal infections from malignancy. It is also not as sensitive as an MRI scan in diagnosing epidural abscesses.

11.3 Differential Diagnosis of Spinal Infections

11.3.1 Spinal Trauma

Osteoporotic vertebral compression fractures are a frequently encountered clinical problem, and their prevalence is on the rise with an ever-increasing ageing population. Vertebral fractures are the most common skeletal injury resulting from osteoporosis, with an estimated incidence of 700,000 per year in the United States [24]. They are more prevalent in the elderly, which is also the patient group likely to be susceptible to spinal infections.

Three fracture patterns, wedge, crush, and biconcave, have been described in the osteoporotic spine [25] (Fig. 11.4a and b).

The most common pattern is the wedge fracture [26]. Fractures commonly occur in the thoracolumbar region. Radiographs show the osteopenia characteristic in these patients. The vertebral body shows a fracture with loss of height and wedging and occasionally with retropulsion of osseous fragments into the spinal canal. The

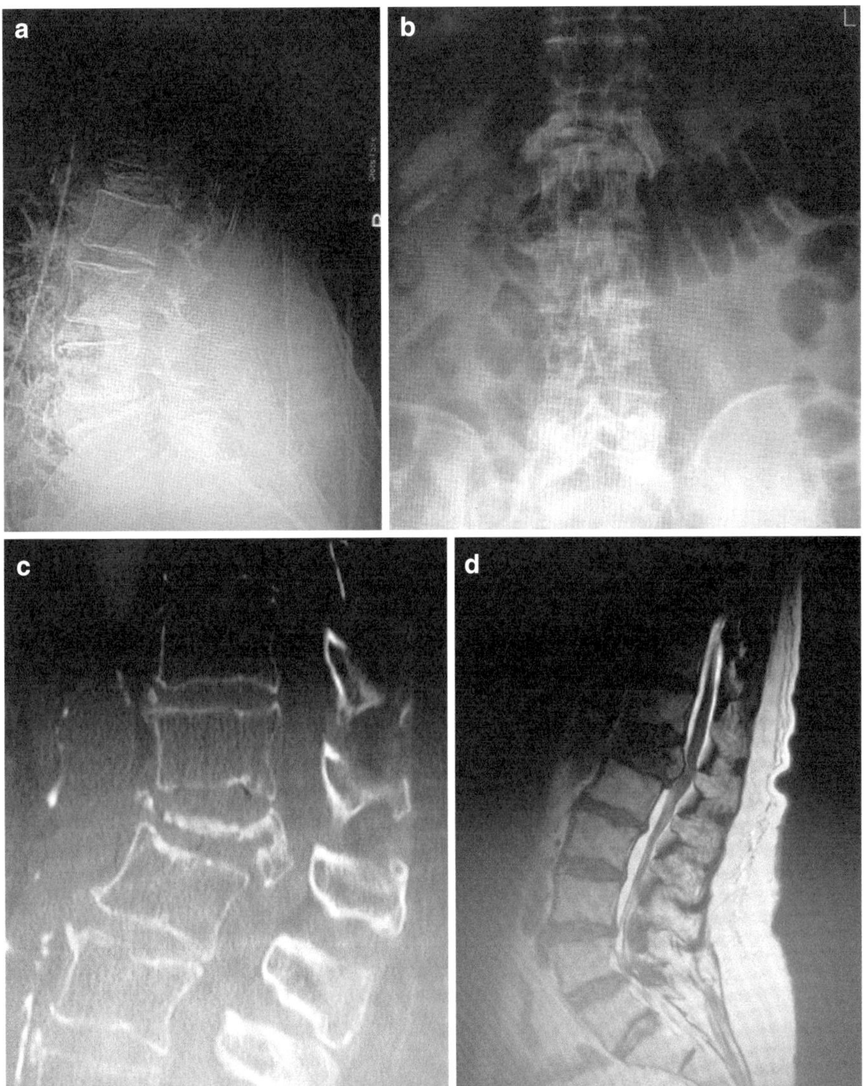

Fig. 11.4 (**a**, **b**) A 78-year-old with osteoporotic fracture of T12. The appearances result in vertebra plana which may mimic TB of the vertebral body. (**c**, **d**) CT scan and T2 weighted sagittal MRI scan image of the patient with osteoporotic fracture. The discs are preserved which rules out discitis. CT scan reveals the bone loss and vertebra plana

collapse of the vertebral body results in the appearance of "vertebra plana." These features may mimic those of tuberculosis and even plasmacytoma (Fig. 11.4c and d).

Magnetic resonance imaging of the spine is probably the best modality for determining fracture age, and differentiating it from spinal infections. In the acute period following a vertebral fracture, magnetic resonance imaging shows a geographic pattern of low-intensity-signal changes on T1-weighted images and high-intensity-signal changes on T2-weighted. The absence of edema in the pedicles and a relative paucity of soft tissue reaction adjacent to the fracture would differentiate an osteoporotic fracture from infections (Fig. 11.4d). The discs adjacent to the fracture are normally spared and may have a spurious appearance of widening due to the collapse of the vertebral body. Osteoporotic compression may also show intravertebral vacuum phenomenon [22].

As the fracture becomes chronic, a linear area of low-intensity signal change replaces the geographic area on T1-weighted images. As healing continues, the linear pattern is replaced by restoration of fatty marrow. Sagittal short tau inversion recovery (STIR) sequences are helpful; they show high-intensity signal changes in areas of edema from acute or healing fractures [27].

11.3.2 Degenerative Disc Disease (DDD)

Degenerative disc disease remains the commonest cause of non-specific low back pain affecting the adult population. Pain from degenerative disc disease usually tends to be activity related. It is not associated with constitutional symptoms such as fever or loss of appetite, and hematological parameters of WBC, ESR, and CRP remain unaffected in degenerative disc disease. However radiological features of DDD may mimic those of spinal infections particularly on MRI scans [21]. DDD is often associated with a loss of disc height and sclerosis of end plates on plain radiographs, which may resemble infectious discitis. However gas within the disc space is suggestive of degeneration rather than infection (Fig. 11.1c).

Modic et al. described three patterns of vertebral marrow abnormalities on MRI scans in DDD [28]. In Modic type 1 pattern, the disc adjacent marrow exhibits a low signal on T1 weighted sequences and high signal on T2 weighted images (Fig. 11.1a and b). Type II pattern is characterized by a high osseous signal in T1 and isointense or slightly hyperintense signal on T2 weighted MRI sequences, and Type III has a low signal in T1 and T2 sequences. Type I, indicative of early disc degeneration, may mimic infectious discitis. A major distinguishing feature between infectious and degenerative pathologies will be that the degenerative disc tends to be dehydrated and therefore dark on T2 weighted sequences (Fig. 11.1b).

Charran et al. described a radiological entity referred to as "destructive discovertebral disc disease" (DDDD) characterised by vertebral mal-alignment, severe disc resorption, and "bone sand" formation secondary to vertebral fragmentation [29]. The authors postulated that the condition was predisposed by segmental instability/mal-alignment of the spine in a setting of severe disc degeneration and coexisting metabolic bone disease. The presence of fragmented bone referred to as "bone sand" by the authors was deemed to be the hallmark of DDDD. All these features may resemble ongoing infection, but intervertebral vacuum phenomenon on CT would separate DDDD from an infective process along with hematological tests.

11.3.3 Spinal Tumors

Primary bone tumors of the spine and metastatic vertebral lesions may all mimic spondylitis. The skeleton is the third commonest site for metastases, and the axial skeleton is the preferred site over the appendicular skeleton.

Metastases and primary tumors usually arise within the vertebral body often leading to pathological fractures. Tumors in children mimicking spinal infection include Ewing's sarcoma and leukemia [14, 30]. Constitutional symptoms of back pain and fever and elevation of ESR and CRP in these conditions often raise the diagnosis of spinal infection. Vertebra plana may be seen on plain radiographs in patients with Ewing's sarcoma. About 6% of patients with leukemia may have vertebral collapse. All of these features mimic spinal infection [14].

Another condition in children mimicking vertebral TB is eosinophilic granuloma [14]. Langerhans cell histiocytosis, also known as eosinophilic granuloma, is a self-limiting process that produces focal destruction of bone and may mimic spinal infective pathology in children. Vertebral involvement occurs in 7.8% to 25% [31]. The thoracic and cervical spine appear to be the most commonly affected areas. The most common presenting complaint is pain. The pain may be associated with pyrexia and even an elevated WBC count and ESR in a minority of patients resulting in infection being in the differential diagnosis [14]. Radiographically, vertebra plana is characteristic of Langerhans cell histiocytosis, with partial or complete collapse of the vertebra resulting in a "coin-on-edge" appearance. Different grades of vertebra plana have been described [31, 32]. Vertebra plana may mimic spinal TB and plasmacytoma, and histological diagnosis may be needed to differentiate between these conditions. Typical radiological features that have been described and may aid in differentiating this condition from TB and other infections include the absence of osteolysis, preservation of the pedicles and posterior elements, non-involvement of the adjacent disc spaces, the absence of adjacent paravertebral soft tissue shadow, and affection of only one vertebra [31] (Fig. 11.5a, b, c, and d).

In adults myeloma may present with vertebral collapse. Metastatic spine disease in adults may also mimic spinal infections. An important differentiating feature, between neoplasms and infections, on the MRI is the preservation of discs in neoplasms, whereas an infective process will involve the disc space. Thus the adage "Good disc, bad news; bad disc, good news" is a good way of highlighting the fact that neoplasms within the spine seldom affect the disc space, whereas pyogenic infections inevitably destroy the disc space [2] (Fig. 11.5).

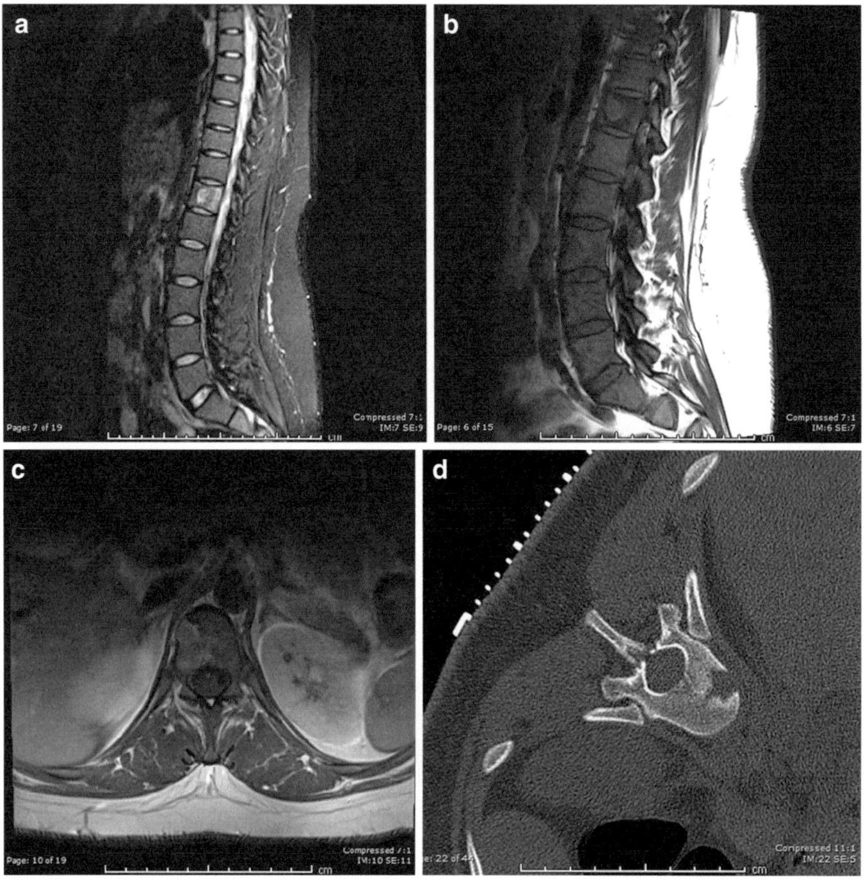

Fig. 11.5 (**a** and **b**) Sagittal MRI scan of an 18-year-old with an eosinophilic granuloma at T12. Note the preservation of discs which tends to rule out infection as a potential cause of the lesion. (**c** and **d**) Axial MRI scan and CT scan of the above patient. Note paucity of soft tissue reaction

11.3.4 Charcot Joint of Spine

First described by Mitchel in 1831 and then by Charcot in 1868, neuropathic arthropathy, also known as Charcot arthropathy, refers to progressive and severe joint destruction that results from underlying disorders of the nervous system [33].

Traumatic spinal cord injury is currently the commonest etiology for Charcot arthropathy of the thoracolumbar spine. Mobile segments caudad to the stabilized segment of the spine are typically affected, with physiotherapy being the source of repeated movement in paraplegic patients [34]. Other described causes include congenital insensitivity to pain and diabetes mellitus. Congenital insensitivity to pain is a group of hereditary sensory and autonomic neuropathies causing a lack of deep pain sensation, leading to progressive painless destruction of multiple large joints.

Imaging may help to distinguish between spondylodiscitis and neuropathic arthropathy. Neuropathic spinal arthropathy usually shows significant osseous debris and joint disorganization and involves the facet joints in addition to the end plates. The MRI features may superficially mimic multifocal infective spondyloarthritis, although the latter does not usually simultaneously involve the facet joints [35] (Fig. 11.6a–d).

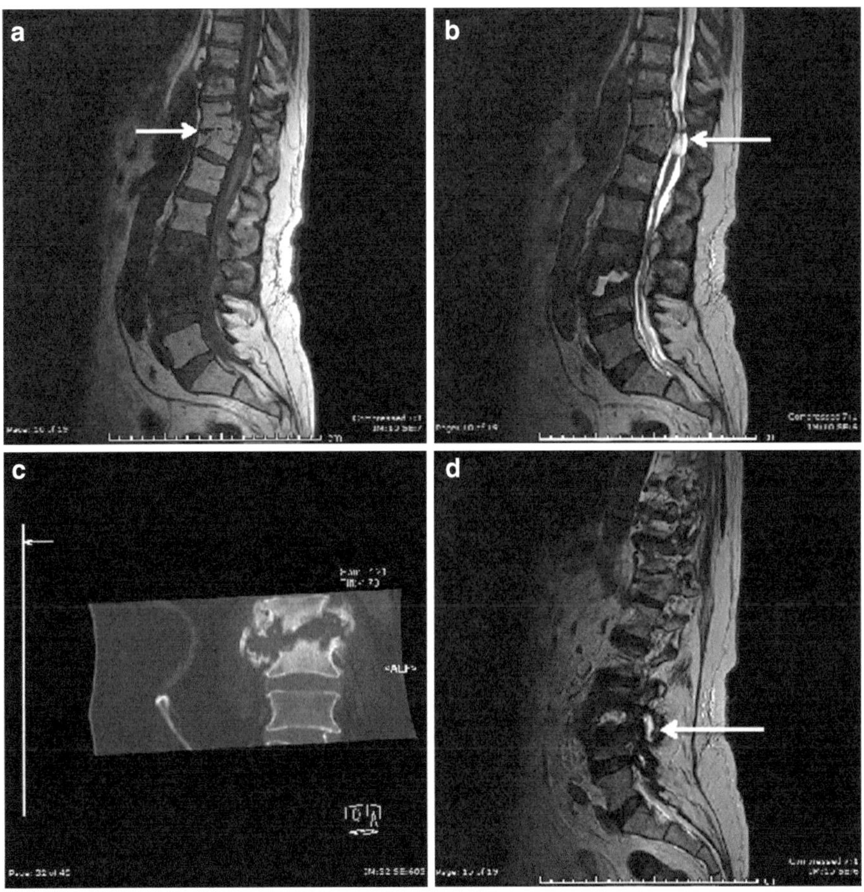

Fig. 11.6 (**a**, **b**, **c**, **d**) Case of traumatic spinal cord injury (highlighted by the solid white arrows) revealing Charcot changes at L3/4 with marked destruction of adjacent vertebral bodies and disorganization of the disc space mimicking discitis. Figure 11.6d shows disorganization within the facet joint (arrow) often seen in Charcot arthropathy

11.4 Conclusion

Spinal infections pose a significant clinical and diagnostic dilemma to the treating clinician. The protean clinical manifestations and varied imaging findings make diagnosis challenging. Very often the diagnosis is established on the basis of symptoms and hematological and radiological findings accompanied by corroboration of microbiology and histological data.

Acknowledgments The authors would wish to express their sincerest thanks to Dr. Jaspreet Singh, Consultant Radiologist at the Robert Jones and Agnes Hunt Orthopaedic Hospital, Oswestry, for his kind contribution of the imaging utilized in this chapter.

References

1. Duarte RM, Vaccaro AR. Spinal infection: state of the art and management algorithm. Eur Spine J. 2013;22:2787–99.
2. Tyrrell PN, Cassar-Pullicino VN, McCall IW. Spinal infection. Eur Radiol. 1999;9(6):1066–77.
3. Jain AK, Rajasekaran S, Jaggi KR, et al. Tuberculosis of the Spine. Current Concepts Review. J Bone Joint Surg Am. 2020;102:617–28.
4. An HS, Seldomridge JA. Spinal infections: diagnostic tests and imaging studies. Clin Orthop. 2006;444:27–33.
5. Tsiodras S, Falagas ME. Clinical assessment and medical treatment of spine infections. Clin Orthop. 2006;444:38–50.
6. Zimmerli W. Vertebral osteomyelitis. N Engl J Med. 2010;362(11):1022–9.
7. Colmenero JD, Jimenez-Mejias ME, Sanchez-Lora FJ, et al. Pyogenic, tuberculous, and brucellar vertebral osteomyelitis: a descriptive and comparative study of 219 cases. Ann Rheum Dis. 1997;56:709–15.
8. Hadjipavlou AG, Mader JT, Necessary JT, et al. Hematogenous pyogenic spinal infections and their surgical management. Spine. 2000;25(13):1668–79.
9. Carragee EJ. Pyogenic vertebral osteomyelitis. J Bone Joint Surg Am. 1997;79:874–80.
10. Govender S. Spinal infections. J Bone Joint Surg Br. 2005;87(B):1454–8.
11. Butler JS, et al. Nontuberculous pyogenic spinal infection in adults: a 12-year experience from a tertiary referral center. Spine. 2006;31(23):2695–700.
12. Kapeller P, Fazekas F, Krametter D, et al. Pyogenic infectious spondylitis: clinical, laboratory and MRI features. Eur Neurol. 1997;38:94–8.
13. Priest DH, Peacock JE Jr. Haematogenous vertebral osteomyelitis due to Staphylococcus aureus in the adult: clinical features and therapeutic outcomes. South Med J. 2005;98:854–62.
14. Dormans JP, Moroz L. Infection and tumors of the spine in children. J Bone Joint Surg. 2007. Suppl 1;89(A):79–97.
15. Wenger DR, Bobechko WP, Gilday DL. The spectrum of intervertebral disc space infection in children. J Bone Joint Surg Am. 1978;60:100–8.
16. Digby JM, Kersley JB. Pyogenic nontuberculous spinal infection. J Bone Joint Surg Br. 1979;61:47–55.
17. Emery SE, Chan DP, Woodward HR. Treatment of hematogenous pyogenic vertebral osteomyelitis with anterior debridement and primary bone grafting. Spine. 1989;14:284–91.
18. Rath SA, Neff U, Schneider O, Richter HP. Neurosurgical management of thoracic and lumbar vertebral osteomyelitis and discitis in adults: a review of 43 consecutive surgically treated patients. Neurosurgery. 1996;38:926–33.

19. Schulitz KP, Assheuer J. Discitis after procedures on the intervertebral disc. Spine. 1994;19:1172–7.
20. Fernandez M, Carrol CL, Baker CJ. Discitis and vertebral osteomyelitis in children: an 18-year review. Pediatrics. 2000;105:1299–304.
21. Rothman SLG. The diagnosis of spinal Infections. Orth Clin North America. 1996;27(1):15–31.
22. José M, Mellado L, del Palomar P, et al. MR imaging of spinal infection: atypical features, interpretative pitfalls and potential mimickers. Eur Radiol. 2004;14:1980–9.
23. Smids C, Kouijzer IJ, Vos FJ, et al. A comparison of the diagnostic value of MRI and ^{18}F-FDG-PET/CT in suspected spondylodiscitis. Infection. 2017;45(1):41–9.
24. Melton LJ 3rd, Lane AW, Cooper C, et al. Prevalence and incidence of vertebral deformities. Osteoporos Int. 1993;3:113–9.
25. Eastell R, Cedel SL, Wahner HW, et al. Classification of vertebral fractures. J Bone Miner Res. 1991;6:207–15.
26. Oda K, Shibayama Y, Abe M, Onomura T. Morphogenesis of vertebral deformities in involutional osteoporosis. Age-related, three-dimensional trabecular structure. Spine. 1998;23:1050–6.
27. Link TM, Guglielmi G, van Kuijk C, et al. Radiologic assessment of osteoporotic vertebral fractures: diagnostic and prognostic implications. Eur Radiol. 2005;15(8):1521–32.
28. Modic MT, Steinberg PM, Ross JS, et al. Degenerative disc disease: assessment of changes in vertebral body marrow with MR imaging. Radiology. 1988;166:193–9.
29. Charran K, Tony G, Lalam R, Tyrrell PNM, et al. Destructive discovertebral degenerative disease of the lumbar spine. Skelet Radiol. 2012;41:1213–21.
30. Venkateswaran L, Rodriguez-Galindo C, Merchant TE, et al. Primary Ewing tumor of the vertebrae: clinical characteristics, prognostic factors, and outcome. Med Pediatr Oncol. 2001;37:30–5.
31. Yeom JS, Lee CK, Shin HY, Lee CS, Han CS, Chang H. Langerhans' cell histiocytosis of the spine. Analysis of twenty-three cases. Spine. 1999;24:1740–9.
32. Garg S, Mehta S, Dormans JP. Langerhans cell histiocytosis of the spine in children. Long-term follow-up. J Bone Joint Surg Am. 2004;86:1740–50.
33. Chan RLS, Chan CH, Chan HF, et al. The many facets of neuropathic arthropathy. BJR Open. 2019;1(1):20180039.
34. Standaert C, Cardenas DD, Anderson P. Charcot spine as a late complication of traumatic spinal cord injury. Arch Phys Med Rehabil. 1997;78:221–5.
35. Lacout A, Lebreton C, Mompoint D, et al. CT and MRI of spinal neuroarthropathy. Am J Roentgenol. 2009;193:W505–14.

Chapter 12
TB Spine in Children

Karthick Rangasamy and Nirmal Raj Gopinathan

Abstract The child's spine is not the replica of a miniature adult. The characteristics and sequelae of paediatric spinal tuberculosis are different from an adult one. The disrupted growth potential following tuberculosis infection may cause the spinal deformity to progress as the child grows. Due to this dynamic behaviour, the child should be monitored till skeletal maturity even after healing. Most of these cases can be managed by chemotherapy and rest alone, and surgery is indicated for specialized situations only. In children, spinal tuberculosis is the most common cause of kyphotic deformity. The kyphotic deformity of more than 60° and those having instability require surgical stabilisation. Nowadays, all global posterior reconstruction is preferred for thoracic and lumbar caries spine surgery.

Keywords Tuberculosis · Spine · Children · Kyphosis · Paediatric tuberculosis Infection · Deformity · Caries spine

12.1 Introduction

Compared to adults, tuberculosis (TB) spine in children poses a different challenge due to the growth of vertebrae during the active and healed phase. Because of the cartilaginous and soft texture of vertebrae in children, the rate of destruction is quick, and there is a risk of rapid onset neurological deficits during the active phase of the disease. The growth potential may also be altered if the immature diseased vertebra is surgically intervened. In the healed disease of a growing vertebra, as the child grows, the deformity might progress, and it not only alters the biomechanics in the axial skeleton but also the neural structures in its vicinity are at risk. Due to this dynamic behaviour, the children should be monitored regularly till skeletal maturity [1].

K. Rangasamy (✉) · N. R. Gopinathan
Department of Orthopaedic surgery, Post Graduate Institute of Medical Education and Research (PGIMER), Chandigarh, India

S. S. Dhatt, V. Kumar (eds.), *Tuberculosis of the Spine*,
https://doi.org/10.1007/978-981-16-9495-0_12

According to the 2020 WHO Global tuberculosis report, children constitute 12% of all TB cases. The overall incidence of TB in India is found to be 193 per one lakh population. An estimate of 3.3% new TB cases and also 18% of previously treated cases were found to be multidrug-resistant (MDR)/rifampicin resistant (RR) TB [2]. The children are having a higher proportion of extrapulmonary TB (EPTB) (20–25%) in comparison to the overall incidence of extrapulmonary TB (16%) [3, 4]. Skeletal TB contributes to 10% of EPTB, and spinal TB constitutes about 50% of skeletal TB. The incidence of TB spine in children is variable across different parts of Asia with a reported incidence of 58% in children among all spine tuberculosis in Korea, 26% in Hong Kong, and one-third of all patients as reported from Chennai (South India) [5–9]. TB spine is primarily a medical disease, and it needs early attention and treatment in children to prevent complications.

12.2 Development of Vertebral Column

Embryologically, the vertebral column develops from three primary ossification centres: one for the vertebral body and two for the posterior elements. These centres have central ossified bone with the surrounding cartilage. The secondary ossification centres are present on the spinous process tip, transverse process, facets, and on ring apophysis of both the superior and inferior vertebral body endplate. As the child grows, along with vertebrae the intervertebral disc and annulus also expand. The longitudinal growth of thoracic and lumbar vertebrae occurs at a rate of 0.8–1.1 mm/year. The thoracic disc and lumbar disc grow at a rate of 0.2–0.6 mm/year and 0.3–0.8 mm/year, respectively. The growth of the axial column is contributed by each vertebral ring apophysis at the rate of 0.5 mm/year, and hence every vertebra confers growth on an average of 1 mm/year. The pace of growth is not uniform, and it is accelerated during infancy and again during prepubertal age with steady growth in between (2–10 years of age) [5].

12.3 Pathophysiology

The infection is caused by the *Mycobacterium tuberculosis* complex, which includes around 60 species. Among all the species, *Mycobacterium tuberculosis* (the most common), *Mycobacterium bovis*, *Mycobacterium africanum*, and Mycobacterium microti are generally known to affect humans [10]. Spinal TB infection is usually a secondary infection from a primary focus through the hematogenous dissemination of bacilli. In 50% of TB spine in children, the primary remains unknown [11]. The site of primary infection could be in the lungs, mediastinal lymph nodes, mesentery, gastrointestinal tract, genitourinary system, or any viscera. In children, the anterior type of spinal TB is common as a result of the deposition of bacilli on the anterior aspect of the vertebral body through the end arterioles [12] (Fig. 12.1). The anterior

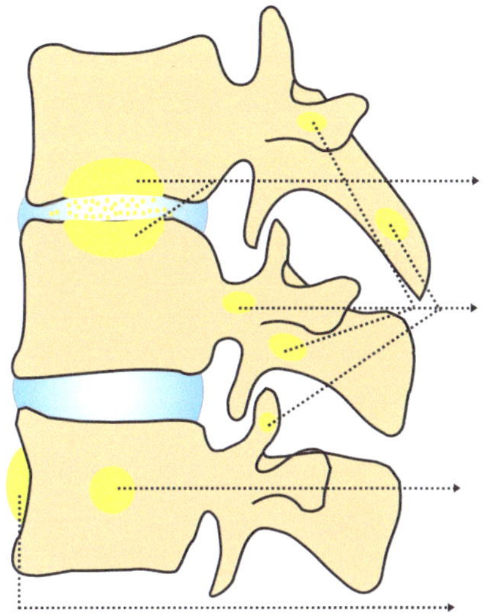

Fig. 12.1 Types of vertebral lesions in tuberculosis

involvement also occurs by extension from the abscess underneath the anterior longitudinal ligament and periosteum. Concerning histopathology, TB is characterized by granulomatous inflammation with infiltration of lymphocytes and epithelioid cells, which amalgamate to form the classical Langhans giant cells and results in caseous necrosis of infected tissues which may track along the path of least resistance to form a cold abscess (Fig. 12.2). A tubercular lesion healed in kyphotic deformity may progress as the child grows and can present with late-onset paraplegia.

12.4 Clinical Presentation

In contrast to pyogenic infections, spinal TB is usually characterised by insidious onset and is gradually progressive. The children usually present late because of non-specific symptoms, and this leads to delayed diagnosis. Backache or axial pain is the usual complaint. The pain is sometimes accompanied by night cries, muscle spasms, or deformity. The child is usually pale, and listless. In the upper cervical spine TB, the child can present with torticollis due to severe muscle spasms. Otherwise, the child might walk by supporting the head using both hands. The spinal TB manifests according to the site, severity, and the duration of disease, and also depending upon the occurrence of complications like an abscess, neurological deficits, and deformity. The thoracolumbar junction is the most affected region in the spinal column followed by the lumbar spine and cervical spine [13, 14] (Fig. 12.3). Moon et al. [4] in their retrospective analysis of 124 children with TB spine found that thoracic lesions were seen in 42.7%, cervical in 29.1%, lumbar/lumbosacral in 25%, and cervicodorsal lesions in 3.2% of their case series.

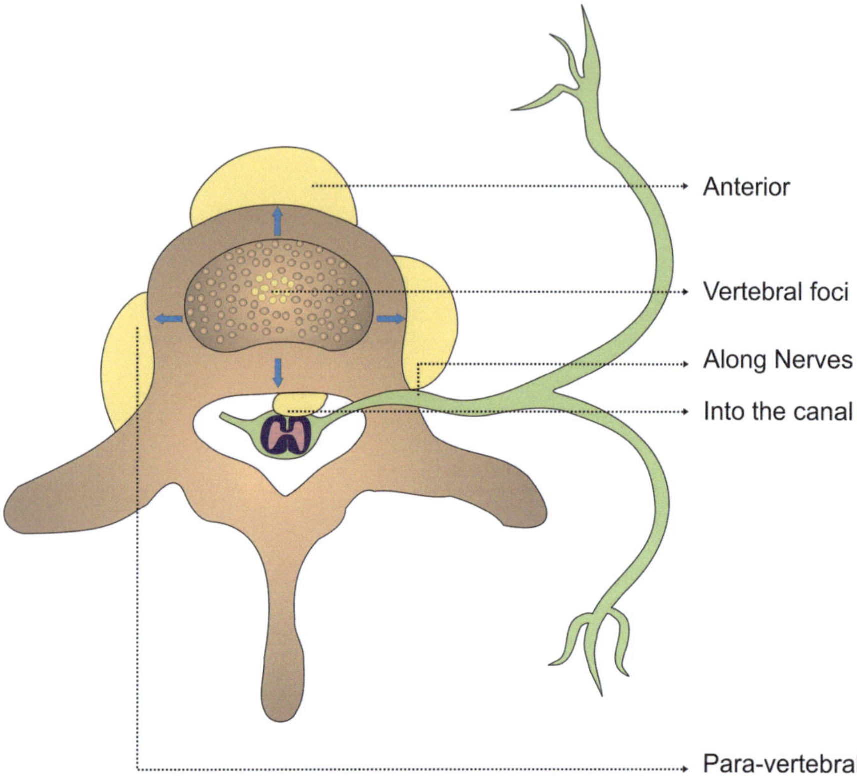

Fig. 12.2 Different directions of tracking of pus from a vertebral focus

Clinically, knuckle or angular deformity can be seen in the back with or without local/distant cold abscess. The paravertebral cold abscesses are seen in about 50% of spinal TB among children [1]. The retropharyngeal abscess track from cervical TB may produce dysphagia or respiratory stridor. The lumbar cold abscess might track along the psoas sheath resulting in a pseudo flexion deformity of the hip. Rest pain is usually pathognomonic, and the intensity of which is dependent on the severity of bone destruction and also instability [15]. The constitutional symptoms like weight loss, anorexia, malaise, night sweats, and fever are more associated with pulmonary TB rather than spinal TB [16].

The two types of neurological deficits that occur in the TB spine are (1) early-onset paraplegia which commonly occurs within the initial 2 years of active disease and (2) late-onset paraplegia which develops many years following the initial disease or perhaps due to continued collapse of the healed vertebrae (Figs. 12.4 and 12.5). Direct compression by the presence of an abscess, sequestrum, granulation tissue, or due to instability can result in early-onset paraplegia. Stretching of the spinal cord over the internal gibbus (even after healing of TB) is the commonest cause of late-onset paraplegia [17]. Usually, the neurological symptoms of these slow-growing infections manifest late due to the gradual cord compression during

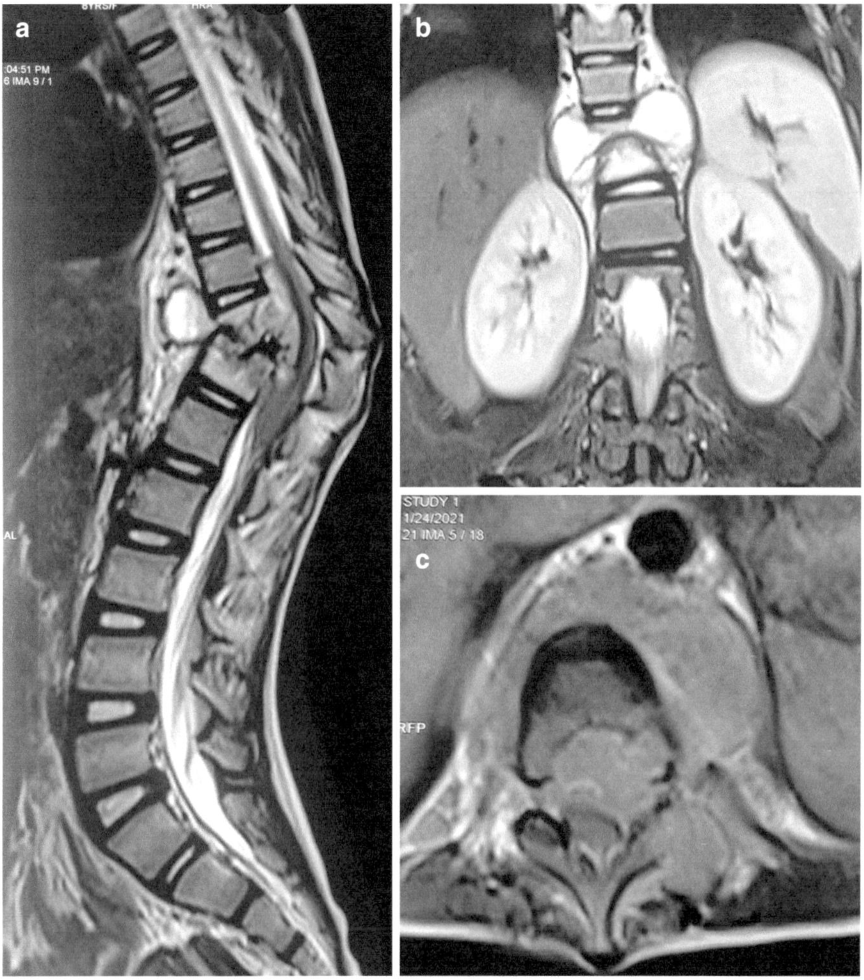

Fig. 12.3 (**a**–**c**) An 8-year-old child having caries spine at lower dorsal spine with vertebral collapse; the pus extends anteriorly and also compressing spinal cord posteriorly with early-onset paraplegia

which the neural structure gains adaptability thus resulting in late presenting deficits even after two-third to three-fourth of canal compromise [18, 19].

Tuli SM classified the neurological deficits in spinal TB which was further modified by Jain and Sinha into five stages [20]. The stage advances as the severity of the cord getting compressed increases and poor prognosis are noted in advanced stages (stage V).

- Stage I: The patient/child is unaware of the neural deficit, and only the clinician detects the presence of plantar reflex-extensor, and/or ankle clonus.

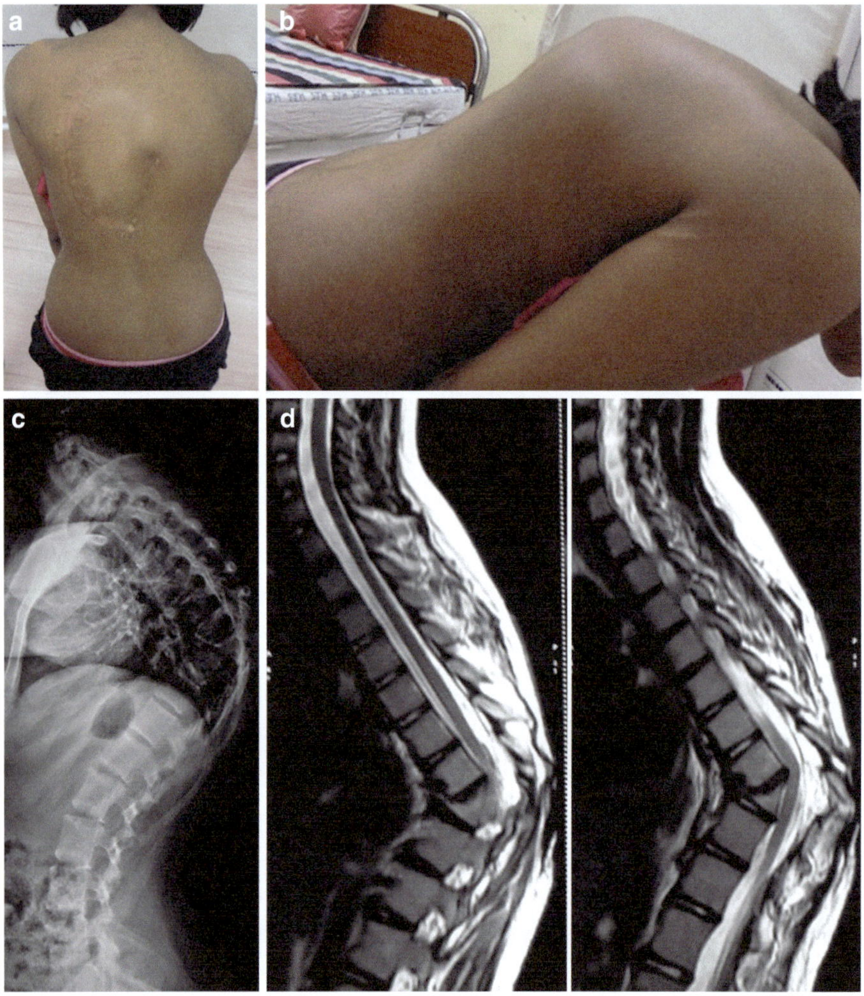

Fig. 12.4 (**a–d**) A 13-year-old child presented with progressive kyphotic deformity (apex at D7D8) with spastic paraparesis developed after 5 years of anterolateral decompression without instrumentation and multidrug chemotherapy. (Picture credit: Dr. Ashish Dagar, New Delhi)

- Stage II: The patient suffers spasticity along with the motor deficit but still ambulatory. The anticipated motor score in patients with quadriparesis ranges between 60 and 100. The anticipated motor score in paraparesis ranges between 80 and 100. The lateral column sensory impairment is noted at all root levels.
- Stage III: The patient is bedridden with spasticity. The anticipated motor score is between 0 and 30 in quadriplegics and between 50 and 80 in paraplegics. The sensory scoring remains the same as in stage II.

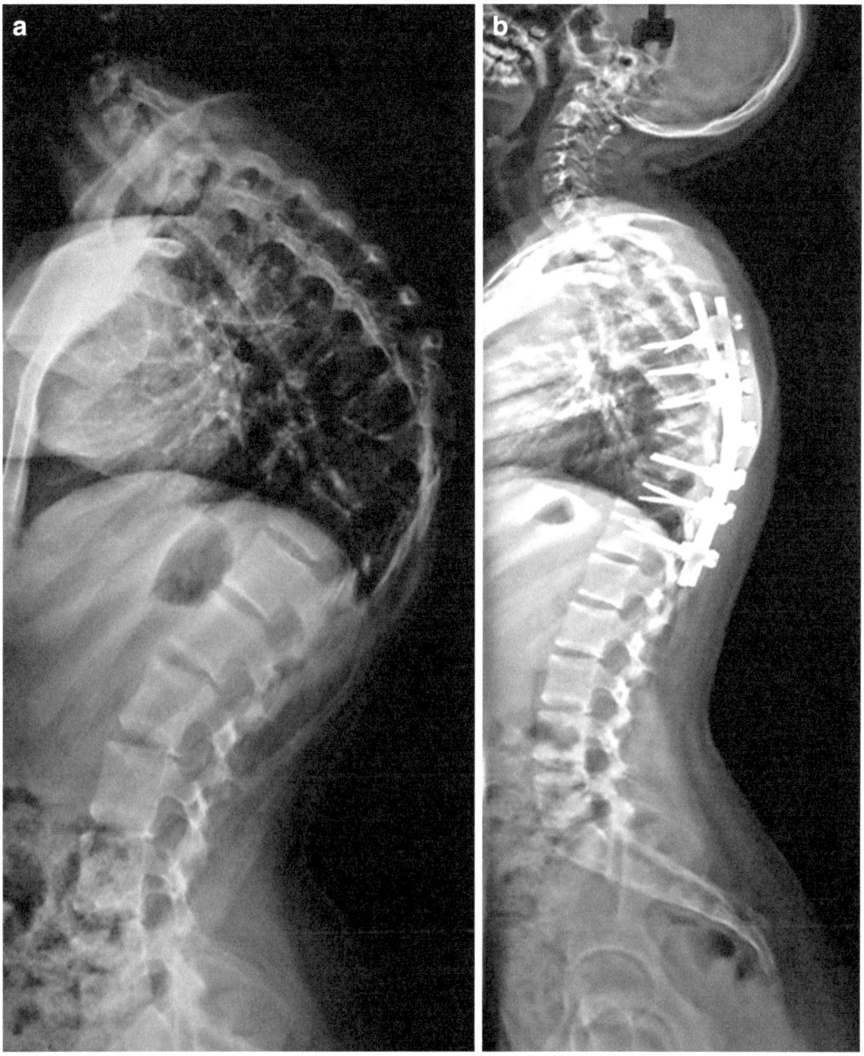

Fig. 12.5 Comparing (**a**) before and after (**b**) kyphotic deformity correction by pedicle subtraction osteotomy and pedicle screw fixation. (Picture credit: Dr. Ashish Dagar, New Delhi)

- Stage IV: The patient is bedridden with severe sensory loss and/or pressure sores. The motor score anticipated in a quadriplegic is 0 and in a paraplegic, is 50. Sensory impairment of both the lateral, as well as the posterior column, is seen.
- Stage V: Same signs like in stage IV and/or with bowel and bladder involvement, and/or flexor spasms/flaccid quadriplegia/paraplegia. There is usually loss of motor power or sensations below the affected level.

Even if some amount of motor power or sensations are preserved, it will be still considered as stage V when there is a presence of bladder/bowel involvement or flexor spasm.

12.5 Deformity

The TB spine is mainly an anterior disease, and the destruction of the vertebral body results in anterior collapse and kyphotic deformity. When compared to adults, the kyphotic deformity in the skeletally immature children might progress despite healed status. The progression of deformity depends upon the age, the level of tubercular lesion, and also the number of vertebrae affected. Factors like differential destruction of vertebral ring apophysis due to the active disease or through surgical debridement, disproportional loading of the spine, and also the altered vascularity influence the progress of kyphotic deformity over time [5]. The children should be monitored regularly for appearance/increase in kyphotic angle or any neurological deficit till skeletal maturity. The vertebral collapse patterns in TB cases of the growing spine were different at each spine level due to the different anatomical orientation of facet joints and the location of transverse processes. The anatomical orientation of the cervical spine prevents early vertical collapse and allows anterior slip to occur, while thoracic spine orientation leads to early kyphotic collapse and lumbar spine anatomical orientation favours early vertical collapse although this will be altered by age of child, growth cartilage status, and severity of bone destruction [4].

The clinical manifestation depends upon the number of vertebrae affected resulting in knuckle (1 vertebra), angular kyphosis/gibbus (2 vertebrae), or rounded kyphosis (more than 3 vertebrae). Jain et al. described that the kyphosis deformity of >60° angulation had a more chance of developing neurological deficit and should be surgically stabilized [21]. Due to inherent lordosis, the cervical and lumbar spine tolerate the vertebral loss very well in comparison to thoracic and thoracolumbar junction lesions. Rajasekaran noted that about 44% of kyphotic deformity spontaneously improves, 39% deformity progresses (worsens), and the kyphus remained static in 17% of children after the healing of the lesion [22].

Rajasekaran in his follow-up of TB spine in children for 15 years had described the signs of instability. The four radiological "spine at risk" signs are subluxation of the facet joint, retropulsion, lateral translation, and toppling sign (defined by a line drawn along the anterior surface of caudal normal vertebra crossing the mid-point of the anterior surface of the cranial normal vertebral bone) (Fig. 12.6). He suggested that children with an instability score of 2 or more had disruption of the posterior facet and advised surgical intervention in such situations [22, 23]. The severe type of kyphotic collapse known as "buckling collapse" occurs when the kyphotic angle is more than 120°. The risk factors are the age of the child <7 years at the time of infection, loss of more than 2 vertebral bodies, thoracolumbar spine involvement, and the presence of radiographic "spine at risk" signs [23].

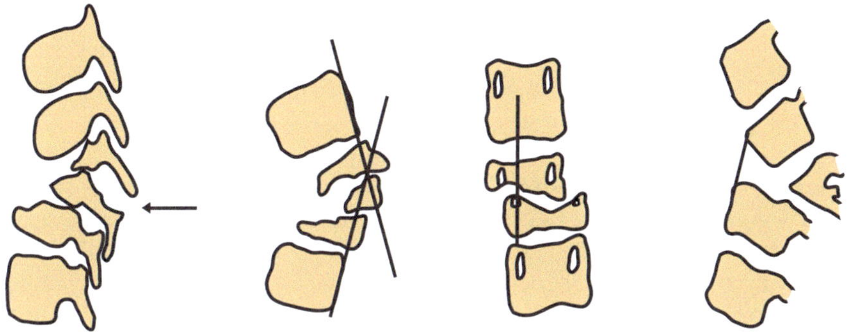

Fig. 12.6 Radiological "spine at risk" signs in children as described by Rajasekaran

Rajasekaran [22, 23] also described three types of curves in children based on the progression of the deformity and they are:

- Type 1 curves – where curvature increases until skeletal maturity and surgical intervention were required.
- Type 2 curves – where the deformity decreased with growth progression.
- Type 3 curves – where there was only minimal change in the deformity either during the active or healed phases of the disease.

The progressive kyphosis causes an increase in the stretching of the spinal cord over the internal gibbus that leads to late-onset paraplegia. Also, in younger children, the severe kyphotic deformity with further progression interferes with the growth of the thoracic cavity and leads to decreased pulmonary function [1].

Pearls

Buckling collapse:

Kyphotic angle >120°.

Risk factors are:

- Age of the child <7 years at the time of infection.
- Loss of >2 vertebral bodies.
- Thoracolumbar spine involvement.
- Presence of radiographic "spine at risk" signs.

12.5.1 Cervical Spine TB in Children

The cervical TB spine is uncommon, the incidence ranging from 3% to 5% of spinal TB [24–26]. The cervical spine TB may involve the atlantoaxial complex region, mid-cervical spine, or cervical-dorsal junction. The younger children are more prone to develop spinal TB in the upper cervical region due to its anatomy and biomechanics (Fig. 12.7). The fulcrum for normal cervical spine motion in children who are <8 years old is at the level of C2–C3 disc space. Increased mobility occurs at this space because of the disproportionally larger head, laxity of ligaments, poor control of muscles, and also due to the horizontal orientation of the upper cervical spine facet joints to a certain extent. After 10 years of age, the fulcrum of mobility moves towards the mid-cervical region, and the incidence of TB in older children is more here [26]. Cervico-dorsal junction involvement is usually rare but if develops, presents with a severe deformity due to involvement of transition zone of the mobile lordotic cervical spine with fixed kyphotic thoracic one. Tubercular lesions in the atlantoaxial region exhibit the potential to develop

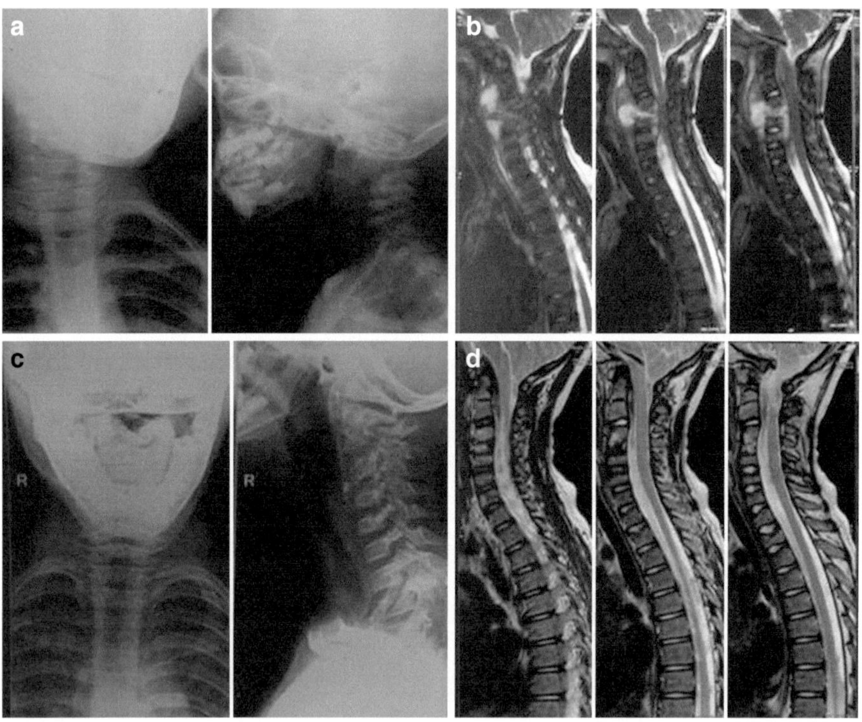

Fig. 12.7 A 5-year-old child with cervical spine (mid-cervical) TB (**a** and **b**) managed by multi-drug chemotherapy showing healed lesion (**c** and **d**) with an 18-month follow-up. (Picture credit: Dr. Anil Agarwal, Chacha Nehru Bal Chikitsalaya, New Delhi)

instability as well as neurological deficit and which may require surgical stabilization/fusion. Govender et al. retrospectively reviewed the outcome among the 58 children diagnosed with cervical spine TB. They found the improved functional outcome of cervical TB with anti-TB chemotherapy alone, and they performed surgery only for children developing neurologic deficit, atlantoaxial instability (atlantodental interval (ADI) of >5 mm in the flexion/extension view), or in those with progressive deformity [26].

12.6 Investigations

Erythrocyte sedimentation rate (ESR), although sensitive (60% to 90%), has low specificity in detecting TB. ESR can be used as a prognosticative marker for monitoring therapeutic responses to anti-TB chemotherapy. C-reactive protein (CRP) is more specific for acute infections like pyogenic rather than TB. It can also be used to monitor the treatment response. Although the Mantoux test (40% to 55% sensitivity and 75% specificity) has been recommended as a low-cost test in developing countries, its accuracy is questionable in endemic countries or immunodeficient children. It can be used to detect latent TB infections (LTBI) (Fig. 12.8). Interferon-gamma (IFN-gamma) assay (50% to 65% sensitivity and 85% specificity) is also not useful in endemic regions but can help in detecting LTBI. The children with LTBI have a lifetime risk of 24% in developing (symptomatic) TB disease, and the risk increases to 43% among the infants [27–30].

The culture of specimens obtained from infected tissue is considered the gold standard for confirming the diagnosis. But low sensitivity of culture makes histopathological examination showing typical granuloma with caseous necrosis and staining showing acid-fast bacilli (AFB) as the reference standards for diagnostic

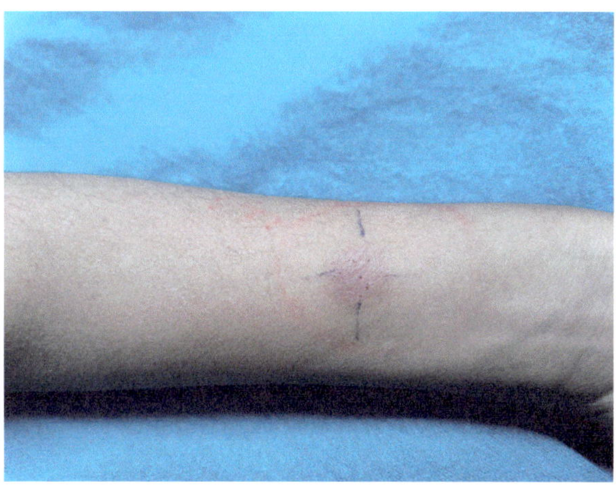

Fig. 12.8 Mantoux test: Tuberculin skin test measured after 48–72 hours after injection. The diameter of induration (not erythema) to be measured. Value ≥15 mm in a child with no risk factors considered significant

modalities. The conventional culture on Lowenstein-Jenson (LJ) medium usually took 4 to 6 weeks, and BACTEC radiometric culture assay took a minimum of 2 weeks for reports. Molecular diagnostics are used frequently to get rapid results. The sensitivity and specificity of polymerase chain reaction (PCR) are 75% and 97%, respectively, whereas of GeneXpert MTB/RIF is 82.9% and 98%, respectively. The newer Xpert MTB/RIF Ultra with 87.8% sensitivity and 94.8% specificity is useful in the early detection of paucibacillary and HIV-associated infection, particularly in smear-negative, culture-positive specimens, among the paediatric population and also in extrapulmonary specimens [31].

12.6.1 Imaging

Plain radiograph: The radiograph got not much role in detecting early lesions. The radiolucent lesion to visualize on radiograph needs 30% bone mineral loss. Disc space narrowing and rarefaction of endplates appear once the disease progresses. As 60 to 70% have associated pulmonary TB, the chest radiograph is mandatory.

Computed tomography (CT): CT detects vertebral destruction well before a radiograph. Cervicodorsal junctions are poorly visualized in radiograph so TB in this region requires CT or MRI. But in children, radiation exposure is a matter of concern. Also, it helps in percutaneous CT guided biopsy for diagnosis.

Magnetic Resonance Imaging (MRI): It remains the imaging modality of choice because it detects the tubercular infection earlier. Gadolinium (contrast) enhanced MRI is useful in the differentiation of TB from all other infective spondylodiscitis. MRI helps in the best visualisation of the disease extent in soft tissue, the abscess spread, as well as the neural compression. Whole spine screening detects skip lesions in the spine.

Positron emission tomography (PET): The disease activity can be assessed in real-time with the help of 18F-fluorodeoxyglucose (18F-FDG) labelled PET based on the rationale the 18F-FDG known to accumulates in the macrophages at the inflammatory sites.

All these investigations can't help in differentiating neoplasm from spine infections. So, the biopsy is mandatory for the confirmation of the diagnosis or for ruling out a neoplasm [31].

12.7 Treatment

TB spine is primarily a medical disease, and surgery is indicated only in specialized situations. The goal of TB treatment is to heal the disease with minimal residual deformity and without any neurological sequelae (Fig. 12.9).

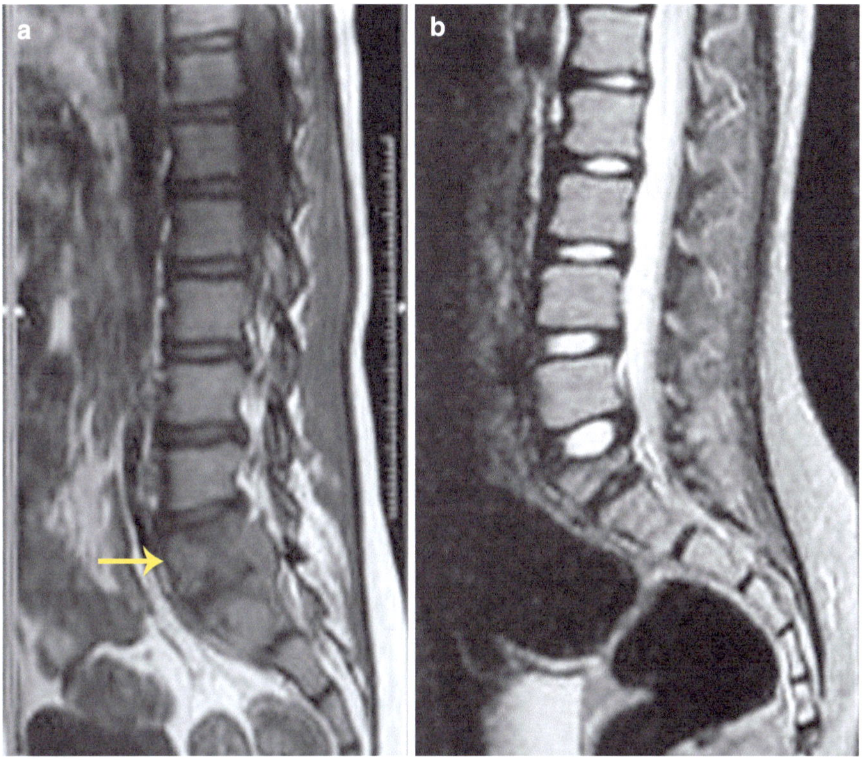

Fig. 12.9 A 7-year-old child with (**a**) lumbosacral TB (L5-S1) managed by multidrug chemotherapy showing healed lesion (**b**) with an 18-month follow-up. (Picture credit: Dr. Anil Agarwal, Chacha Nehru Bal Chikitsalaya, New Delhi)

12.7.1 Chemotherapy

In both complicated and uncomplicated TB, the mainstay of treatment remains to be multidrug chemotherapy. Usually, to start with 4 drug chemotherapy and the dosage is adjusted as per the child's weight. Drug dosage is decided according to the four categories of weight which are <10 kg group, 10–17 kg group, 18–25 kg group, and > 25 kg group. In a child weighing <10 kg, isoniazid and rifampicin are prescribed as 75 mg each along with pyrazinamide 250 mg and ethambutol 200 mg/day. The drugs are given in double, triple, and quadruple dosages for the above-listed weight categories (10–17 kg, 18–25 kg, and > 25 kg), respectively. During the middle of treatment, the child's weight should be monitored to adjust for the dosage of drugs [5]. Before starting the drugs like ethambutol and streptomycin paediatrician consultation should be sought to avoid toxicity in children. The duration of chemotherapy is debated for a long time, ranging from 9 months to 18 months.

Chatterjee and Banta [1] from India recommended 12 months of multidrug chemotherapy and suggested repeating an MRI at 12 months, and if it shows complete healing, chemotherapy can be stopped. With the emergence of drug-resistant strains, one should do drug sensitivity testing and tissue diagnosis to detect MDR TB early so that second-line drugs can be added. Along with chemotherapy, bracing/orthosis also forms an important part of treatment to ensure the restriction of diseased vertebrae movements.

12.7.2 Surgical Management

Treatment aims to achieve healing of the disease and at the same time maintaining the stability, the sagittal alignment of the spine, and also prevention of deformity progression. The indications for surgical treatment are the absence of response to chemotherapy or disease recurrence, neurological deficit remaining static or worsening even after starting chemotherapy, severe weakness at the time of presentation, devastating pain, instability, and deformities. Most of the cold abscesses are treated by chemotherapy alone. Large abscesses causing compressive effect (retropharyngeal abscess causing dysphagia, large psoas abscess causing pseudo hip flexion deformity) and tissue diagnosis required for diagnostic dilemma/suspected MDR-TB are other indications for surgery.

Pearls

Indications for surgery:

- Absence of response to chemotherapy.
- Recurrent disease.
- Static or progressive neurological deficit despite a course of multidrug chemotherapy.
- Severe neurological weakness at the time of presentation.
- Devastating pain.
- Instability.
- Deformity (kyphosis >60°).

In children, debridement alone does not prevent the progression of deformity or improve healing rates, as it may lead to growth plate damage and rapid deformity progression. Debridement, as well as fusion with or without instrumentation, can be carried out through anterior approach, posterior approach, global reconstruction by the posterior approach, or combined procedures [31]. Nowadays, with the help of a preop CT scan, the anatomy and diameter of pedicles are calculated before surgery, and the pedicle screw fixation is preferred in children. The posterior instrumentation using pedicle screws helps in stronger fixation and simultaneous correction of sagittal plane deformity to the desired angle. Jain et al. [5] advocated the use of hartshill rectangle in very young children (<5 years of age) whose pedicle diameter is very small. Following surgery for the next 3 to 4 months, instrumentation is protected with Minerva jacket till anterior and posterior fusion is achieved.

The early diagnosis of spinal TB with subsequent prevention of the neuro deficits and prevention of progression of kyphosis is the best way of managing a child with spinal TB. Moon et al. [4] in their retrospective case series of 124 children, 14.5% (18/124) had neurological deficits. 14 children were managed by chemotherapy alone, and 4 children underwent additional focal debridement and decompression surgery. Later on, all children showed healed status and neural recovery.

In the past, anterior debridement along with radical excision of the tubercular lesion in addition to anti-tubercular therapy (ATT) was performed. In contrast to pyogenic organisms, the tubercle bacilli do not have the property of adherence to metals nor the formation of biofilm [32]. Various approaches used are:

Anterior approach: TB is primarily an anterior disease, but performing an anterior debridement alone will fail to prevent the progression of the deformity. Rajasekaran noted graft slippage, absorption, subsidence, and fracture in 59% of cases who had undergone anterior body fusion without any instrumentation [31]. The extrapleural anterolateral approach allows a single-stage correction of kyphosis in the thoracic/thoracolumbar spine by providing exposure to anterior and posterior elements at the same time. The avoidance of opening of retroperitoneal space and chest cavity makes it less morbid.

Posterior approach: Due to its familiarity and shorter learning curve, it is the most commonly performed approach. The advantages are providing adequate exposure for the circumferential decompression of the spinal cord, better correction of the deformity using pedicle screws, and also the possibility of extending the instrumentation further. Transpedicular decompression and posterior instrumentation prevent the deformity progression as well as the neurological sequelae. Posterior instrumentation/fusion alone before growth spurts in children may lead to the crankshaft phenomenon due to continued growth in the anterior column. Combined fusion is recommended to prevent it.

Combined approach: Anterior decompression with fusion along with posterior instrumentation can be done simultaneously or in a staged manner. Anterior decompression allows removal of disease foci, direct neural decompression, and anterior reconstruction using bone grafts or cages. The posterior approach has the advantage of better deformity correction, reducing stress on anteriorly placed grafts, and prevention of progression of the sagittal plane deformity.

Global reconstruction by posterior approach alone: This is the preferred approach nowadays, and global reconstruction can be achieved by the posterior approach alone. Various posterior and posterolateral approaches such as transpedicular, transfacetal, extrapleural approaches or costotransversectomy are used to reach the anterior and lateral spinal column safely. Transpedicular and transfacetal approaches are easier and facilitate to reach anterior in the lumbar spine, but costotransversectomy is required in the thoracic spine [31].

12.7.3 Kyphotic Correction Surgery in Healed TB

Kyphotic deformity correction is a difficult task in healed lesions rather than in active disease, and it is a challenging task for even experienced surgeons because of the higher risk of neural damage associated with it. So, it should not be done for cosmetic purposes alone. Chemotherapy alone cures most of the cases; however, 3 to 5% of the cases advance to ≥60° kyphosis and they need surgery [33]. The presence of myelomalacia in preop MRI is a sign of poor prognosis, and it should be explained to parents before surgery.

The combined approach includes anterior decompression by corpectomy, posterior column shortening, as well as posterior instrumentation and anterior and posterior grafting. The options of posterior approach deformity correction procedures are transpedicular decancellation procedure, posterior vertebral column resection and closing opening wedge osteotomy, pedicle subtraction osteotomy (Fig. 12.10), and posterior closing wedge osteotomy. Rajasekaran et al. [34] noted an average kyphosis correction from 69.2° preoperative to 32.4° postoperatively by closing opening

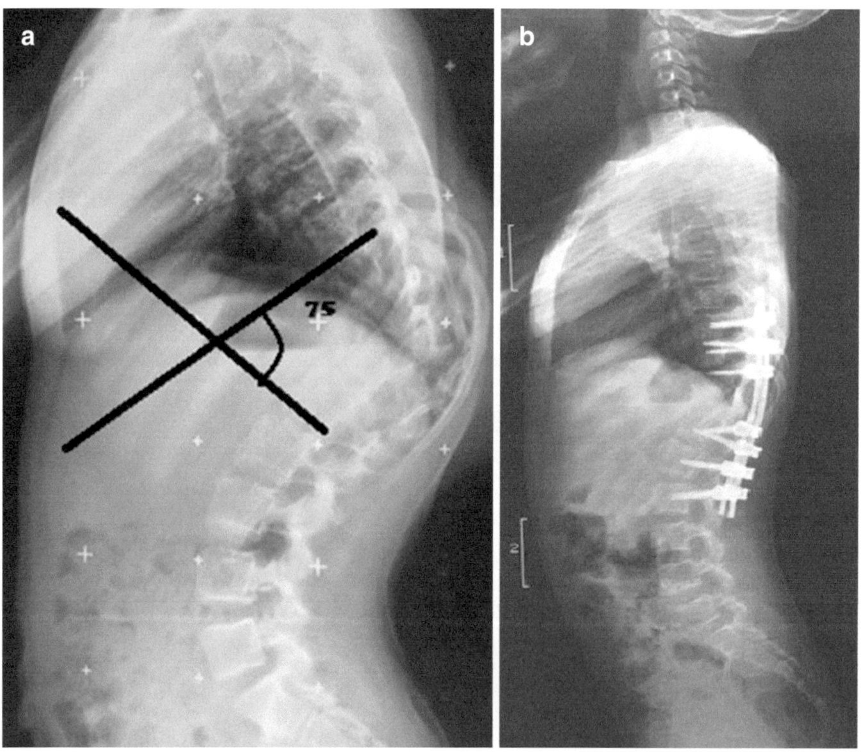

Fig. 12.10 An 11-year-old had healed TB with (**a**) kyphotic angle >60° (D10-D12) and was corrected by pedicle subtraction osteotomy with pedicle screw fixation (**b**) (Picture credit: Dr. Ashish Dagar, New Delhi)

wedge osteotomy. The intra-op neural monitoring should be advocated in difficult cases especially deformity correction in healed tuberculosis. In late-onset paraplegia cases, anterior decompression with fusion along with anterior transposition of the cord is advocated. The internal gibbus removal can be done either through the anterior transthoracic transpleural approach or through the extrapleural anterolateral approach [5].

12.8 Summary

TB spine is primarily a medical disease, and in children, an uncomplicated disease can be treated by multidrug chemotherapy along with rest and bracing. The spine deformity may progress as the child grows, and they must be placed under follow-up until their skeletal maturity. Prevention of late-onset paraplegia is better than its treatment. Surgery is indicated only for specialized situations, and it should be tailored individually. The current trend is all global posterior reconstruction for the thoracic and lumbar spine, and anterior debridement along with fusion is preferred for lower cervical spine TB.

References

1. Chatterjee S, Banta A. The spectrum of tuberculosis of the spine in pediatric age group: a review. Childs Nerv Syst. 2018;34(10):1937–45. https://doi.org/10.1007/s00381-018-3891-x.
2. World Health Organization. Global tuberculosis report 2020.
3. Maltezou HC, Spyridis P, Kafetzis DA. Extra-pulmonary tuberculosis in children. Arch Dis Child. 2000;83(4):342–6.
4. Moon MS, Kim SS, Lee BJ, Moon JL. Spinal tuberculosis in children: retrospective analysis of 124 patients. Indian J Orthop. 2012;46:150–8.
5. Jain AK, Sreenivasan R, Mukunth R, Dhammi IK. Tubercular spondylitis in children. Indian J Orthop. 2014;48(2):136–44. https://doi.org/10.4103/0019-5413.128747.
6. A controlled trial of ambulant out-patient treatment and in-patient rest in bed in the management of tuberculosis of the spine in young Korean patients on standard chemotherapy a study in Masan, Korea. First report of the Medical Research Council Working Party on Tuberculosis of the Spine. J Bone Joint Surg Br. 1973;55:678–97.
7. A controlled trial of anterior spinal fusion and debridement in the surgical management of tuberculosis of the spine in patients on standard chemotherapy: A study in Hong Kong. Br J Surg. 1974;61:853–66.
8. A 10-year assessment of a controlled trial comparing debridement and anterior spinal fusion in the management of tuberculosis of the spine in patients on standard chemotherapy in Hong Kong. Eighth Report of the Medical Research Council Working Party on Tuberculosis of the Spine. J Bone Joint Surg Br. 1982;64:393–8.
9. A 10-year assessment of controlled trials of inpatient and outpatient treatment and of plaster-of-Paris jackets for tuberculosis of the spine in children on standard chemotherapy. Studies in Masan and Pusan, Korea. Ninth report of the Medical Research Council Working Party on Tuberculosis of the Spine. J Bone Joint Surg Br. 1985;67:103–10.

10. Jain AK, Dhammi IK. Tuberculosis of the spine: a review. Clin Orthop Relat Res. 2007;460:39–49.
11. Teo HE, Peh WC. Skeletal tuberculosis in children. Pediatr Radiol. 2004;34(11):853–60.
12. Tyagi R. Spinal infections in children: a review. J Orthop. 2016;13(4):254–8.
13. Pertuiset E, Beaudreuil J, Liote F, et al. Spinal tuberculosis in adults: a study of 103 cases in a developed country, 1980–1994. Medicine (Baltimore). 1999;78:309–20.
14. Kulchavenya E. Extrapulmonary tuberculosis: are statistical reports accurate? Ther Adv Infect Dis. 2014;2:61–70.
15. Su SH, Tsai WC, Lin CY, et al. Clinical features and outcomes of spinal tuberculosis in southern Taiwan. J Microbiol Immunol Infect. 2010;43:291–300.
16. Hayes AJ, Choksey M, Barnes N, Sparrow OC. Spinal tuberculosis in developed countries: difficulties in diagnosis. J R Coll Surg Edinb. 1996;41:192–6.
17. Tuli SM. Tuberculosis of the skeletal system. JP Medical Ltd. 2016;
18. Hoffman EB, Crosier JH, Cremin BJ. Imaging in children with spinal tuberculosis–a comparison of radiography, computed tomography and magnetic resonance imaging. JBJS. 1993;75B:233–9.
19. Jain AK, Agarwal AN, Mehrotra G. Correlation of canal encroachment with neurological deficit in tuberculosis of spine. Int Orthop. 1999;23(2):85–6.
20. Jain AK, Sinha S. Evaluation of paraplegia grading systems in tuberculosis of the spine. Spinal Cord. 2005;43(6):375–80.
21. Jain AK. Treatment of tuberculosis of the spine with neurologic complications. Clin Orthop Relat Res. 2002;398:75–84.
22. Rajasekaran S. The natural history of posttubercular kyphosis in children. Radiological signs which predict late increase in deformity. J Bone Joint Surg Br. 2001;83:954–62.
23. Rajasekaran S. Buckling collapse of the spine in childhood spinal tuberculosis. Clin Orthop Relat Res. 2007;460:86–92.
24. Behari S, Nayak SR, Bhargava V, Banerji D, Chhabra DK, Jain VK. Craniocervical tuberculosis: protocol of surgical management. Neurosurgery. 2003;52:72–81.
25. Fang D, Leong JC, Fang HS. Tuberculosis of the upper cervical spine. J Bone Joint Surg Br. 1983;65:47–50.
26. Govender S, Ramnarain A, Danaviah S. Cervical spine tuberculosis in children. Clin Orthop Relat Res. 2007;460:78–85. https://doi.org/10.1097/BLO.0b013e31806a915f.
27. Cohn DL, O'Brien RJ, Geiter LJ, Rockville MD, Gordin FM, Hershfield E, et al. Targeted tuberculin testing and treatment of latent tuberculosis infection. Am J Respir Crit Care Med. 2000;161(4):221–47.
28. Horsburgh CR Jr. Priorities for the treatment of latent tuberculosis infection in the United States. N Engl J Med. 2004;350(20):2060–7.
29. Hoskyns W. Paediatric tuberculosis. Postgrad Med J. 2003;79(931):272–8.
30. Walls T, Shingadia D. Global epidemiology of paediatric tuberculosis. J Infect. 2004;48(1):13–22.
31. Rajasekaran S, Soundararajan DCR, Shetty AP, Kanna RM. Spinal Tuberculosis: Current Concepts. Global Spine J. 2018;8(4 Suppl):96S–108S. https://doi.org/10.1177/2192568218769053.
32. Oga M, Arizona T, Takasita M, Sugioka Y. Evaluation of the risk of instrumentation as a foreign body in spinal tuberculosis. Clinical and biologic study Spine (Phila Pa 1976). 1993;18:1890–4.
33. Rajasekaran S. Natural history of Pott's kyphosis. Eur Spine J. 2013;22(suppl 4):634–40.
34. Rajasekaran S, Vijay K, Shetty AP. Single stage closing-opening wedge osteotomy of spine to correct severe post-tubercular kyphotic deformities of the spine: a 3-year follow-up of 17 patients. Eur Spine J. 2010;19:583–92.

Chapter 13
The Medical Management of Spinal Tuberculosis

K. S. Sri Vijay Anand and Rishi M. Kanna

Abstract Anti-tubercular drugs have revolutionized the treatment of tuberculosis and have significantly reduced the mortality rates making them the mainstay in the management of uncomplicated spinal tuberculosis. The unique features of *Mycobacterium tuberculosis*, use of multiple drugs, development of drug resistance, and prolonged duration of treatment make anti-tubercular therapy challenging. The first-line drugs are the most potent, least toxic, and cheaper drugs in comparison to the second-line drugs. Side effects are common; therefore, a thorough knowledge of the pharmacological properties of drugs is essential. The current guidelines recommend daily dosing of fixed drug combinations. Though 9 to 12 months of therapy have been proven to be effective, there is still no consensus on treatment duration yet. In the light of emerging drug resistance, the second-line drugs are used frequently, and there is an unmet need for newer drugs with better safety profiles. Immunomodulators have the potential to be a valuable adjuvant to anti-tubercular drugs in increasing cure rates, decreasing the duration of therapy, and thereby decreasing drug resistance. Increased drug-sensitivity testing and ensuring compliance to anti-tubercular therapy is the key in mitigating the pandemic of tuberculosis and is fundamental to WHO's "End TB" strategy.

Keywords Spinal tuberculosis · Anti-tubercular drugs · Drug resistance · Immunomodulation

13.1 Introduction

The treatment of tuberculosis has evolved over time from the sanitorium-based treatment in the pre-anti-tubercular era to the current era of multidrug anti-tubercular therapy. The invention of anti-tubercular drugs can be considered a significant milestone in the era of modern medicine. In the pre-anti-tubercular era, tuberculosis was

---

K. S. Sri Vijay Anand · R. M. Kanna (✉)
Department of Spine Surgery, Ganga Hospital, Coimbatore, India

S. S. Dhatt, V. Kumar (eds.), *Tuberculosis of the Spine*,
https://doi.org/10.1007/978-981-16-9495-0_13

responsible for one in four deaths earning the sobriquet "Captain of all these men of death" [1]. The advent of multidrug anti-tubercular drugs and directly observed treatment and short-course therapy (DOTS) has revolutionized tuberculosis management and has decreased the mortality rates from 30 to 50% in the pre-anti-tubercular era to less than 1% in drug-sensitive cases. The cure rates have also improved from 30–44% to 83–96.8% [2]. Currently, multidrug anti-tubercular drugs remain the mainstay in treating uncomplicated spinal tuberculosis, with surgical management reserved for cases with instability or neurological compromise.

Unlike other pyogenic infections of the human body, the pharmacological management of tuberculosis has certain unique features such as the combination of multiple drugs, different phases of treatment, and long duration of therapy. Hence it is termed as chemotherapy akin to the treatment guidelines pursued for cancer management. The reason for this can be ascribed to the unique features of the tubercular mycobacterium, including a thick mycobacterial cell wall with limited permeability, the slow multiplication of bacteria, the capacity to adapt in vivo to different environments, and the ability for rapid development of resistance [3]. Though multidrug anti-tubercular therapy's efficacy and success have been proven, the controversies regarding the dosing and duration of the treatment are unresolved. The emergence of drug resistance poses a new challenge in controlling the pandemic and necessitates newer drugs and strategies. This chapter aims to provide a thorough review of the anti-tubercular drugs.

13.2 History and Evolution of Anti-tubercular Treatment

Though tuberculosis has infected humans since time immemorial, the scientific treatment is less than a century old. Historic treatment modalities including manual pressure and traction (Hippocrates, 450 BC), advocacy of fresh air, milk, and sea voyages (Galen,174 AD), King's touch (twelfth–eighteenth century), removal of the scrofulous gland (Guy de Chauliac, 1363), and rest as fundamental treatment (Hugh Owen Thomas, 1875) evidently had dismal outcomes. Earlier surgical attempts before the anti-tubercular era often had catastrophic results with high mortality. The first successful sanatorium-based treatment was reported by Hermann Brehmer in 1854, and this trend continued till the advent of anti-tubercular drugs in the 1940s [4].

Streptomycin (SM) and para-aminosalicylic acid (PAS) were among the first anti-tubercular drugs to be invented. Para-aminosalicyclic acid was rediscovered for its use in tuberculosis by Swedish chemist Jörgen Lehmann in 1944. Around the same time, streptomycin was derived from fungi *Actinomycetes* by American microbiologists Selman Waksman and Albert Schatz for its use in tuberculosis. The first randomized control study by the British medical research council (1950) comparing the efficacy of these two drugs found the combination therapy to be effective in achieving cure rates and preventing resistance [5]. This study laid the foundation for multidrug anti-tubercular therapy. Isonicotinyl-hydrazine (INH) was first synthesized by Hans Meyer and Josef Malley in 1912. However, its anti-tubercular activity was discovered only in 1951 by Harry Yale of New Jersey. The introduction of the three-drug regimen (PAS, SM, INH) significantly improved cure rates and reduced resistance; however, the treatment lasted for 24 months [6]. Ethambutol was introduced in the early 1960s and successfully replaced PAS, which was poorly tolerated. It further reduced the duration of treatment to 18 months. The next significant advance was the introduction of rifampicin (RIF) derived from *Streptomyces mediterranei.* The efficacy of rifampicin was proved in two major trials and offered predictable cure rates of >95% in a short duration of 9 months [7, 8]. The treatment duration was further shortened to 6 months by the introduction of pyrazinamide (PZA) [9]. These five (INH, RIF, EMB, PZA, SM) are the first-line drugs that form the backbone of modern anti-tubercular therapy. Osteoarticular tuberculosis is the second commonest form of tuberculosis after pulmonary infection, and the vertebral column is affected preferentially compared to other bones and joints due to its hyper-vascularity. Osteoarticular tuberculosis has reduced bacterial load ($<10^4$ colony forming units per ml) in the infected tissues. Thus, pharmacological treatment regimes that are effective for pulmonary TB will work for spinal tuberculosis as well [10].

13.3 Principles of Multidrug Anti-tubercular Therapy

Unlike conventional infections, the tubercular infection needs multidrug chemotherapy for various micro-biological reasons, as detailed below:

1. In vivo, the mycobacteria are found in four different forms: (1) extracellular rapidly dividing, (2) extracellular slowly dividing, (3) intracellular intermittently dividing, and (4) dormant bacilli [11]. Therefore, it necessitates the use of multiple drugs effective against different bacterial forms. While isoniazid, ethambutol, and streptomycin are effective against rapidly multiplying bacilli, rifampicin acts on slowly multiplying bacilli, and pyrazinamide kills the intracellular bacilli within macrophages [12].
2. The slow-growing nature of mycobacteria is both a boon and bane. While the disease progression is slow, it renders the drugs that act on rapid multipliers ineffective, limiting the therapeutic options. Hence, there is a need to use drugs for a longer period of time (typically months).
3. The limited permeability of mycobacterial cell wall and intra-macrophage bacilli makes the drug permeability low [3]. Hence, specific drugs that penetrate macrophages and thick bacterial cell wall are an essential part of the treatment.
4. Mycobacteria are notorious for developing rapid drug resistance to monotherapy. Mycobacterial mutations leading to isoniazid resistance can be found at a rate of 1in 10^6 and 1 in 10^8 to rifampicin. The resistance to both can be found in

1 in 10^{14}. Hence to subvert the development of resistance, a minimum of two drugs are used in combination [10].

5. Most anti-tubercular drugs except thiacetazone have a long duration of action known as "lag-effect." This property enabled intermittent drug dosing and was fundamental to the success of DOTS [13, 14].

13.4 First-Line Drugs

Despite decades of intensive research, very few drugs have proven to be efficacious. The five first-line drugs (INH, RIF, EMB, PZA, SM) are the most effective and least toxic among the available anti-tubercular drugs, and hence judicious use with an emphasis on compliance is recommended to prevent the development of resistance. Prolonged therapy with multiple drugs could predispose to a range of adverse effects and complications. Therefore a thorough knowledge of pharmacokinetics, drug interactions, and side effect profile is necessary along with periodic monitoring to ensure a safe and successful treatment.

13.4.1 Isoniazid (INH)

Isoniazid is a keystone in the management and prophylaxis of tuberculosis. INH is a prodrug that produces an array of radicals (most notable-iso-nicotinoyl radical) upon activation by the catalase-peroxidase KatG. These radicals bind nicotinamide adenine dinucleotide (NAD) to form an INH-NAD adduct that inhibits InhA, the enoyl-ACP reductase of the fatty acid synthase type II system (FASII), resulting in the inhibition of mycolic acid biosynthesis and, ultimately, cell death [15].

INH is particularly active against fast-growing mycobacteria [16]. It acts on both intracellular and extracellular bacilli and can cross the blood-brain barrier. Upon entering the bacterial cell, INH kills only dividing bacteria, with no action on mycobacteria in the stationary phase [17]. During the initial 1–4 days, INH is bacteriostatic, after which the action is bactericidal and correlates with its loss of acid fastness property [18, 19]. Resistance to INH involves multiple genes in several pathways. The most common cause for resistance is a mutation in the *katG* gene, followed by other genes such as *inhA, ahpC, kasA, ndh* [20, 21]. The recommended dosage is 5 mg/kg in adults and 10 mg/kg in children. The adverse effects include peripheral neuropathy, lethargy, hepatitis and rarely convulsions, psychosis, and lupus-like syndrome. Pyridoxine (10–25 mg/day) is recommended along with it to counteract the risk of peripheral neuropathy. INH is a cytochrome P450 inhibitor and known to increase the plasma concentrations of drugs such as anti-convulsants, benzodiazepines, acetaminophen, and oral anti-coagulants.

13.4.2 Rifampicin (RIF)

Rifampicin, a rifamycin derivative, acts by binding to the β-subunit of the RNA polymerase and inhibiting messenger RNA's elongation [22, 23]. It is active against rapid multipliers and slow metabolizing bacilli, both intracellular and extracellular [24]. This effectiveness on bacilli with sporadic metabolism offers a "sterilizing effect." The recommended dosage is 10 mg/kg in adults and 15–20 mg/kg in children. Dose-related hepatotoxicity can occur, and the maximum dosage should not exceed 600 mg/day. Other adverse effects include orange-red discoloration of urine, flu-like syndrome, abdominal syndrome, rarely purpura, and hemolytic anemia. Rifampicin is an inducer of cytochrome P450 and warrants dosage adjustments of other drugs metabolized in the liver such as oral hypoglycemics, anti-convulsants, anti-fungals, protease inhibitors, and non-nucleoside reverse transcriptase inhibitors, cardiac drugs, etc. The mutations in the 81 bp of *rpoB* gene (codons 507-533) that code for the β-subunit of the RNA polymerase is the most common cause of rifampicin resistance [25].

13.4.3 Pyrazinamide (PZA)

Pyrazinamide is a structural analogue of nicotinamide and a prodrug converted to its active form pyrazinoic acid by an amidase encoded by the gene *pncA* [26]. It has been postulated that PZA inhibits membrane transport, trans-translation, and coenzyme A synthesis needed for the bacteria to survive [27]. The key characteristic of PZA is its activity against non-replicating persisters in an acidic, inflammatory environment. It is most effective during the initial two months of treatment while acute inflammatory changes persist. It offers an excellent "sterilizing effect" and plays a vital role in shortening chemotherapy duration. The recommended dosage is 25 mg/kg in adults and 35 mg/kg in children. Heptotoxicity, hyperuricemic arthralgia, exanthema, and pruritis are the known adverse effects. Dose adjustments are needed in patients on cyclosporine and gout treatment. The main mechanisms for pyrazinamide resistance in *M. tuberculosis* are due to mutations in *pncA* with loci in the 561 bp region of the open reading frame or in a 82 bp region of its putative promoter [28, 29].

13.4.4 Ethambutol (EMB)

Ethambutol is active only against replicating bacilli (bacteriostatic), where it inhibits the enzyme arabinosyltransferases and prevents the biosynthesis of the mycobacterial cell wall arabinogalactan [30]. Other mechanisms include impairment of glycerol metabolism as well as RNA synthesis. The recommended dosage is 15 mg/kg in adults and 15–25 mg/kg in children. The most notable adverse effect is dose-dependent retrobulbar neuritis. Often the central fibers are affected, resulting in loss of visual acuity, scotomas, and inability to distinguish green or red color. When detected early and the drug is discontinued, the effects are reversible. Other adverse effects include abdominal pain, eosinophilia, peripheral neuritis, myocarditis, and hypersensitivity. The drug is contraindicated in children for the difficulty in testing visual acuity reliably. Dose adjustments are needed in patients with reduced creatinine clearance (<30 mL/min). The most common mutation for resistance to ethambutol is located in codon 306 of *embB* gene encoding arabinosyltransferase [31].

13.4.5 Streptomycin (SM)

Streptomycin is an aminocyclitol glycoside derived from *Streptomyces griseus*. Administered as an intramuscular injection, it is particularly active against actively multiplying bacilli present in cavities. It acts by inhibiting the initiation of the translation of ribosomal protein S12 and the 16S rRNA coded by the genes *rpsL* and *rrs*, respectively [32, 33]. The key characteristic is its action in alkaline pH. Streptomycin is recommended at a dosage of 15 mg/kg in adults and 15–25 mg/kg in children. The adverse effects include ototoxicity, vestibulotoxicity, nephrotoxicity, rashes, eosinophilia, and fever. The most common mutation conferring resistance to streptomycin is a substitution in codon 43 from lysine to arginine in *rpsL* [34].

Streptomycin can cross the placenta and cause ototoxicity and nephrotoxicity in the fetus, hence not recommended in pregnancy. All the other first-line drugs (INH, RIF, PZA, ETB) can safely be used in pregnancy. The pharmacokinetics of children differ from adults. Children metabolize drugs faster, and the serum concentration of drugs is much less compared to adults and therefore need a higher body weight dose (mg/kg).

The dosage, minimum inhibitory concentration (MIC), and adverse effects of the first-line anti-tubercular drugs are listed in Table 13.1.

13.5 Second-Line Drugs, Adverse Effects, Monitoring

The emerging drug resistance to first-line drugs has necessitated the use of second-line drugs frequently. The second-line drugs have less efficacy, more toxicity, and costlier than the first-line drugs. Fluoroquinolones, injectable aminoglycosides, ethionamide, and cycloserine are the common second-line drugs used.

Table 13.1 Dosing and pharmacological properties of first-line anti-tubercular drugs

Drug	Dosage Adult mg/Kg	Dosage Children Mg/kg	Minimum inhibitory concentration (MIC). μg/ml for mycobacteria	Property	Differential action	Adverse effect
Isoniazid	5 (max 300 mg)	10 mg/kg (range 7–15 mg/kg); maximum dose 300 mg/day	0.02–0.2	Bactericidal	Effective against extracellular rapid multipliers	Hepatotoxicity Vitamin B6 deficiency Peripheral Neuropathy Lupus-like syndrome
Rifampicin	10 (max 600 mg)	15 mg/kg (range 10–20 mg/kg); maximum dose 600 mg/day	0.05–0.1	Bactericidal	Effective against extracellular rapid multipliers and slow multipliers	Hepatotoxicity (dose-related) Thrombocytopenia Neutropenia Orange/red discoloration of bodily fluids CYP450 Inducer
Pyrazinamide	25	35 mg/kg (range 30–40 mg/kg)	6.25–50	Bactericidal	Effective against intracellular mycobacteria in acidic medium	Hepatotoxicity Hyperuricemia Arthralgia
Ethambutol	15	Children 20 (15–25)*	1–5	Bacteriostatic	Effective against rapid extracellular multipliers	Optic neuropathy Hepatotoxicity Peripheral neuropathy
Streptomycin	15	20 mg/kg (range 15–25 mg/kg	2–8	Bactericidal	Effective against rapid multipliers in alkaline pH	Ototoxicity Vestibulotoxicity Nephrotoxicity

13.5.1 Fluoroquinolones

The fluoroquinolones (FQs) are broad-spectrum antibiotic and have excellent in vitro and in vivo activity against *M. tuberculosis* [35, 36]. They are bactericidal, and the mechanism of action is by inhibiting DNA synthesis. Ciprofloxacin, ofloxacin, levofloxacin, and moxifloxacin are commonly used fluoroquinolones. The recommended dosage is 400–600 mg/day. Adverse effects are relatively infrequent (0.5–10%) and limited to headache, gastrointestinal intolerance, rashes, and dizziness. The most common mechanism for drug resistance is a mutation in DNA gyrase, the cellular target for FQ's [37].

13.5.2 Aminoglycosides

The injectable aminoglycosides amikacin (AMK), kanamycin (KAN), and capreomycin (CAP) are an integral part of treatment in multidrug-resistant tuberculosis. These are derived from *Streptomyces* and are bactericidal. The mechanism of action of AMK and KAN is inhibition of protein translation, whereas capreomycin inhibits mRNA–tRNA translocation by binding to 70S ribosome [38]. The dosage for all three drugs is 15 mg/kg/day administered as a single dose. Adverse effects include renal toxicity, ototoxicity, and electrolyte disturbances (hypokalemia, hypocalcemia, hypomagnesemia), and regular monitoring of hearing and renal function is recommended. Resistance to AMK and KAN is associated with changes in the 16S rRNA, and cross-resistance between these drugs is prevalent [39]. Resistance to capreomycin is associated with a mutation in TlyA (encodes 2'-O-methyltransferase involved in methylation) [40] and correlates with increased treatment failure rates and mortality [41].

13.5.3 Cycloserine

Cycloserine is obtained from *Streptomyces orchidaceus* and is bacteriostatic. It inhibits mycobacterial cell wall synthesis. Recommended dose is 1 g/day administered as a single dose. Adverse effects include psychosis, headache, and seizures, and the drug is to be avoided in patients with psychiatric illness and renal insufficiency [42]. It possesses excellent gastric tolerance and has less cross-resistance with other drugs making it a viable candidate in the treatment of multidrug-resistant (MDR) and extreme drug-resistant (XDR) TB [43].

13.5.4 Ethionamide/Prothionamide

Ethionamide/prothionamide are bacteriostatic and are derived from isonicotinic acid. The mechanism of action is similar to INH by inhibiting Inh A of mycolic acid synthesis [44]. The drug is taken as single dose of 1gm/day. The side effects include severe gastrointestinal intolerance, hepatitis, peripheral neuropathy, hypothyroidism, and depression. Cross-resistance between the two drugs is prevalent.

13.5.5 Para-aminosalicylic Acid (PAS)

PAS was one of the earliest anti-tubercular drugs introduced. However, it was replaced due to rapid resistance and gastric intolerance. Other adverse effects include hypothyroidism, hepatic dysfunction, and hypersensitivity. The recommended dosage is 12gm in single or two divided doses.

The other drugs that are used as second-line drugs but with limited efficacy include Linezolid, Thioacetazone, Clofazimine, Clarithromycin, Imipenam, etc.

13.6 Newer Drugs

In the light of increasing drug-resistance to *M. tuberculosis*, there is an unmet need for newer drugs acting via novel targets with better efficacy, with the least drug interactions and toxicity profile.

13.6.1 Bedaquiline

Bedaquiline is a novel class of anti-tubercular drug introduced in 2012. It is highly sensitive for mycobacterial ATP synthase and inhibits its activity by binding to its subunit c [45]. It is advocated for use in MDR and XDR-TB in combination with other second-line drugs. Development of cross-resistance with other anti-tuberculosis is minimal due to its unique mechanism of action. The reported side effects include nausea, arthralgia, headache, hemoptysis, chest pain, anorexia, rash, and elevation of hepatic transaminases. The notable adverse effect is QT prolongation and hence not be used with other QT-prolonging drugs [46]. Low-level resistance to bedaquline and cross-resistance to clofazimine has been reported due to mutations in the *rv0678* gene encoding the MmpL5 efflux pump repressor [47]. It is available through RNTCP in India from 2019.

13.6.2 Delamanid

Delamanid is a prodrug (dihydro-nitroimidazooxazole derivative) upon activation by the enzyme deazaflavin-dependent nitroreductase (Rv3547), which inhibits the synthesis of mycobacterial cell wall components [48]. The adverse effect includes headache, nausea, dizziness, and QT prolongation [49]. The safety profile is good, with no notable interactions with other anti-TB drugs and the least toxicity. Given the variable results in studies comparing the efficacy of the drug [50], WHO recommends its use only in a more extended MDR regimen if no suitable alternative could be found [51].

13.7 Immunomodulators

The very fact that only 5% of those infected develop clinical disease indicates that host immunity plays a vital role in curtailing tubercular infection [1, 52]. The major components of host defense against tubercular infection include specific T-cell immunity, macrophage activation, and granuloma formation, which are mediated by the cytokines produced by CD 4 cells. The depletion of CD4 cells and related impaired immune responses have been well documented in tubercular infection. In the absence of novel potent anti-tubercular drugs, host-directed therapy using immunomodulators offers a promising avenue for adjuvant therapy in drug-sensitive and drug-resistant tuberculosis. The application and benefits of immunomodulation in tuberculosis include as follows: (1) limits non-productive tissue-damaging inflammatory responses, (2) stimulates host immunity, and offers an earlier cure. An earlier cure enables a shortened duration of treatment, thereby reducing non-compliance and a resultant increase in drug resistance, (3) helps in killing intracellular bacilli and persisters in a granuloma, (4) offers immune memory preventing recrudescence (5) as an adjuvant in drug-resistant tuberculosis where limited therapeutic options are available (6) in an immunocompromised host (6) When failure to respond to a standard treatment regime.

Various drugs, cytokines, mycobacterial products, and whole mycobacteria have been evaluated for their role as possible immunomodulators with varied success. The earliest attempt of immunotherapy was by Robert Koch himself using tuberculin but was unsuccessful. The only vaccine against tuberculosis available is Bacille Calmette-Guérin (BCG), which has only limited efficacy. *Mycobacterium vaccae* has been used as an immunomodulator. A meta-analysis of 54 studies using an intradermal injection of *M. vaccae* reported increased sputum conversion in pulmonary TB. RUTI is a vaccine made of detoxified cellular fragments of *M. tuberculosis*, delivered in liposomes. Phase II trials have demonstrated therapeutic potential as an adjuvant immunomodulator [53].

In the pre-anti-tubercular era, exposure to sunlight and vitamin D was the standard treatment. The role of vitamin D beyond calcium metabolism is well recognized. Vitamin D possesses anti-MTB activity mediated via the classical nuclear receptor (nVDR) [54]. *Mycobacterium tuberculosis*-infected monocytes upregulate the expression of VDR [55]. Vitamin D induces the gene expression of cathelicidin antimicrobial peptide (CAMP), the precursor of the active antimicrobial agent, cathelicidin (LL-37) [56, 57]. Cathelicidin exerts its antibacterial activity by its ability to bind and disrupt bacterial cell wall phosphatidylglycerol monolayers by promoting autophagy and increased reactive oxygen species production (ROS) [58, 59].

Eicosanoids regulation has been linked with clinically relevant immunomodulation. Cyclooxygenase-2 (COX2) regulates the production of pro-inflammatory cytokines and inflammation via prostaglandin E2 (PGE2) production [60]. Leukotrienes are involved in the initiation of inflammation [61]. A balance between concentrations of lipoxin A4 (LXA4) and leukotriene B4 is essential as overproduction of LXA4 may cause immunosuppression. NSAIDs such as Aspirin and Ibuprofen inhibit COX-2 and result in increased LXA4 and decreased TNF-α, thus reducing the inflammation [60, 62]. Zileuton, 5-Lipoxygenase inhibitor, blocks leukotriene production, facilitating COX2 activation and PGE2 synthesis [63]. In experimental models, zileuton successfully decreased the IFN- α, β levels, and the mycobacterial load [64]. The WHO recommends routine inclusion of NSAIDs as adjunctive therapy to the standard TB treatment regimen to reduce antibiotic-related joint pain. However, the use of NSAID as preventative treatment remains unclear.

Levamisole, an antihelminth, is an immunostimulant that stimulates antibody formation, enhances T-cell activation and proliferation, and promotes chemotaxis and phagocytosis [65, 66].

13.7.1 Cytokines

Cytokines are small proteins that play a profound role in the immune system. Various cytokines with different functions have been proposed to be of benefit in tuberculosis. IFN-γ, secreted by Th1 cells, upregulates class I and II antigen-presentation pathways and induces macrophages' microbicidal effector functions [67, 68]. IFN-α and IFN-ω are known to activate macrophages and influence the function of dendritic and Th1 cells [69, 70]. GM-CSF stimulates antimicrobial activities in both macrophages and neutrophils [71]. IL-12 and IFN-γ synergistically enhance the activation state of macrophages and induce T and NK cells to produce IFN-γ. IL-4 and TGF-β possess anti-inflammatory properties. IL-7, IL-11, and IL-17 modulate cytokine production by monocyte and macrophages. IL-16 is a chemoattractant to CD4+, T cells, and monocytes. The levels of IL-6 have been correlated with disease severity and prognosis, and its decline correlates with clinical recovery. Blockade of the IL-6/IL-6R pathway is proposed to serve as a potential target for immunomodulation.

Immune checkpoint inhibition has been proven to be of benefit in cancer therapy. Programmed cell death 1 (PD-1) [72–74], cytotoxic T lymphocyte-associated antigen 4 (CTLA-4) [75, 76], lymphocyte-activation gene 3 (LAG3), and T cell immunoglobulin and mucin domain3 (TIM3) [77, 78] are the molecules that are being investigated for immune checkpoint inhibition in tuberculosis. They act on target cells leading to expansion and dampening of antigen-specific effector T cell responses. Besides, they regulate the secretion of a myriad of cytokines, including IFN-γ, TNF-α, type 1 interferons, GM-CSF, IL-2, IL-7, and IL-15.

Immunomodulation has been a subject of increased interest in the past decade, and numerous drugs are being investigated. However, it is beyond the scope of this chapter to elaborate on all the drugs. Very few studies have investigated the role of immunomodulation in osteoarticular/spinal tuberculosis. Arora et al. in their study used levamisole, BCG, and DT vaccine in patients with poor or delayed response to standard anti-tubercular chemotherapy [79]. They found that CD4 counts are a reliable indicator of host immunity, and their level correlated well with recovery. Saurabh et al. also reported a similar correlation between peripheral T-cell count and clinical responsiveness [74] in a more recent prospective study.

13.8 RNTCP and DOTS

Revised National TB Control Program (RNTCP) was started in 1993 and expanded to the entire nation in 2006 with an objective to achieve and maintain a TB treatment success rate of at least 85% among new sputum positive (NSP) patients and to achieve and maintain detection of at least 70% of the estimated new sputum positive people in the community. RNTCP uses the World Health Organization (WHO) recommended Directly Observed Treatment Short Course (DOTS) strategy and offers free diagnostic services and treatment. In 2020, RNTCP was renamed as National Tuberculosis Elimination Program (NTEP) with the goal of ending TB by 2025 (5 years ahead of global target) using four strategic pillars "Detect-Treat-Prevent-Build."

Directly Observed treatment short-course (DOTS) is a specific strategy, endorsed by the WHO, to improve treatment adherence by requiring health workers, volunteers, or family members to observe and record patients taking each dose. It categorizes patients into two and recommends treatment regimes. The first WHO endorsed DOTS-Plus programs began in 2000. During the intensive phase, a health care worker supervises drug intake by the patient, and during the continuation phase, the patient is issued with a multiblister pack of which the first dose is taken in front of the health care worker, and the patient returns the empty blister pack next week to get next week medicines (Table 13.2). However, as per the current RNTCP guidelines, there are only two categories: (1) drug-sensitive (including previously treated) and (2) drug-resistant tuberculosis.

Since 2017, in RNTCP, the weekly thrice dosage method has been discontinued, and all patients are given daily drug regimens (Table 13.3) as the weekly dosing increased the chances for drug resistance, relapse, and adverse drug reactions [80, 81]. In RNTCP, TB drugs for the entire course of treatment are supplied in an

Table 13.2 DOTS in India

Category	Type of patient	Regimen
New cases **Category I** **(Red box)**	New sputum smear-positive New sputum smear-negative **New extra-pulmonary(spinal/ osteoarticular)** New others	$2(HRZE)_3$ $+4\ (HR)_3$
Previously treated Category II **(Blue box)**	Sputum smear-positive relapse Sputum smear-positive failure Sputum smear-positive treatment after default Others	$2(HRZES)_3 + 1(HRZE)_3$ $+5\ (HR)_3$

The number before the letters refers to the number of months of treatment, and the subscript refers to the number of doses per week
H-Isoniazid (600 mg), R-Rifampicin (weigh <60 kg-450 mg, weight > 60 yrs-600 mg), Z-Pyrazinamide (1500 mg), E-Ethambutol (1200 mg), S-Streptomycin (age < 50 yrs-750 mg, age > 50 yrs-500 mg)

Table 13.3 RNTCP: New guidelines versus old [82]

Recent guidelines	Old guidelines
Daily regimen	Intermittent regimen
Ethambutol in continuation phase of both Cat I and Cat II regimen	Ethambutol in the continuation phase of only Cat II regimen
Fixed-dose combination as per weight band	No fixed-dose as per weight band
No need for extension of the intensive phase	Extension of intensive phase if sputum smear-positive at the end of intensive phase
Follow-up clinical and laboratory investigation	Follow-up laboratory only
Long-term follow-up up to 2 years	No long-term follow-up

individual patient wise box. Each box contains two pouches. One is for the intensive phase, and the other is for the continuation phase. The patient, wise boxes are color-coded, red boxes for new patients (category 1), and blue boxes for previously treated patients (category 2) (Table 13.4). Pediatric TB patients have separate boxes (Table 13.5). The drugs are issued as a fixed-dose combination (FDC) where two or more drugs are combined in a single pill or tablet at fixed doses. FDC significantly increase adherence and simplify the delivery of DOTS. Fixed-dose combinations of four drugs (Isoniazid, Rifampicin, Pyrazinamide, and Ethambutol), three drugs (Isoniazid, Rifampicin, and Ethambutol), and two drugs (Isoniazid and Rifampicin) are available under RNTCP for five weight bands. The central TB division of India recommends a treatment duration of 12 months, extendable up to 18 months for

Table 13.4 Fixed-dose combination for adults

Weight category	Number of tablets to be consumed	
	Intensive phase	Continuation phase
	HRZE	**HRE**
	75/150/400/275	**75/150/275**
25–34 kg	2	2
35–49 kg	3	3
50–64 kg	4	4
65–75 kg	5	5
>75 kg kg	6	6

Table 13.5 Fixed-dose combination for children

Weight category	Number of tablets to be consumed			
	Intensive phase		Continuation phase	
	HRZ	**E**	**HR**	**E**
	50/75/150	**100**	**50/175**	**100**
4–7 kg	1	1	1	1
8–11 kg	2	2	2	2
12–15 kg	3	3	3	3
16–24 kg	4	4	4	4
25–29 kg	3 + 1A	3	3 + 1A	3
30–39 kg	2 + 2A	2	2 + 2A	2

A = Adult FDC, HRZE-75/150/400/275, HRE-75/150/275

spinal tuberculosis based on clinico-radiological correlation. The first 2 months of intensive phase (HRZE) is followed by continuation phase for 10 months (HRE). The extension of the continuation phase in spinal tuberculosis for a prolonged period is based on expert opinion rather than evidence, and when in doubt regarding treatment response, drug-resistance should be suspected, and a multi-disciplinary approach with an inclusion of an expert in the management of drug-resistant TB is warranted.

13.9 WHO Guidelines

The current WHO recommendations advocate the use of four-drug combination therapy (Isoniazid, Rifampicin, Pyrazinamide, and Ethambutol) during the initiation phase (2 months) and two drug regimens (Isoniazid, Rifampicin) during the continuation phase (10 months) [83]. The same duration of treatment is recommended for children also [84]. In populations with known or suspected high levels of isoniazid resistance, HRE is recommended in the continuation phase as an alternative to HR to reduce drug-resistance development (conditional recommendation, insufficient evidence, expert opinion) [85]. Another recent recommendation was against the use of category II for patients who require retreatment. Patients who had defaulted, failure of treatment, or recurrence have a higher risk of drug resistance and therefore recommend drug sensitivity testing before deciding on the treatment regimen [85, 86].

13.10 Endpoint of Treatment

While multidrug chemotherapy's efficacy is proven, controversy exists regarding the ideal duration of treatment and endpoint. Recent studies evaluating the efficacy of short-course ATT (6 to 9 months) in comparison to 12 months regimen found it to be effective, with no relapses noted at the end of 2 years [87]. The authors have used and recommended a short course regimen (2 months intensive phase, HRZE; 7 months continuation phase, HRE). However, better-designed studies with a large population are required before adopting to a short course regimen.

Radiological healing usually lags behind the clinical response. The decision to stop anti-tubercular therapy or to continue ATT beyond the minimum stipulated time of 9–10 months can be made based on a combination of findings. The findings that suggest healing but does not imply include (1) Clinical well-being—decrease in pain, return to normalcy, weight gain (2) Plain radiographs showing fusion of involved segments and sclerosis of vertebral bodies, (3) decrease in ESR, (4) MRI shows resolution of vertebral edema and abscess (Fig. 13.1). All these factors need to be taken into account before stopping anti-tubercular therapy. It cannot be over-emphasized that the key to successful treatment in tuberculosis is to do drug-sensitivity testing in all possible patients and ensuring compliance.

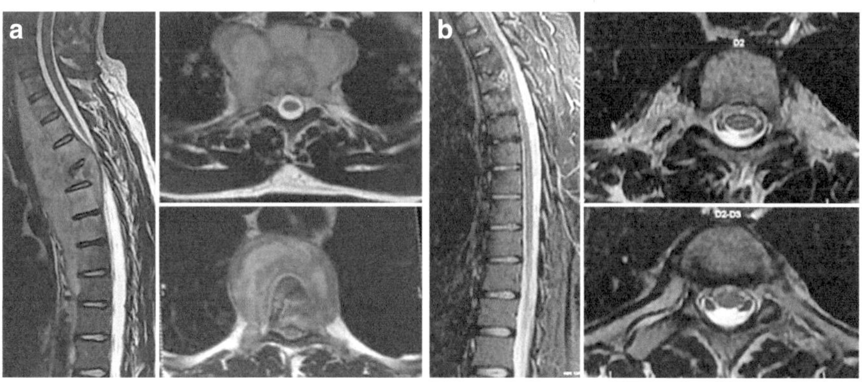

Fig. 13.1 (**a**) Pre-treatment MRI T2-T3 TB spondylodiscitis with a large prevertebral, epidural abscess, vertebral edema, and destruction. (**b**) MRI images after 9 months of multidrug-anti-tubercular therapy show a significant reduction in vertebral edema and complete resolution of abscess, suggesting good healing response

13.11 Conclusion

Multi-drug therapy has significantly revolutionized the treatment of spinal tuberculosis. More patients seek treatment early in the course of the disease, and this has improved the outcomes. The four first-line drugs are the mainstay of treatment. Drug side effects are common and should be closely monitored. In drug-resistant cases, serious efforts of isolating the bacilli in culture and drug sensitivity assessment are critical for good functional outcomes.

Conflict of Interest None of the authors has any conflict of interest.

References

1. Daniel TM. The history of tuberculosis. Respir Med. 2006 Nov;100(11):1862–70.
2. Tuli SM. Tuberculosis of the skeletal system. JP Medical Ltd. 2016;
3. Raviglione MC, O'Brien RJ. Tuberculosis (Chapter 158: pages 1006-1020). Fauci AS, Braunwald E, Kasper DL, Hauser SL, Longo DL, Jamison JL, Loscalzo J Eds Harrison's Principles of Internal Medicine, 17th Edition McGraw-Hill, Inc, New York, USA. 2008.
4. Daniel TM. Hermann Brehmer and the origins of tuberculosis sanatoria. Int J Tuberc Lung Dis. 2011 Feb;15(2):161–2, i.
5. Group BMJP. Treatment of pulmonary tuberculosis with streptomycin and para-amino-salicylic acid: a medical research council investigation. Br Med J. 1950 Nov 11;2(4688):1073–85.
6. Group BMJP. Various combinations of isoniazid with streptomycin or with P.A.S. in the treatment of pulmonary tuberculosis: seventh report to the medical research council. Br Med J. 1955 Feb 19;1(4911):435–45.
7. Controlled clinical trial of four 6-month regimens of chemotherapy for pulmonary tuberculosis. Second report. Second East African/British Medical Research Council Study. Am Rev Respir Dis. 1976 Sep;114(3):471–5.
8. Controlled trial of 6-month and 8-month regimens in the treatment of pulmonary tuberculosis: the results up to 24 months. Tubercle. 1979 Dec;60(4):201–10.
9. British Thoracic Society. A controlled trial of 6 months' chemotherapy in pulmonary tuberculosis Final report: results during the 36 months after the end of chemotherapy and beyond. Br J Dis Chest. 1984 Jan;1(78):330–6.
10. Toman K, Organization WH. Toman's tuberculosis: case detection, treatment, and monitoring : questions and answers. World Health Organization; 2004. 350.
11. Five-year follow-up of a controlled trial of five 6-month regimens of chemotherapy for pulmonary tuberculosis. Hong Kong Chest Service/British Medical Research Council. Am Rev Respir Dis. 1987 Dec;136(6):1339–42.
12. Controlled trial of 2, 4, and 6 months of pyrazinamide in 6-month, three-times-weekly regimens for smear-positive pulmonary tuberculosis, including an assessment of a combined preparation of isoniazid, rifampin, and pyrazinamide. Results at 30 months. Hong Kong Chest Service/British Medical Research Council. Am Rev Respir Dis. 1991 Apr;143(4 Pt 1):700–6.
13. Grumbach F, Canetti G, Grosset J, le Lirzin M. Late results of long-term intermittent chemotherapy of advanced, murine tuberculosis: limits of the murine model. Tubercle. 1967 Mar;48(1):11–26.
14. Lotte A, Hatton F, Perdrizet S, Rouillon A. A concurrent comparison of intermittent (Twice-Weekly) Isoniazid Plus Streptomycin and daily Isoniazid plus PAS in the domiciliary treatment of Pulmonary Tuberculosis; Tuberculosis Chemotherapy Centre. Madras Bull World Health Organ. 1964;31:247–71.

15. Vilchèze C, Jacobs WR. The mechanism of isoniazid killing: clarity through the scope of genetics. Annu Rev Microbiol. 2007;61:35–50.
16. Pansy F, Stander H, Donovick R. In vitro studies on isonicotinic acid hydrazide. Am Rev Tuberc. 1952 Jun;65(6):761–4.
17. Mitchison DA, Selkon JB. The bactericidal activities of antituberculous drugs. Am Rev Tuberc. 1956 Aug;74(2 Part 2):109–16.
18. Middlebrook G. Sterilization of tubercle bacilli by isonicotinic acid hydrazide and the incidence of variants resistant to the drug in vitro. Am Rev Tuberc. 1952 Jun;65(6):765–7.
19. Schaefer WB. The effect of isoniazid on growing and resting tubercle bacilli. Am Rev Tuberc. 1954 Jan;69(1):125–7.
20. Unissa AN, Subbian S, Hanna LE, Selvakumar N. Overview on mechanisms of isoniazid action and resistance in Mycobacterium tuberculosis. Infect Genet Evol. 2016 Nov;1(45):474–92.
21. Hazbón MH, Brimacombe M, Bobadilla del Valle M, Cavatore M, Guerrero MI, Varma-Basil M, et al. Population genetics study of isoniazid resistance mutations and evolution of multidrug-resistant Mycobacterium tuberculosis. Antimicrob Agents Chemother. 2006 Aug;50(8):2640–9.
22. Blanchard JS. Molecular mechanisms of drug resistance in Mycobacterium tuberculosis. Annu Rev Biochem. 1996;65:215–39.
23. Campbell EA, Korzheva N, Mustaev A, Murakami K, Nair S, Goldfarb A, et al. Structural Mechanism for Rifampicin Inhibition of Bacterial RNA Polymerase. Cell. 2001 Mar 23;104(6):901–12.
24. Mitchison DA. Basic mechanisms of chemotherapy. Chest. 1979 Dec;76(6 Suppl):771–81.
25. Ramaswamy S, Musser JM. Molecular genetic basis of antimicrobial agent resistance in Mycobacterium tuberculosis: 1998 update. Tuber Lung Dis. 1998;79(1):3–29.
26. Konno K, Feldmann FM, McDermott W. Pyrazinamide susceptibility and amidase activity of tubercle bacilli. Am Rev Respir Dis. 1967 Mar;95(3):461–9.
27. McDermott W, Tompsett R. Activation of pyrazinamide and nicotinamide in acidic environments in vitro. Am Rev Tuberc. 1954 Oct;70(4):748–54.
28. Scorpio A, Lindholm-Levy P, Heifets L, Gilman R, Siddiqi S, Cynamon M, et al. Characterization of pncA mutations in pyrazinamide-resistant Mycobacterium tuberculosis. Antimicrob Agents Chemother. 1997 Mar;41(3):540–3.
29. Juréen P, Werngren J, Toro J-C, Hoffner S. Pyrazinamide resistance and pncA gene mutations in Mycobacterium tuberculosis. Antimicrob Agents Chemother. 2008 May;52(5):1852–4.
30. Takayama K, Armstrong EL, Kunugi KA, Kilburn JO. Inhibition by ethambutol of mycolic acid transfer into the cell wall of Mycobacterium smegmatis. Antimicrob Agents Chemother. 1979 Aug;16(2):240–2.
31. Telenti A, Philipp WJ, Sreevatsan S, Bernasconi C, Stockbauer KE, Wieles B, et al. The emb operon, a gene cluster of Mycobacterium tuberculosis involved in resistance to ethambutol. Nat Med. 1997 May;3(5):567–70.
32. Moazed D, Noller HF. Interaction of antibiotics with functional sites in 16S ribosomal RNA. Nature. 1987 Jun 4;327(6121):389–94.
33. Finken M, Kirschner P, Meier A, Wrede A, Böttger EC. Molecular basis of streptomycin resistance in Mycobacterium tuberculosis: alterations of the ribosomal protein S12 gene and point mutations within a functional 16S ribosomal RNA pseudoknot. Mol Microbiol. 1993 Sep;9(6):1239–46.
34. Almeida Da Silva PE, Palomino JC. Molecular basis and mechanisms of drug resistance in Mycobacterium tuberculosis: classical and new drugs. J Antimicrob Chemother. 2011 Jul 1;66(7):1417–30.
35. Bartlett JG, Dowell SF, Mandell LA, File TM, Musher DM, Fine MJ. Practice guidelines for the management of community-acquired pneumonia in adults. Infectious Diseases Society of America. Clin Infect Dis. 2000 Aug;31(2):347–82.
36. Wang J-Y, Hsueh P-R, Jan I-S, Lee L-N, Liaw Y-S, Yang P-C, et al. Empirical treatment with a fluoroquinolone delays the treatment for tuberculosis and is associated with a poor prognosis in endemic areas. Thorax. 2006 Oct;61(10):903–8.

37. Ginsburg AS, Grosset JH, Bishai WR. Fluoroquinolones, tuberculosis, and resistance. Lancet Infect Dis. 2003 Jul;3(7):432–42.
38. Stanley RE, Blaha G, Grodzicki RL, Strickler MD, Steitz TA. The structures of the anti-tuberculosis antibiotics viomycin and capreomycin bound to the 70S ribosome. Nat Struct Mol Biol. 2010 Mar;17(3):289–93.
39. Alangaden GJ, Kreiswirth BN, Aouad A, Khetarpal M, Igno FR, Moghazeh SL, et al. Mechanism of resistance to amikacin and kanamycin in Mycobacterium tuberculosis. Antimicrob Agents Chemother. 1998 May;42(5):1295–7.
40. Via LE, Cho S-N, Hwang S, Bang H, Park SK, Kang HS, et al. Polymorphisms associated with resistance and cross-resistance to aminoglycosides and capreomycin in mycobacterium tuberculosis Isolates from South Korean patients with drug-resistant tuberculosis. J Clin Microbiol. 2010 Feb;48(2):402–11.
41. Migliori GB, Lange C, Centis R, Sotgiu G, Mütterlein R, Hoffmann H, et al. Resistance to second-line injectables and treatment outcomes in multidrug-resistant and extensively drug-resistant tuberculosis cases. Eur Respir J. 2008 Jun 1;31(6):1155–9.
42. WHO | Guidelines for the programmatic management of drug-resistant tuberculosis [Internet]. WHO. World Health Organization; [cited 2021 Jan 30]. Available from: https://www.who.int/tb/publications/tb-drugresistant-guidelines/en/
43. WHO | Companion handbook to the WHO guidelines for the programmatic management of drug-resistant tuberculosis [Internet]. WHO. World Health Organization; [cited 2021 Jan 30]. Available from: http://www.who.int/tb/publications/pmdt_companionhandbook/en/
44. Banerjee A, Dubnau E, Quemard A, Balasubramanian V, Um KS, Wilson T, et al. inhA, a gene encoding a target for isoniazid and ethionamide in Mycobacterium tuberculosis. Science. 1994 Jan 14;263(5144):227–30.
45. Koul A, Dendouga N, Vergauwen K, Molenberghs B, Vranckx L, Willebrords R, et al. Diarylquinolines target subunit c of mycobacterial ATP synthase. Nat Chem Biol. 2007 Jun;3(6):323–4.
46. Provisional CDC Guidelines for the Use and Safety Monitoring of Bedaquiline Fumarate (Sirturo) for the Treatment of Multidrug-Resistant Tuberculosis [Internet]. [cited 2021 Jan 30]. Available from: https://www.cdc.gov/mmwr/preview/mmwrhtml/rr6209a1.htm?s_cid=rr6209a1_e
47. Veziris N, Bernard C, Guglielmetti L, Du DL, Marigot-Outtandy D, Jaspard M, et al. Rapid emergence of Mycobacterium tuberculosis bedaquiline resistance: lessons to avoid repeating past errors. European Respiratory Journal [Internet] 2017 Mar 1 [cited 2021 Jan 30];49(3). Available from: https://erj.ersjournals.com/content/49/3/1601719
48. Xavier AS, Lakshmanan M. Delamanid: A new armor in combating drug-resistant tuberculosis. J Pharmacol Pharmacother. 2014;5(3):222–4.
49. Blair HA, Scott LJ. Delamanid: a review of its use in patients with multidrug-resistant tuberculosis. Drugs. 2015 Jan;75(1):91–100.
50. von Groote-Bidlingmaier F, Patientia R, Sanchez E, Balanag V, Ticona E, Segura P, et al. Efficacy and safety of delamanid in combination with an optimised background regimen for treatment of multidrug-resistant tuberculosis: a multicentre, randomised, double-blind, placebo-controlled, parallel group phase 3 trial. Lancet Respir Med. 2019 Mar 1;7(3):249–59.
51. WHO | WHO position statement on the use of delamanid for multidrug-resistant tuberculosis [Internet]. WHO. World Health Organization; [cited 2021 Jan 30]. Available from: http://www.who.int/tb/publications/2018/Position_Paper_Delamanid/en/
52. American Thoracic Society. Diagnostic standards and classification of tuberculosis. Am Rev Respir Dis. 1990 Sep;142(3):725–35.
53. Nell AS, D'lom E, Bouic P, Sabaté M, Bosser R, Picas J, et al. Safety, tolerability, and immunogenicity of the novel antituberculous vaccine RUTI: randomized, placebo-controlled phase II clinical trial in patients with latent tuberculosis infection. PLoS One. 2014 Feb 26;9(2):e89612.
54. Ji Y, Wang X, Donnelly RJ, Uskokovic MR, Studzinski GP. Signaling of monocytic differentiation by a non-hypercalcemic analog of vitamin D3, 1,25(OH)2-5,6 trans-16-ene-vitamin

D3, involves nuclear vitamin D receptor (nVDR) and non-nVDR-mediated pathways. J Cell Physiol. 2002 May;191(2):198–207.
55. Liu PT, Stenger S, Li H, Wenzel L, Tan BH, Krutzik SR, et al. Toll-like receptor triggering of a vitamin D-mediated human antimicrobial response. Science. 2006 Mar 24;311(5768):1770–3.
56. Martineau AR, Wilkinson KA, Newton SM, Floto RA, Norman AW, Skolimowska K, et al. IFN-γ- and TNF-independent vitamin D-inducible human suppression of mycobacteria: the role of cathelicidin LL-37. J Immunol. 2007 Jun 1;178(11):7190–8.
57. Sørensen OE, Follin P, Johnsen AH, Calafat J, Tjabringa GS, Hiemstra PS, et al. Human cathelicidin, hCAP-18, is processed to the antimicrobial peptide LL-37 by extracellular cleavage with proteinase 3. Blood. 2001 Jun 15;97(12):3951–9.
58. Yuk J-M, Shin D-M, Lee H-M, Yang C-S, Jin HS, Kim K-K, et al. Vitamin D3 induces autophagy in human monocytes/macrophages via cathelicidin. Cell Host Microbe. 2009 Sep 17;6(3):231–43.
59. Yang C-S, Shin D-M, Kim K-H, Lee Z-W, Lee C-H, Park SG, et al. NADPH oxidase 2 interaction with TLR2 is required for efficient innate immune responses to mycobacteria via cathelicidin expression. J Immunol. 2009 Mar 15;182(6):3696–705.
60. Agarwal S, Reddy GV, Reddanna P. Eicosanoids in inflammation and cancer: the role of COX-2. Expert Rev Clin Immunol. 2009 Mar;5(2):145–65.
61. Tobin DM, Ramakrishnan L. TB: the Yin and Yang of lipid mediators. Curr Opin Pharmacol. 2013 Aug;13(4):641–5.
62. Vilaplana C, Marzo E, Tapia G, Diaz J, Garcia V, Cardona P-J. Ibuprofen therapy resulted in significantly decreased tissue bacillary loads and increased survival in a new murine experimental model of active tuberculosis. J Infect Dis. 2013 Jul 15;208(2):199–202.
63. Berger W, De Chandt MTM, Cairns CB. Zileuton: clinical implications of 5-Lipoxygenase inhibition in severe airway disease. Int J Clin Pract. 2007 Apr;61(4):663–76.
64. Mayer-Barber KD, Andrade BB, Oland SD, Amaral EP, Barber DL, Gonzales J, et al. Host-directed therapy of tuberculosis based on interleukin-1 and type I interferon crosstalk. Nature. 2014 Jul 3;511(7507):99–103.
65. Chatterjee S, Nutman TB. Helminth-induced immune regulation: implications for immune responses to tuberculosis. PLoS Pathog. 2015 Jan 29;11(1):e1004582.
66. Abate E, Belayneh M, Idh J, Diro E, Elias D, Britton S, et al. Asymptomatic helminth infection in active tuberculosis is associated with increased regulatory and Th-2 responses and a lower sputum smear positivity. PLoS Negl Trop Dis [Internet]. 2015; Aug 6 [cited 2021 Jan 20];9(8). Available from: https://www.ncbi.nlm.nih.gov/pmc/articles/PMC4527760/
67. Schroder K, Hertzog PJ, Ravasi T, Hume DA. Interferon-gamma: an overview of signals, mechanisms and functions. J Leukoc Biol. 2004 Feb;75(2):163–89.
68. Condos R, Raju B, Canova A, Zhao B-Y, Weiden M, Rom WN, et al. Recombinant gamma interferon stimulates signal transduction and gene expression in alveolar macrophages in vitro and in tuberculosis patients. Infect Immun. 2003 Apr 1;71(4):2058–64.
69. Giosué S, Casarini M, Alemanno L, Galluccio G, Mattia P, Pedicelli G, et al. Effects of aerosolized interferon-alpha in patients with pulmonary tuberculosis. Am J Respir Crit Care Med. 1998 Oct;158(4):1156–62.
70. Palmero D, Eiguchi K, Rendo P, Castro Zorrilla L, Abbate E, González Montaner LJ. Phase II trial of recombinant interferon-alpha2b in patients with advanced intractable multidrug-resistant pulmonary tuberculosis: long-term follow-up. Int J Tuberc Lung Dis. 1999 Mar;3(3):214–8.
71. Pedral-Sampaio DB, Netto EM, Brites C, Bandeira AC, Guerra C, Barberin MG, et al. Use of Rhu-GM-CSF in pulmonary tuberculosis patients: results of a randomized clinical trial. Braz J Infect Dis. 2003 Aug;7(4):245–52.
72. Jurado JO, Alvarez IB, Pasquinelli V, Martínez GJ, Quiroga MF, Abbate E, et al. Programmed death (PD)-1:PD-ligand 1/PD-ligand 2 pathway inhibits T cell effector functions during human tuberculosis. J Immunol. 2008 Jul 1;181(1):116–25.

73. Hassan SS, Akram M, King EC, Dockrell HM, Cliff JM. PD-1, PD-L1 and PD-L2 Gene expression on T-cells and natural killer cells declines in conjunction with a reduction in PD-1 protein during the intensive phase of tuberculosis treatment. PLoS One. 2015;10(9):e0137646.
74. Singh A, Mohan A, Dey AB, Mitra DK. Inhibiting the programmed death 1 pathway rescues Mycobacterium tuberculosis-specific interferon γ-producing T cells from apoptosis in patients with pulmonary tuberculosis. J Infect Dis. 2013 Aug 15;208(4):603–15.
75. Merlo A, Saverino D, Tenca C, Grossi CE, Bruno S, Ciccone E. CD85/LIR-1/ILT2 and CD152 (cytotoxic T lymphocyte antigen 4) inhibitory molecules down-regulate the cytolytic activity of human CD4+ T-cell clones specific for Mycobacterium tuberculosis. Infect Immun. 2001 Oct;69(10):6022–9.
76. García Jacobo RE, Serrano CJ, Enciso Moreno JA, Gaspar Ramírez O, Trujillo Ochoa JL, Uresti Rivera EE, et al. Analysis of Th1, Th17 and regulatory T cells in tuberculosis case contacts. Cell Immunol. 2014 Jun;289(1–2):167–73.
77. Sada-Ovalle I, Chávez-Galán L, Torre-Bouscoulet L, Nava-Gamiño L, Barrera L, Jayaraman P, et al. The Tim3-galectin 9 pathway induces antibacterial activity in human macrophages infected with Mycobacterium tuberculosis. J Immunol. 2012 Dec 15;189(12):5896–902.
78. Sada-Ovalle I, Ocaña-Guzman R, Pérez-Patrigeón S, Chávez-Galán L, Sierra-Madero J, Torre-Bouscoulet L, et al. Tim-3 blocking rescue macrophage and T cell function against Mycobacterium tuberculosis infection in HIV+ patients. J Int AIDS Soc [Internet]. 2015; Oct 19 [cited 2021 Jan 18];18(1). Available from: https://www.ncbi.nlm.nih.gov/pmc/articles/PMC4612469/
79. Arora A, Nadkarni B, Dev G, Chattopadhya D, Jain AK, Tuli SM, et al. The use of immunomodulators as an adjunct to antituberculous chemotherapy in non-responsive patients with osteo-articular tuberculosis. J Bone Joint Surg. 2006 Feb 1;88-B(2):264–9.
80. Chang KC, Leung CC, Yew WW, Ho SC, Tam CM. A nested case-control study on treatment-related risk factors for early relapse of tuberculosis. Am J Respir Crit Care Med. 2004 Nov 15;170(10):1124–30.
81. Chang KC, Leung CC, Grosset J, Yew WW. Treatment of tuberculosis and optimal dosing schedules. Thorax. 2011 Nov 1;66(11):997–1007.
82. Chaudhuri. Recent changes in technical and operational guidelines for tuberculosis control programme in India–2016: A paradigm shift in tuberculosis control [Internet]. [cited 2021 Mar 15]. Available from: https://www.jacpjournal.org/article.asp?issn=2320-8775;year=2017;volume=5;issue=1;spage=1;epage=9;aulast=Chaudhuri
83. India WHOCO for. Index-TB guidelines: guidelines on extra-pulmonary tuberculosis in India. 2016 [cited 2021 Jan 29.]; Available from: https://apps.who.int/iris/handle/10665/278953
84. Organization WH. Rapid advice : treatment of tuberculosis in children [Internet]. World Health. Organization. 2010; [cited 2021 Jan 29]. Available from: https://apps.who.int/iris/handle/10665/44444
85. WHO | Guidelines for treatment of drug-susceptible tuberculosis and patient care (2017 update) [Internet]. WHO. World Health Organization; [cited 2021 Jan 29]. Available from: http://www.who.int/tb/publications/2017/dstb_guidance_2017/en/
86. Azhar GS. DOTS for TB relapse in India: A systematic review. Lung India. 2012 Apr 1;29(2):147.
87. Nene AM, Patil S, Kathare AP, Nagad P, Nene A, Kapadia F. Six versus 12 months of anti tubercular therapy in patients with biopsy proven spinal tuberculosis: a single center, open labeled, prospective randomized clinical trial-A Pilot study. Spine (Phila Pa 1976). 2019 Jan 1;44(1):E1–6.

Chapter 14
Multidrug Resistance and Extensively Drug-Resistant Tuberculosis: Diagnosis and Management Protocols

Vinay Jasani, Ahmed Abdelaal, and Mohamed Mohamed

Abstract Since the inception of the first antituberculous chemotherapeutic agent, drug resistance has been one of the most challenging problems facing the global fight to control tuberculosis. Drug resistance to antituberculous chemotherapy is a spectrum which includes mono-drug resistance (e.g. rifampicin resistance), multi-drug resistance (MDR), extensively drug resistant (XDR), and finally total drug resistance (TDR). Clinical suspicion of drug resistance is a crucial step in managing tuberculosis patients. Nevertheless, the diagnosis of MDR/XDR is purely a microbiological diagnosis, based on bacteriological and molecular testing. Surveillance programs for drug resistance among tuberculosis patients, the development of advanced diagnostic tools, and the subsequent formulation of management algorithms have rendered detection and cure of such a formidable challenge a possibility.

Keywords Tuberculosis · Spine · Multidrug resistance · Extensively drug resistant MDR · XDR

14.1 Definitions and Historical Perspective

Tuberculosis (TB) and tuberculous spondylitis (TB spine) is a disease that has been affecting humans over millennia. Features consistent with TB meningitis have been postulated in *Homo erectus* fossils from Turkey [1]. Tuberculous spondylitis has been identified using DNA analysis in Eastern Mediterranean human remains dating back to 9000 BCE [2]. The modern progression of this ancient affliction is the emergence of multidrug-resistant TB, a global health concern.

V. Jasani (✉) · A. Abdelaal · M. Mohamed
Department of Spine Surgery, University Hospital of North Midlands NHS Trust, Newcastle under Lyme, UK
e-mail: Vinay.jasani@uhnm.nhs.uk

S. S. Dhatt, V. Kumar (eds.), *Tuberculosis of the Spine*,
https://doi.org/10.1007/978-981-16-9495-0_14

Table 14.1 Drug resistance categories

Monoresistance describes resistance to only one first-line anti-TB drugs. Rifampicin resistance (RR) or isoniazid resistance with rifampicin susceptibility (Hr) are examples of monoresistance.
Multidrug resistance (MDR) is used to describe mycobacteria exhibiting resistance to both rifampicin and isoniazid.
Extensively drug resistant (XDR) was coined in 2006 to describe strains of MDR-TB resistant to fluoroquinolone and at least one of the three second-line injectable drugs (capreomycin, kanamycin, and amikacin) [6].
Rifampicin resistance (RR) describes resistance to rifampicin, whether this is monoresistance, MDR, or XDR.

Antimicrobial resistance is defined as the condition when infective organisms change over time and no longer respond to medicines making infections more difficult to treat and increasing the risk of disease spread, severe illness, and death [3]. Mycobacterium TB can be classified into drug-sensitive infections amenable to treatment with first line of anti-TB treatment (ATT), or drug-resistant infections.

The discovery of streptomycin by Waksman in 1943 marked the beginning of the modern era in the treatment of tuberculosis (TB). Its first use in the treatment of TB bone and joint lesions was published by Bosworth in 1950 [4]. However, the biological phenomenon of drug resistance was soon observed in the laboratory when patients started to excrete bacilli that were resistant to streptomycin [5]. With the emergence of new anti-TB drugs over the following decade, it became clear that a combination of multiple agents of a longer duration was needed to prevent the potential for resistance to a single agent.

Examining the evolution of drug resistance in TB reveals two distinct patterns: primary and secondary. Primary resistance is defined as infection with a drug-resistant organism in a previously untreated patient. Resistance developing during the course of treatment in a patient with an initially drug-sensitive infection is termed secondary resistance. These two patterns require different approaches in the management of patients as well as in managing an epidemic.

The World Health Organization (WHO) has recently described different types of drug resistance classified in categories based on drug susceptibility testing (DST) of clinical isolates confirmed to be *M. tuberculosis* [3]. These categories are summarised in Table 14.1.

14.2 Incidence

According to the WHO global TB report in 2020, there were an estimated 465,000 (range, 400,000–535,000) incident cases of rifampicin-resistant TB, of which 78% had multidrug-resistant TB. The burden of multidrug- or rifampicin-resistant TB (MDR/RR-TB) as a share of the number of TB cases remains stable. In 2019, an estimated 3.3% of new TB cases (primary resistance) and 18% of previously treated cases (secondary resistance) had MDR/RR-TB [3].

Data on resistance to fluoroquinolones have been collected over the past 15 years in some countries. Among these countries, the proportion of MDR-TB cases with resistance to any fluoroquinolone for which testing was done was approximately 20%. However, these figures should be interpreted with caution as they are likely to be underestimated.

The geographical distribution of cases of MDR-TB shows that approximately 50% of the global burden is accounted for by 3 countries. The countries are India (27%), China (14%), and the Russian Federation (8%). The highest incidences of new and previously treated MDR-TB cases at the country level are in several of the former Soviet Union countries (above 20% in new cases and above 50% in previously treated cases) [3]. Globally, a significant proportion of MDR-TB cases have never been treated for TB before, implying human to human transmission [7].

Periodic national surveys conducted every 5 years represent the most common approach to investigating the burden of drug resistance in resource-limited countries. However, since the launch of the Global Project on Anti-TB Drug Resistance Surveillance in 1994, the establishment of continuous surveillance systems has offered the benefits of rapid detection of outbreaks, real-time monitoring of the effectiveness of interventions, and an understanding of trends.

TB spine specifically accounts for 0.5% of the burden of all TB cases. If we extrapolate from limited data on global estimates of MDR-TB, the likelihood is of 1000–5000 cases of MDR-TB spine annually. A prevalence study in India over 9 years identified a 4.9% prevalence MDR-TB spine and 0.4% XDR TB spine in a retrospective cohort of 730 cases of TB spine [8]. A number of published reports include children with MDR / XDR TB spine. Although the exact incidence of MDR/XDR TB spine in children is unknown, approximately 3% of all childhood TB is MDR [9].

14.3 Causes of Drug Resistance

In an attempt to overcome the problem of the emergence of drug resistance to single agents, multiple drugs became the key in the treatment of TB. Initial combination chemotherapy regimens required 18 months of treatment. Unsurprisingly, compliance to treatment protocols was one of the major challenges to treatment. Trials by the Medical Research Council (MRC) of the UK showed that shorter courses could be equally effective in spinal TB [10]. This has paved the way for the introduction of the directly observed treatment short course (DOTS) by the WHO as part of the global initiative to control TB. The implementation of these regimens worldwide, even in resource-limited settings, ensured adherence to treatment protocols by providing supervised treatment by a healthcare worker.

Despite the global efforts and the advances gained in surveillance and preventative measures, drug resistance in TB patients continues to be a major challenge to treatment. Potential factors facilitating the global emergence of drug-resistant TB include the following:

- *Inappropriate treatment regimens:* Arbitrary treatment protocols contribute to the development of drug resistance. In 2010, Udwadia et al. evaluated prescription patterns between private practitioners in Mumbai, India [11]. They found that only six out of 106 practitioners who responded used the correct drug protocol. The lackadaisical overuse of the antibiotics in TB has led to the sequential accumulation of resistance mutations of the mycobacteria in patients who are receiving inadequate treatment.
- *Spread of resistant strains:* Current surveillance systems in different countries indicate that 3.3% of new TB cases in 2019 had RR/MDR-TB as compared to 18% of the previously treated cases [3]. Lin et al. in 2011 examined the spatiotemporal distribution of TB patients with different drug resistance phenotypes. They noticed increased geographical aggregation of MDR in TB patients without previous treatment. They attributed the emergence of transmissible drug-resistant strains as a possible cause [12].
- *Facility-based transmission:* Despite better adherence to treatment, patients who began their TB therapy in a hospital setting or who were hospitalised during the course of their treatment had a significantly higher risk of developing drug resistance than those who were treated as outpatients [13]. Similarly, being a prisoner while receiving TB therapy was strongly associated (OR 4.4) with developing drug resistance [14].
- *Amplifier effect of DOTS:* The implementation of the DOTS strategy in the presence of drug resistance can paradoxically exacerbate the problem, a phenomenon described as the amplifier effect of short course chemotherapy [6]. Failure to recognise pre-treatment resistance to one first-line agent and the continued repeated use of DOTS results in developing resistance to all first-line anti-TB drugs [15].

In addition, there does seem to be a genetic susceptibility in humans with strong associations between HLA-DRB1*08032-DQB1*0601, HLA-DRB1*13, and HLA-DRB1*14 and MDR-TB [16, 17].

On a cellular level, *Mycobacterium tuberculosis* is characterised by a low mutation rate (about 2×10^{-10}mutations/bacterial population/generation). Despite this, the case load of MDR and XDR TB due to mutations is considerable worldwide. Both mathematical and clinical models have shown that the actual rate of drug-resistant mutations is higher than in theoretical predictions. The selection pressure of incomplete treatment or variable drug penetrance in lesions resulting in sublethal drug doses seems to be a driver for mutations as in other bacterial species [18]. The diverse gene mutations causing MDR and XDR TB have been sequenced and identified (Table 14.2).

Table 14.2 Genes associated with drug resistance and mutation frequency for each gene in clinical isolates of Mycobacterium tuberculosis

Drug	Gene	Mutation frequency in isolates %
Rifampicin	rpoB encoding for b-subunit of RNA polymerase	90–100
Isoniazid	katG encoding for catalase-peroxidase inhA encoding for fatty acid enoyl acyl carrier protein reductase A (Inh)	40–97 8–64
Ethambutol	embB encoding for arabinosyl transferase	47–89
Pyrazinamide	pncA encoding for pyrazinamidase	44–97
Streptomycin	rrs encoding for 16S rRNA subunit rpsL encoding for S12 ribosomal protein gidB encoding for 7-methylguanosine methyltransferase	12–26 40–68 5–13
Amikacin, kanamycin, capreomycin	rrs encoding for 16S rRNA	40–90
Kanamycin	eis encoding for aminoglycoside acetyltransferase	28–80
Capreomycin	tlyA encoding for 20-O- methyltransferase	4–13
Ofloxacin, levofloxacin, moxifloxacin, gatifloxacin	gyrA encoding for DNA gyrase subunit A gyrB encoding for DNA gyrase subunit B	70–90 0–11
Ethionamide	inhA encoding for fatty acid enoyl acyl carrier protein reductase A (InhA) ethA encoding for EthA ethR encoding for transcriptional repressor EthR, NADH-ACP	33–62 46–72 0–4

Table 14.3 Clinical risk factors for MDR-TB

Failure to respond to a first-line DOTS regimen (WHO Category I or II)
Relapse after a full course of treatment with a first-line regimen
Treatment after defaulting from treatment with a first-line regimen
Exposure to a known case of MDR-TB
Exposure to TB in institutions with high prevalence of MDR-TB, such as a prison or hospital
Living in areas or countries with high prevalence of MDR-TB
HIV coinfection
Failure of bony healing, new active sites or abscesses and or continued sinus discharge after 4–5 months of multiple antitubercular treatment

14.4 Diagnosis of MDR and XDR

Clinical suspicion is important in diagnosing drug resistance to anti-TB medications during the course of treatment (Table 14.3). The most significant indicator of the development of drug resistance is failure of treatment. Additionally, drug-resistant TB should always be suspected in those with social contact with MDR or

XDR patients because of the risk of new infection with a resistant strain. Similarly, healthcare workers who are involved in treating patients with TB via the DOTS strategy are at higher risk. Also, there is a higher prevalence of MDR and XDR TB among HIV patients. The WHO currently recommends HIV testing for all patients of all ages who present with symptoms suggestive of TB, irrespective of the epidemiological setting.

For MDR/XDR TB spine, clinical features would include spinal pain, deformity, and/or neurological compromise as would be manifest in non-drug resistant TB spine. It would be the failure to respond to treatment that would be the additional diagnostic feature triggering a suspicion for MDR/XDR TB spine.

Additional diagnostic adjuncts specific to TB spine aim to improve an understanding of the impact of the disease on that individual and help any interventional planning including biopsy.

Basic laboratory tests including full blood count and erythrocyte sedimentation rate are valuable as in non-drug resistant TB. An assessment of nutritional status should also be established to allow optimisation.

Imaging studies of value would include weight-bearing radiographs to assess deformity (whole spine standing images are preferable where available). Magnetic resonance imaging of the whole spine will provide evidence of skip lesions, the extent of abscess cavity, bony destruction and compromise of the space available for the neural elements, and healing progress. Computerised tomography of the affected area of the spine may also provide additional information on bony destruction as well as planning for biopsy or surgery.

For osseous and spine TB, it has been suggested that after 4–5 months of multiple antitubercular treatment, failure of progressive clinical or radiological bony healing, formation of additional active tubercular foci, increase in size or appearance of new cold abscesses, and continued discharge of sinuses all point to MDR/XDR-TB [19, 20].

However, the final definitive diagnosis of drug resistance must be based on drug susceptibility testing (DST) and is not a clinical or radiological diagnosis. Two methods are available for testing drug resistance of mycobacterium tuberculosis: phenotypic (or culture-based) and genotypic (or molecular).

As TB spine is usually paucibacillary, traditional cultures using Lowenstein Jensen medium can have a low yield (50%) and a long time until diagnosis (around 3–6 weeks). Other culture methods including BACTEC-46, BACTEC MGIT-96, and Septi-Chek AFB have shorter times to detection (12–15 days) and over 90% yield if smear positive [21]. Once the culture is positive, DST can be carried out on the culture over a 3-week period. Due to the low yield and long time to results, molecular methods are being favoured over culture methods.

Molecular methods have revolutionised the diagnosis of MDR/XDR TB. These methods use polymerase chain reaction techniques to detect drug-resistance mutations of the mycobacterium DNA or RNA [22]. They are much faster and have higher sensitivity than culture-based methods. Hence, it is not routinely necessary to confirm the results of a positive molecular DST with culture-based DST. Increasing access to molecular testing is one of the main components of the WHO's End TB

Strategy. In 2010, WHO endorsed the use of Xpert®MTB/RIF (Cepheid, Sunnyvale, USA) gene probe for RR as it has good sensitivity and specificity and at the same time can provide a rapid confirmation of TB and RR in less than 2 hours. Due to low sensitivity in smear-negative and HIV-positive patients, the Xpert®MTB/RIF Ultra (Cepheid, Sunnyvale, USA) was developed as the next-generation assay to overcome these limitations. These assays have been recommended for diagnosing extrapulmonary TB and rifampicin resistance by the WHO in 2020.

Line-probe assays (to look for multiple drug resistance) are also available. Hain Genotype®MTBDRplus is another WHO-endorsed test that has high sensitivity and specificity for TB and resistance to rifampicin and isoniazid. Line-probe assays such as Genotype®MTBDRsl provide the only currently available molecular routine test to detect resistance to fluoroquinolones, injectable drugs, and ethambutol. Nipro NTM þ MDRTB detection kit 2 endorsed by the WHO in 2016 detects resistance to rifampicin, isoniazid, pyrazinamide, and fluoroquinolones.

Next-generation sequencing and targeted-gene sequencing are developing advanced molecular diagnostics which can study the genotype of the bacteria in a single run. Some of these techniques are being trialled to detect drug resistance in TB.

For TB spine, these assays would generally need to be performed on tissue samples or cultures unless concurrent pulmonary TB provided sputum samples.

In the latest consolidated guidelines on the management of drug-resistant TB, the WHO strongly recommends the use of molecular DST as an initial test to detect at least rifampicin resistance before the initiation of therapy for TB [3]. Although molecular testing is still not widely available in resource-limited countries, increasing availability might allow for this "universal DST" to screen for drug resistance in all patients undergoing any TB treatment. The WHO recommends that any MDR-TB patient should also be additionally tested for XDR.

Tissue sampling is imperative when MDR/XDR TB spine is suspected. CT-guided biopsy gives the best diagnostic yield and should be considered first unless surgery is a priority intervention for other reasons, in which case an open biopsy can be undertaken. CT-guided biopsy has a diagnostic yield of 60–75.8% for TB generally, including MDR/XDR TB [23, 24]. Samples of pus and granulation tissue seem to have higher phenotypic and genotypic yield when compared with necrotic caseous tissue [25]. Pus and granulation tissue samples should be sent for AFB smear, liquid culture, histological analysis, and molecular testing.

Diagnostic tools are summarised in Table 14.4.

Table 14.4 Diagnostic flow for MDR/XDR TB spine

Clinical suspicion – document ALL previous drug regimen
Standing spine radiograph
MRI whole spine with sagittal STIR, T1 and T2 sequences; T1 and T2 axials of abnormal areas. Contrast-enhanced studies may provide additional information
CT scan of affected part
Percutaneous (CT-guided) or open biopsy for pus and granulation tissue
DST (culture methods, molecular testing, and/or sequencing technologies)

Effective treatment varies according to the drug resistance patterns as described previously. Failure to identify resistance to a particular agent carries the potential risk of prescribing ineffective treatment and amplifying drug resistance, with a subsequent decrease in the likelihood of successful treatment outcome.

14.5 Medical Treatment

A discussion of treatment of MDR-TB should include a discussion about prevention. The factors giving rise to MDR-TB outlined previously would logically be the factors to tackle it to prevent drug resistance. Principles of medical management of MDR/XDR are summarised in Table 14.5.

Rapid diagnosis and completion of multidrug treatment of TB can help prevent resistance developing. Contact tracing and even isolation of established MDR/XDR cases could also help prevent spread of drug resistance [26]. HIV/AIDS patients with TB should be diagnosed and treated as soon as possible as they lack immunity and are at greater risk of developing drug resistance.

The mainstay of treatment after establishing a diagnosis is going to be medical. Drug treatment was initially not successful due to the use of drugs developed decades previously with side effects that are hard to tolerate. There are now newer drugs developed specifically for MDR-TB with the goal of improving outcomes. Bedaquiline and delamanid are examples of drugs only approved in the last 8 years that are now pivotal in the management of MDR/XDR TB.

There are some principles relevant to the treatment of MDR/XDR generally that should be extrapolated to the treatment of MDR/XDR TB spine. Individualised treatment based on DST after sampling is important. Molecular testing gives the most rapid results with rifampicin resistance being reliably determined within 2 hours by Xpert®MTB/RIF. Line-probe assays can detect mutations commonly associated with resistance to rifampicin, isoniazid, fluoroquinolones, and second-line injectable agents within a few days.

If DST for second-line TB medicines is not yet available, the clinician needs to estimate the likelihood of effectiveness of the medicines used, informed by the patient's history of use of second-line TB medicines, the drug-resistance pattern of the contact or index case, and recent representative drug-resistance surveillance data.

Table 14.5 General principles for medical treatment of MDR/XDR

A thorough history and documentation of drugs used (including doses and duration if possible) is imperative
Drug sensitivity testing, available from a reliable laboratory, should be used to guide therapy
Regimens should consist of minimum 4 new drugs not used previously
Never add a single drug to a failing regimen— "Addition Syndrome"
Treatment end points should be individualised and can be 18 to 24 months

In general, drugs used in a failed first-line regimen should be considered to be ineffective regardless of recent DST results [6].

The classification of medicines used in MDR-TB treatment regimens was revised following the update of the WHO guidelines on drug-resistant TB treatment in 2018 [27]. These medicines are categorised into groups A, B, and C as follows (Table 14.6):

TB spine lesions tend to be paucibacillary with more dormant bacteria which makes it harder to eradicate. As in all osseous TB, the emphasis is on multiple drug treatment and prolonged treatment in an effort to prevent dormant bacterial populations replicating.

There are few trials of drug treatment regimes in any extrapulmonary MDR-TB, let alone MDR/XDR TB spine. More data specific to MDR/XDR TB spine are required to optimise treatment and outcomes. MDR/XDR TB spine in children is also not well researched. Success with linezolid, clofazimine, and quinoline in combinations with other second- and third-line agents has been reported in limited case reports [28, 29]. Bedaquiline has revolutionised the treatment of pulmonary MDR-TB in allowing all-oral and shorter regimes. It is effective against dormant and replicating mycobacterium which makes it a promising agent for MDR/XDR TB spine. However, reports of bedaquiline resistance are already published making the widespread use of this agent a concern [30, 31].

Currently, the recommendation is that the treatment of MDR/XDR TB spine in all age groups follows that of pulmonary TB as per the WHO updates in 2020. These are outlined as follows (Table 14.7):

Novel adjuncts for treating MDR have been reported, but the evidence is low and further studies are warranted before general use is recommended. These include immunomodulators such as interferon gamma, autologous bone marrow-derived mesenchymal stromal cells, vitamin D, and BCG injections. Specific to TB spine, Jain et al. reported on adjuncts of levamisole, BCG injections, and antitubercular therapy with some success [32].

Monitoring of treatment for pulmonary MDR includes regular sputum sampling. Regular sampling is not something that is easily achievable in MDR/XDR TB spine. The main recommended methods of monitoring are liver function tests and renal function tests, erythrocyte sedimentation rates (ESR), and plain radiographs. Repeat MRI is also important to assess healing by demonstrating resolving pre- and paravertebral abscess and bony oedema. Gillam et al. described the changes with time and healing of TB spine. They highlighted that calcification or fatty replacement of oedema is seen as high signal intensity on T1-weighted images in the periphery of the vertebra, which then extends inwards as healing progresses. In addition, there

Table 14.6 WHO categories of drugs for MDR-TB

Group A medicines to be prioritised**:** levofloxacin, moxifloxacin, bedaquiline, linezolid
Group B medicines to be used next**:** clofazimine, cycloserine, terizidone
Group C medicines to be included to complete the regimen**:** ethambutol, delamanid, pyrazinamide, imipenem-cilastin, meropenem, amikacin, ethionamide, prothionamide, P-aminosalicylic acid

Table 14.7 WHO recommendations for MDR-TB treatment

Drug resistance pattern	Treatment regime
Rifampicin-susceptible, isoniazid-resistant tuberculosis (Hr-TB)	Rifampicin, ethambutol, pyrazinamide, and levofloxacin for a duration of 6 months (No need for streptomycin or other injectables)
MDR / Rifampicin-resistant (MDR / RR) TB Short all-oral regime (Only if not been exposed to treatment with second-line TB medicines used in this regimen for more than 1 month and in whom resistance to fluoroquinolones has been excluded)	Bedaquiline, levofloxacin/moxifloxacin, clofazimine, ethionamide, ethambutol, isoniazid (high dose), and pyrazinamide for 4 months (with the possibility of extending to 6 months if the patient remains sputum smear positive or culture positive at the end of the fourth month), followed by 5 months of treatment with levofloxacin/moxifloxacin, clofazimine, ethambutol, and pyrazinamide. Bedaquiline use in this regimen is for 6 months
MDR / Rifampicin-resistant (MDR / RR) TB Longer regime for patients not suitable for short regime including quinolone resistance or unreliable DST	In MDR/RR-TB patients on longer regimens, all three Group A agents and at least one Group B agent should be included to ensure that treatment starts with at least four TB agents likely to be effective, and that at least three agents are included for the rest of the treatment if bedaquiline is stopped. If only one or two Group A agents are used, both Group B agents are to be included. If the regimen cannot be composed with agents from Groups A and B alone, Group C agents are added to complete it. 18 months total duration
MDR with additional fluoroquinolone resistance BUT NOT FOR extrapulmonary TB including TB spine	Bedaquiline, pretomanid, and linezolid 6–9 months
MDR / RR-TB with HIV coinfection	Antiretroviral therapy is recommended for all patients with HIV and drug-resistant TB requiring second-line anti-tuberculosis drugs irrespective of CD4 cell count, as early as possible (within the first 8 weeks) following initiation of anti-tuberculosis treatment

will be a diminishing gadolinium enhancement with healing [33]. The MRI changes may lag behind biological responses by 3 months. In situations where further confirmation is required, fluorodeoxyglucose positron emission tomography (FDG PET) scan can be helpful by demonstrating reduced activity [32]. The ultimate sign of healing is achievement of bony fusion across infected sites.

In 2016, Central Tuberculosis Division of India stated in their document that the standard of care is to obtain follow-up serial X-rays every 3 months or so and, based on clinical response, repeat MRI at 6, 9, 12, and 18 months with imaging features to be interpreted in light of clinical response. Follow-ups are suggested about every 6 months for a total of 2 years. The endpoint must be determined on a case-by-case basis [34].

14.6 Surgical Treatment

As is the case for medical treatment, there are no established evidence-based protocols for surgical intervention in MDR/XDR TB spine. The main indications for surgery remain as those for non-MDR-TB spine. These are instability, deformity, neurology, incapacitant pain, and debridement of unresolving abscess or destruction. Open or percutaneous sampling is often required to diagnose MDR/XDR TB spine in cases which do not seem to be resolving.

Although a metanalysis of pulmonary MDR-TB showed better outcomes with surgery than without [35], similar evidence is not available for MDR/XDR TB spine. There are proponents of early surgical intervention in MDR/XDR TB spine to allow adequate sampling for diagnosis and DST as well as to excise infected tissue to reduce microbiological load and allow better drug penetration [36].

The procedures considered for MDR/XDR TB range from combined anterior and posterior procedures to posterior only procedures. The principles follow the same as those in non-MDR/XDR TB spine. There is no contraindication to instrumentation. Li and Xu have both reported on percutaneous catheter drainage followed by local chemotherapy as well as systemic chemotherapy with success in a small number of patients [37, 38].

14.7 Treatment Outcomes

Overall good success rates and very low mortality rates have been reported on in both children and adults, once the MDR/XDR TB spine is diagnosed and DST-based multidrug chemotherapy commenced.

Mortality rates have only been published in case series, and robust data are not available specific to MDR/XDR TB spine. Larger case series have mortality rates of 0 to 2% [8, 37–39].

A good rate of clinical and radiological healing has been noted in adults and children with MDR/XDR TB using a combination of surgery and 24 months of chemotherapy or 24 months of chemotherapy alone. There is a local recurrence problem of approximately 15–18% which generally seems to respond to local debridement [8, 37–40].

Five predictors for successful outcome of MDR-TB have been postulated. They include progressive clinical improvement at 6 months, radiologic improvement during treatment, disease with *Mycobacterium tuberculosis* strains exhibiting resistance to less than or up to 3 antitubercular drugs, use of less than or up to 4 second-line drugs in treatment, and no change of regimen during treatment [39].

14.8 Conclusion

MDR/XDR TB spine should be identified early by using molecular methods to diagnose TB and drug resistance. A high index of suspicion should be maintained for any TB spine that fails to improve with 4 to 5 months of treatment and in high-risk category patients. Pus or granulation tissue sampling from the spine is highly valuable in these situations followed by molecular testing with line assay probes to diagnose and establish a multidrug medical regime of around 18 months. Surgical intervention may provide good outcomes, but the evidence is still to be established. The usual surgical indications remain. Treatment outcomes are good, but prolonged therapy may be needed, and treatment end points should be individualised.

14.9 Atypical Spinal TB

Typically, spinal TB affects contiguous vertebral segments, with the involvement of the intervertebral discs and the paradiscal parts of the vertebral bodies. Atypical TB spine is name given when TB affects the spine in the absence of a spine deformity and the absence of these typical radiological changes.

Although uncommon, they mimic other low-grade infections (brucella, hydatid disease), haematological and metastatic disease, sickle cell spondylitis, intradural tumours, and even disc prolapse [41–44].

As a consequence, atypical TB spine presents a challenge that often delays the appropriate diagnosis and the initiation of treatment. Yalniz et al. estimated the incidence of atypical spinal TB presentation to be 2.1% in his study involving 184 spinal TB patients [45], while it was estimated to be much higher at 12% in another report [46].

Atypical patterns can be very variable. In their review of 23 cases of atypical spinal TB, Naim-Ur-Rahman et al. describe three patterns of atypical tuberculous spondylitis: neural arch only invasion, a single vertebral body involvement, and a spinal canal mass without bony invasion [46]. In 2017, Wang et al. reported on 8 cases of noncontagious multisegmental spinal TB with no intervertebral disc involvement [47].

Intradural lesions can range from subdural to intramedullary granulomas. Bony lesions may be difficult to identify on imaging or may even be absent [48, 49]. Surgical decompression along with a durotomy to reduce intradural pressure tends to have good outcomes for subdural granulomas. For intramedullary lesions, myelotomy may be necessary to decompress the spinal cord [48]. As the diagnosis may only be made post hoc, the possibility of atypical TB should be kept in mind in areas endemic for TB and samples sent for appropriate laboratory testing including culture. Where a diagnosis can be made without surgical sampling, conservative management with ATT and close observation can be successful [48, 49].

Awareness and an index of suspicion of atypical presentations of spinal TB is imperative for an accurate diagnosis and timely initiation of appropriate management, particularly in a patient with other sites of TB or in countries where TB is prevalent.

References

1. Kappelman J, Alçiçek MC, Kazanci N, Schultz M, Ozkul M, Sen S. First Homo erectus from Turkey and implications for migrations into temperate Eurasia. Am J Phys Anthropol. 2008;135(1):110–6.
2. Hershkovitz I, Donoghue HD, Minnikin DE, Besra GS, Lee OY, Gernaey AM, et al. Detection and molecular characterization of 9,000-year-old Mycobacterium tuberculosis from a Neolithic settlement in the Eastern Mediterranean. PLoS One. 2008;3(10):e3426.
3. World Health Organization. Global tuberculosis report 2020. World Health Organization, Geneva.
4. Bosworth DM, Della Pietram A, Farrell RF, B EM. Streptomycin in tuberculous bone and joint lesions with mixed infection and sinuses. Clin Orthop Relat Res. 1950;2005(437):116–20.
5. PYLE MM. Relative numbers of resistant tubercle bacilli in sputa of patients before and during treatment with streptomycin. Proc Staff Meet Mayo Clin. 1947;22(21):465–73.
6. Seung KJ, Keshavjee S, Rich ML. Multidrug-Resistant Tuberculosis and Extensively Drug-Resistant Tuberculosis. Cold Spring Harb Perspect Med. 2015;5(9):a017863.
7. Zhao Y, Xu S, Wang L, Chin DP, Wang S, Jiang G, et al. National survey of drug-resistant tuberculosis in China. N Engl J Med. 2012;366(23):2161–70.
8. Arockiaraj J, Karthik R, Michael JS, Amritanand R, David KS, Krishnan V, et al. 'Need of the Hour': Early Diagnosis and Management of Multidrug Resistant Tuberculosis of the Spine: An Analysis of 30 Patients from a "High Multidrug Resistant Tuberculosis Burden" Country. Asian Spine J. 2019;13(2):265–71.
9. Jenkins HE. Global Burden of Childhood Tuberculosis. Pneumonia (Nathan). 2016;8
10. A controlled trial of six-month and nine-month regimens of chemotherapy in patients undergoing radical surgery for tuberculosis of the spine in Hong Kong. Tenth report of the Medical Research Council Working Party on Tuberculosis of the Spine. Tubercle. 1986;67(4):243–59.
11. Udwadia ZF, Pinto LM, Uplekar MW. Tuberculosis management by private practitioners in Mumbai, India: has anything changed in two decades? PLoS One. 2010;5(8):e12023.
12. Lin H, Shin S, Blaya JA, Zhang Z, Cegielski P, Contreras C, et al. Assessing spatiotemporal patterns of multidrug-resistant and drug-sensitive tuberculosis in a South American setting. Epidemiol Infect. 2011;139(11):1784–93.
13. Gelmanova IY, Keshavjee S, Golubchikova VT, Berezina VI, Strelis AK, Yanova GV, et al. Barriers to successful tuberculosis treatment in Tomsk, Russian Federation: non-adherence, default and the acquisition of multidrug resistance. Bull World Health Organ. 2007;85(9):703–11.
14. Balabanova Y, Drobniewski F, Fedorin I, Zakharova S, Nikolayevskyy V, Atun R, et al. The Directly Observed Therapy Short-Course (DOTS) strategy in Samara Oblast. Russian Federation Respir Res. 2006;7:44.
15. Seung KJ, Gelmanova IE, Peremitin GG, Golubchikova VT, Pavlova VE, Sirotkina OB, et al. The effect of initial drug resistance on treatment response and acquired drug resistance during standardized short-course chemotherapy for tuberculosis. Clin Infect Dis. 2004;39(9):1321–8.
16. Park M-H, Song E, Park H, Kwon Y, Han S, Shim Y. HLA-DRB1 and DQB1 gene polymorphism is associated with multidrug-resistant tuberculosis in Korean patients. Hum Immunol. 2002;63

17. Sharma SK, Turaga KK, Balamurugan A, Saha PK, Pandey RM, Jain NK, et al. Clinical and genetic risk factors for the development of multi-drug resistant tuberculosis in non-HIV infected patients at a tertiary care center in India: a case-control study. Infect Genet Evol. 2003;3(3):183–8.
18. Nguyen QH, Contamin L, Nguyen TVA, Bañuls AL. Insights into the processes that drive the evolution of drug resistance in. Evol Appl. 2018;11(9):1498–511.
19. Tuli SM. Multidrug resistant tuberculosis: A challenge in clinical orthopedics. Indian J Orthop. 2014;48(3):235–7.
20. Jain AK, Jaggi KR, Bhayana H, Saha R. Drug-resistant Spinal Tuberculosis. Indian J Orthop. 2018;52(2):100–7.
21. Somoskövi A, Ködmön C, Lantos A, Bártfai Z, Tamási L, Füzy J, et al. Comparison of recoveries of mycobacterium tuberculosis using the automated BACTEC MGIT 960 system, the BACTEC 460 TB system, and Löwenstein-Jensen medium. J Clin Microbiol. 2000;38(6):2395–7.
22. Huggett JF, McHugh TD, Zumla A. Tuberculosis: amplification-based clinical diagnostic techniques. Int J Biochem Cell Biol. 2003;35(10):1407–12.
23. Joo EJ, Yeom JS, Ha YE, Park SY, Lee CS, Kim ES, et al. Diagnostic yield of computed tomography-guided bone biopsy and clinical outcomes of tuberculous and pyogenic spondylitis. Korean J Intern Med. 2016;31(4):762–71.
24. Waqas M, Qadeer M, Faiz F, Alvi MA, Bari ME. Computed Tomography-Guided Biopsy for Potts Disease: An Institutional Experience from an Endemic Developing Country. Asian Spine J. 2015;9(3):394–8.
25. Tang L, Feng S, Gao R, Han C, Sun X, Bao Y, et al. A Comparative Study on the Role of Xpert MTB/RIF in Testing Different Types of Spinal Tuberculosis Tissue Specimens. Genet Test Mol Biomarkers. 2017;21(12):722–6.
26. LoBue P. Extensively drug-resistant tuberculosis. Curr Opin Infect Dis. 2009;22(2):167–73.
27. WHO operational handbook on tuberculosis. Module 4: treatment - drug-resistant tuberculosis treatment. Geneva: World Health Organization; 2020. Licence: CC BY-NC-SA 3.0 IGO.
28. Giridharan P, Selladurai E, Balaji S, Pramila SK, Shanmugam S, et al. Drug resistant TB spine in a two year old child: A case report. Indian J Tuberc. 2020;67(3):374–7.
29. Shah SS, Goregaonkar AA, Goregaonkar AB. Extensively Drug-resistant Tuberculosis of the Lumbar Spine in a Six-year-old Child: A Case Report. J Orthop Case Rep. 2017;7(2):40–3.
30. Bloemberg GV, Keller PM, Stucki D, Stuckia D, Trauner A, Borrell S, et al. Acquired Resistance to Bedaquiline and Delamanid in Therapy for Tuberculosis. N Engl J Med. 2015;373(20):1986–8.
31. Veziris N, Bernard C, Guglielmetti L, Le Du D, Marigot-Outtandy D, Jaspard M, et al. Rapid emergence of. Eur Respir J. 2017;49:3.
32. Jain AK, Dhammi IK, Modi P, Kumar J, Sreenivasan R, Saini NS. Tuberculosis spine: Therapeutically refractory disease. Indian J Orthop. 2012;46(2):171–8.
33. Gillams AR, Chaddha B, Carter AP. MR appearances of the temporal evolution and resolution of infectious spondylitis. AJR Am J Roentgenol. 1996;166(4):903–7.
34. Sharma SK, Ryan H, Khaparde S, Sachdeva KS, Singh AD, Mohan A, et al. Index-TB guidelines: Guidelines on extrapulmonary tuberculosis for India. Indian J Med Res. 2017;145(4):448–63.
35. Harris RC, Khan MS, Martin LJ, Allen V, Moore DA, Fielding K, et al. The effect of surgery on the outcome of treatment for multidrug-resistant tuberculosis: a systematic review and meta-analysis. BMC Infect Dis. 2016;16:262.
36. Rajasekaran S, Soundararajan DCR, Shetty AP, Kanna RM. Spinal Tuberculosis: Current Concepts. Global Spine J. 2018;8(4 Suppl):96S–108S.
37. Li L, Zhang Z, Luo F, Xu J, Cheng P, Wu Z, et al. Management of drug-resistant spinal tuberculosis with a combination of surgery and individualised chemotherapy: a retrospective analysis of thirty-five patients. Int Orthop. 2012;36(2):277–83.

38. Xu L, Jian-Zhong X, Xue-Mei L, Bao-Feng G. Drug susceptibility testing guided treatment for drug-resistant spinal tuberculosis: a retrospective analysis of 19 patients. Int Surg. 2013;98(2):175–80.
39. Pawar UM, Kundnani V, Agashe V, Nene A. Multidrug-resistant tuberculosis of the spine--is it the beginning of the end? A study of twenty-five culture proven multidrug-resistant tuberculosis spine patients. Spine (Phila Pa 1976). 2009;34(22):E806–10.
40. Seddon JA, Donald PR, Vlok GJ, Schaaf HS. Multidrug-resistant tuberculosis of the spine in children–characteristics from a high burden setting. J Trop Pediatr. 2012;58(5):341–7.
41. Mittal S, Khalid M, Sabir AB, Khalid S. Comparison of Magnetic Resonance Imaging Findings between Pathologically Proven Cases of Atypical Tubercular Spine and Tumour Metastasis: A Retrospective Study in 40 Patients. Asian Spine J. 2016;10(4):734–43.
42. D'souza MM, Mondal A, Sharma R, Jaimini A, Khanna U. Tuberculosis the great mimicker: 18F-fludeoxyglucose positron emission tomography/computed tomography in a case of atypical spinal tuberculosis. Indian J Nucl Med. 2014;29(2):99–101.
43. Rajgopalan M, Srivastava A, Dhammi IK, Jain AK. Tuberculosis–'The great masquerader' presenting as a dumb-bell-shaped intradural extramedullary tumor in a 20-year-old female. J Clin Orthop Trauma. 2017;8(2):168–70.
44. Pande KC, Pande SK, Babhulkar SS. An atypical presentation of tuberculosis of the spine. Spinal Cord. 1996;34(12):716–9.
45. Yalniz E, Pekindil G, Aktas S. Atypical tuberculosis of the spine. Yonsei Med J. 2000;41(5):657–61.
46. Naim-Ur-Rahman A-AKM, Khan FA. Atypical forms of spinal tuberculosis. Acta Neurochir. 1987;88(1–2):26–33.
47. Wang LN, Wang L, Liu LM, Song YM, Li Y, Liu H. Atypical spinal tuberculosis involved noncontiguous multiple segments: Case series report with literature review. Medicine (Baltimore). 2017;96(14):e6559.
48. Kumar S, Jain AK, Dhammi IK, Aggarwal AN. Treatment of intraspinal tuberculoma. Clin Orthop Relat Res. 2007 Jul;460:62–6.
49. Ramdurg SR, Gupta DK, Suri A, Sharma BS, Mahapatra AK. Spinal intramedullary tuberculosis: a series of 15 cases. Clin Neurol Neurosurg. 2009 Feb;111(2):115–8.

Chapter 15
Complications and Management in Tuberculosis of the Spine

Farah Musharbash, Varun Puvanesarajah, and Amit Jain

Abstract Tuberculosis of the spine is a severe form of extra-pulmonary tuberculosis and poses a challenge to physicians worldwide. Left untreated, it can lead to severe complications with significant patient morbidity. In this chapter, we discuss the most common complications of spinal tuberculosis and their management, including cold abscesses, kyphotic deformity, and neurologic deficits, in addition to the specific challenges posed by late onset symptoms. Adverse reactions to anti-tuberculosis drug therapy as well as medicolegal challenges in treating spinal tuberculosis are also highlighted.

Keywords Spine · Tuberculosis · Complications · Kyphosis · Neurologic deficit · Drug reaction · Cold abscess · Legal · Litigation

15.1 Introduction

Spinal tuberculosis accounts for approximately half of musculoskeletal tuberculosis cases and remains a challenge for physicians worldwide [1]. Left untreated, it can lead to serious sequelae and significant patient morbidity [2]. It usually begins in an insidious fashion as a secondary infection, with the *Mycobacterium tuberculosis* (*M. tuberculosis*) pathogen seeding the anterior aspect of the vertebral body most commonly hematogenously [3–5]. In the early stages, patients often present with varying degrees of axial pain, with multiple studies demonstrating 90–100% of patients reporting back pain as a symptom [6–8]. Constitutional symptoms are only present in about 20–30% of patients, with weight loss being quoted as the most consistent constitutional feature, although fevers, night sweats, and malaise can also be present but are more common in patients with concomitant pulmonary tuberculosis [5, 6, 9].

F. Musharbash · V. Puvanesarajah · A. Jain (✉)
Department of Orthopaedic Surgery, The Johns Hopkins Hospital, Baltimore, MD, USA
e-mail: fmushar1@jhmi.edu; vpuvane1@jhmi.edu; amitjain@jhmi.edu

S. S. Dhatt, V. Kumar (eds.), *Tuberculosis of the Spine*,
https://doi.org/10.1007/978-981-16-9495-0_15

The slow onset of progression often leads to a delayed presentation. This is especially an issue in countries with a high tuberculosis burden, where many patients have limited access to healthcare facilities, resulting in initial presentation at an advanced stage [5, 10]. Although the presentation and natural history of spinal tuberculosis can be variable, it usually presents with three main clinical complications: cold abscesses, neurologic deficits, and kyphotic deformity [3]. The timeline at which these complications arise are variable. Neurologic deficits can present early and late in the disease process, even decades after the initial infection, while kyphotic deformity is usually a late presentation of spinal tuberculosis.

15.2 Cold Abscesses

Cold abscesses are purulent collections that form as a result of caseous necrosis which follows the inflammatory response to the *M. tuberculosis* complex [3, 6]. They are found in 48–70% of patients with spinal tuberculosis and are characterized by slow growth and subligamentous spread [3, 11]. These abscesses often grow unnoticed until their mass effect causes symptoms, frequently leading to a delayed diagnosis. On imaging they are best seen on magnetic resonance imaging (MRI) and computed tomography (CT) scans, although even plain radiography may provide evidence of a cold abscess as a soft tissue shadow, increased cervical prevertebral soft tissue space, or mediastinal widening. At later stages they can fistulize, and their wall can become calcified due to the lack of proteolytic enzymes in *M. tuberculosis* [1, 4, 12].

They are most commonly para-vertebral but can also be found in a pre-vertebral or intra-osseous location [6]. About 90% of abscesses are found in the lower thoracic or lumbar spine, and 10% are found in the cervical and upper thoracic spine [3]. Initial presentation depends largely on the location and size of the cold abscess. Abscesses in the cervical region can be retropharyngeal and lead to dysphagia, hoarseness, or difficulty breathing [5]. Those in the thoracic spine are often fusiform paravertebral and rarely symptomatic. Those in the lumbar region can involve the iliopsoas muscle leading to groin swelling and pseudo-flexion hip deformity, and can even track down below the inguinal ligament into the medial thigh compartment [3, 5, 9].

Historically, management of cold abscesses frequently involved drainage with the goal of reducing disease burden and preventing further complications. However, with modern highly penetrating anti-tuberculosis drug therapy, abscesses are commonly successfully resorbed and eventually fill in with new bone following non-operative therapy [3, 4, 13]. Drainage is indicated however when abscesses lead to dysphagia, respiratory compromise, pseudo-flexion hip deformity, or neurologic deficits. Occasionally, draining a large abscess maybe performed while obtaining a biopsy in order to facilitate drug penetration [5].

15.3 Neurologic Deficits

Neurologic symptoms in the setting of spinal tuberculosis can be seen in approximately 10–20% of patients in developed countries and 20–41% in developing countries [14]. Neurologic deficits are often defined as early-onset or late-onset [3, 14, 15]. Early-onset deficits are those occurring while the disease is active (usually within the first 2 years of active disease) and result from direct or indirect compression by an abscess, granulation tissue, or debris onto the spinal cord parenchyma or instability leading to cord compromise [4, 6]. Late onset deficits are those which occur with healed disease and can present many years and even decades after the initial infection [15]. This is usually attributed to spinal cord damage secondary to a transverse bony ridge at the apex of the kyphotic deformity and dural fibrosis [4, 6]. Less common causes of neurologic deficits include infective spinal artery thrombosis, tuberculosis myelitis, and arachnoiditis [4].

Signs and symptoms can range from radicular pain, weakness, and paresthesias to myelopathy and even para- or tetraplegia if left untreated depending on the involved anatomic location [3, 4]. The mainstay treatment remains medical, as medical treatment effectively treats the majority of neurologic deficits from active disease [5, 16]. However, the original Medical Research Council trials which demonstrate the efficacy of conservative therapy only considered patients with limited disease, mild to moderate neurologic deficits, and mild deformity [17]. Recently, studies have found that decompression may lead to faster pain relief and functional recovery as well as decrease the risk of late-onset neurologic sequelae when compared to medical therapy alone [5, 14, 18]. As such, surgery is indicated in specific situations involving severe or rapidly worsening deficits at presentation, as this can indicate the presence of instability, as well as cases that are unresponsive to anti-tuberculous drug therapy [6, 14].

Prognosis after surgical decompression is generally favorable in patients with active early-onset disease with most showing neurologic recovery [19]. This is thought to be related to the low energy and relatively longer timeframe of cord compression with tuberculosis as opposed to trauma and other pyogenic infections [5, 14].

15.4 Kyphotic Deformity

Kyphosis is a late manifestation of spinal tuberculosis, reported in about 29% of patients. It develops as a result of destruction of the anterior aspect of the vertebral body in the thoracic spine. Collapse of the anterior column can lead to a focal gibbus deformity or a globally rounded kyphosis depending on the number of vertebrae involved [5, 6]. Progression of deformity is dependent on multiple factors including age, involved region, and the extent of disease [9, 11]. In children, kyphosis can worsen during periods of growth even following cure of the disease. In contrast, in adults the final deformity is mostly determined by the extent of vertebral changes during the active disease stage [6]. The spine-at-risk radiographic signs (Fig. 15.1) described by Rajasekaran et al. help identify children at risk of developing progressive kyphosis [9, 20].

Surgery is indicated for a severe established deformity or spinal instability leading to a high risk of future deformity or neurologic deficits [5, 6]. In adults, a kyphosis of >60° is generally managed operatively as these usually progress and are associated with a high risk of late-onset neurologic deficits [21]. In children, however, a lower threshold of 30° is suggested due to the higher risk of future progression [1]. In addition, surgery is indicated when there are signs of spinal instability such as three column disease involvement; loss of >1 thoracic vertebral body or >1.5 lumbar vertebral body; pedicular destruction with posterior arch involvement; or two or more "spine-at-risk" signs in children [6].

Historically, surgery for spinal tuberculosis, including debridement and reconstruction, was performed mostly using an all-anterior approach from the principle that tuberculosis is predominantly an anterior column disease. However, with the development of pedicle screw instrumentation, the posterior approach has become more popular. Studies have demonstrated similar pain and neurologic improvement compared to the anterior approach along with improved deformity correction [22, 23]. In addition, current drug therapy regimens can result in satisfactory resorption of anterior abscesses, which makes a more extensive anterior debridement less necessary and permits use of a posterior approach [3]. Combined approaches can also be used for more complex deformities and can be performed in one or two stages [24].

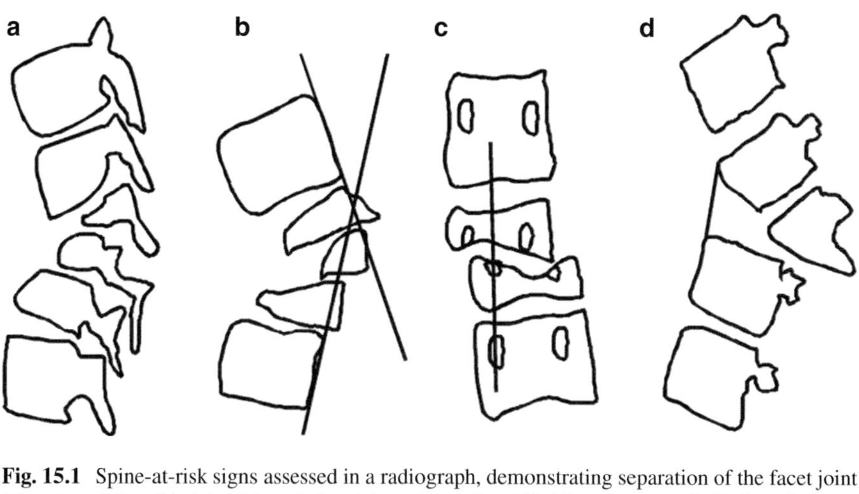

Fig. 15.1 Spine-at-risk signs assessed in a radiograph, demonstrating separation of the facet joint (**a**), retropulsion (**b**), lateral translation (**c**), and toppling (**d**). The presence of >2 signs indicate instability and a high risk of progression in deformity (Reproduced with permission from Jain et al. [9])

15.5 Challenges in Late-Onset Tuberculosis Symptoms

Although tuberculosis can be cured with medical therapy, treatment of late sequelae which are either due to late patient presentation or late symptom onset is challenging and often fraught with complications. Previous studies have demonstrated that in countries with high tuberculosis burden and limited access to healthcare, rates of surgical intervention are higher than in countries with a more developed healthcare system [1]. This reflects the challenge in treating patients who present at later stages of the disease process.

Patients who present with late-onset neurologic deficits at the healed stage of the disease often have a worse prognosis when it comes to neurologic recovery when compared to patients who present with early-onset deficits. This is also true for patients who present with long-standing neurologic deficits that have not been addressed in a prompt matter [14]. In both cases however, surgical decompression may offer the best chance for a potential recovery, but the patient must be advised that recovery is less predictable. In addition, late-onset deficits present a unique diagnostic challenge as one should differentiate whether such a deficit is associated with a healed lesion versus reactivation. Reactivation usually presents with more severe and rapidly developing deficits compared with healed lesions, and detailed review of advanced imaging, including CT and MRI, may reveal disease activity at or around the internal gibbus [14]. Patients with reactivation can be treated with debridement with or without stabilization, while patients with healed disease often require excision of the internal gibbus with or without deformity correction [9]. In addition, patients with reactivation have more favorable outcomes following surgical decompression compared to patients with healed disease [25].

Another challenge is the late development of kyphotic deformities. Deformities of 60° or greater has been observed in approximately 3–5% of patients with spinal tuberculosis treated with medical therapy alone [6]. Deformity correction in healed disease is more difficult and is associated with higher rates of complications compared with active disease. Patients with healed disease who present with a kyphotic deformity greater than 60° often require a combined anterior-posterior approach to correct the deformity, which is a major undertaking compared to a posterior or anterior only approach [9, 14, 24].

15.6 Adverse Drug Reactions

Medical management with anti-tuberculosis drugs remains the mainstay treatment of spinal tuberculosis, which is considered a severe form of extrapulmonary tuberculosis and hence falls under the World Health Organization's (WHO) Category-I treatment. Although protocols may vary by country or institution, the recommended WHO two-phase protocol involves an intensive 2-month phase of isoniazid, rifampicin, ethambutol, and pyrazinamide followed by a continuation phase of isoniazid

Table 15.1 First-line anti-tuberculosis drugs with the most common adverse reactions and their incidences (adapted from Forget et al. [28])

Drug	Reaction (incidence)
Isoniazid	Transaminitis (11%), hepatitis (0.4%), neurologic (1–3%), dermatologic (1%), gastrointestinal (2%), hypersensitivity (0.1–17%)
Rifampicin	Transaminitis (3–9%), hepatitis (1%), dermatologic (0.5–3%), gastrointestinal (1–8%)
Pyrazinamide	Hepatitis (1–5%), dermatologic (2–5%), gastrointestinal (1%)
Ethambutol	Neurologic (0.2–0.3%), dermatologic (0.15%), hepatitis (rare reports)

and rifampicin for a total treatment time of 9 months [4, 26]. Given the relatively long duration of therapy, awareness of adverse drug reactions is paramount, especially with the increasing prevalence of multi-drug resistant tuberculosis leading to the use of second-line drugs which have a greater toxicity profile [6, 27].

Side effects and interactions with other medications are both important considerations. Side effects of common first-line anti-tuberculous drugs and their incidence can be found in Table 15.1 [28]. Transaminitis with asymptomatic elevation of liver function tests up to five times the normal limit is common and can be serially observed without discontinuation of therapy. Neurologic side effects vary, with peripheral neuropathy common with isoniazid treatment and ocular toxicity being the main neurologic adverse effect of ethambutol [29, 30]. Second-line therapies tend to be more toxic. For example, fluoroquinolones are associated with QT prolongation predisposing to torsades de pointes, and aminoglycosides are associated with nephrotoxicity leading to oliguric renal failure [27].

Both rifampicin and isoniazid may also interact with other medications. Rifampicin is a potent inducer of drug metabolism and as a result reduces the level of other medications such as warfarin, contraceptives, corticosteroids, phenytoin, and theophylline, potentially resulting in subtherapeutic anticoagulation, birth control, and seizure prophylaxis. Isoniazid, on the other hand, can increase levels of warfarin, phenytoin, and carbamazepine [31]. The relatively common side effects and multitude of interactions of anti-tuberculosis drug therapy regimens serve to emphasize the importance of proper medical follow-up and monitoring of spinal tuberculosis patients by a multi-disciplinary team.

15.7 Medicolegal Issues

Throughout this chapter, we highlight the importance of early diagnosis and treatment of spinal tuberculosis before complications arise. Along with the immeasurable cost of patient suffering from the complications of delayed treatment, there is also a significant medicolegal cost.

Medicolegal issues arise from both the medical evaluation and therapy of spinal tuberculosis, as well as the complications related to its surgical treatment. Malpractice litigation has been reported when there is a failure to diagnose spinal tuberculosis, delay in starting anti-tuberculosis therapy, incorrect treatment, inadequate monitoring, drug interactions with other medications, and failure to refer to a spinal surgeon [32, 33]. A review by Quraishi et al. from the United Kingdom's National Health Services Litigation Authority database showed that missed spinal infections accounted for 11.8% of all successful claims of alleged negligence with average damages paid out amounting to 433,206 British pounds [34]. As such, adherence to well-established national and international guidelines when evaluating and treating tuberculosis is of utmost importance as it avoids poor outcomes and also helps reduce the incidence of multi-drug resistance [32, 35]. Further, the importance of patient education and informed consent are critical in this setting. For all the aforementioned reasons, it is recommended that the treatment of spinal tuberculosis is undertaken at specialized healthcare centers with proper established protocols and a multi-disciplinary team that is familiar with both the medical and surgical aspects of the disease.

15.8 Conclusion

Tuberculosis of the spine poses a challenge to spinal surgeons worldwide. Left untreated, it can lead to severe complications with significant patient morbidity.

References

1. Ali A, Musbahi O, White VL, Montgomery AS. Spinal tuberculosis: a literature review. JBJS Rev. 2019;7(1):e9.
2. Jain AK. Tuberculosis of the spine: a fresh look at an old disease. J Bone Joint Surg Br Vol. 2010;92(7):905–13.
3. Khanna K, Sabharwal S. Spinal tuberculosis: a comprehensive review for the modern spine surgeon. Spine J. 2019;19(11):1858–70.
4. Garg RK, Somvanshi DS. Spinal tuberculosis: a review. J Spinal Cord Med. 2011;34(5):440–54.
5. Dunn RN, Ben HM. Spinal tuberculosis: review of current management. Bone Joint J. 2018;100(4):425–31.
6. Rajasekaran S, Kanna RM, Shetty AP. Pathophysiology and treatment of spinal tuberculosis. JBJS Rev. 2014;23:2(9).
7. Azzam NI, Tammawy M. Tuberculous spondylitis in adults: diagnosis and treatment. Br J Neurosurg. 1988;2(1):85–91.
8. Pertuiset E, Beaudreuil J, Lioté F, Horusitzky A, Kemiche F, Richette P, Clerc-Wyel D, Cerf-Payrastre I, Dorfmann H, Glowinski J, Crouzet J. Spinal tuberculosis in adults. A study of 103 cases in a developed country, 1980–1994. Medicine. 1999;78(5):309–20.
9. Jain AK, Rajasekaran S, Jaggi KR, Myneedu VP. Tuberculosis of the Spine. JBJS. 2020;102(7):617–28.
10. Kotil K, Alan MS, Bilge T. Medical management of Pott disease in the thoracic and lumbar spine: a prospective clinical study. J Neurosurg Spine. 2007;6(3):222–8.
11. Alavi SM, Sharifi M. Tuberculous spondylitis: risk factors and clinical/paraclinical aspects in the south west of Iran. J Infect Public Health. 2010;3(4):196–200.

12. Rivas-Garcia A, Sarria-Estrada S, Torrents-Odin C, Casas-Gomila L, Franquet E. Imaging findings of Pott's disease. Eur Spine J. 2013;22(4):567–78.
13. Bakhsh A. Medical management of spinal tuberculosis: an experience from Pakistan. Spine. 2010;35(16):E787–91.
14. Jain AK, Kumar J. Tuberculosis of spine: neurological deficit. Eur Spine J. 2013;22(4):624–33.
15. Hodgson AR, Yau A. Pott's paraplegia: a classification based upon the living pathology. Spinal Cord. 1967;5(1):1–6.
16. Pattisson PR, Chir B. Pott's paraplegia: an account of the treatment of 89 consecutive patients. Spinal Cord. 1986;24(2):77–91.
17. Medical Research Council Working Party on Tuberculosis of the S. Twelfth report of the Medical Research Council Working Party on Tuberculosis of the Spine. Controlled trial of short-course regimens of chemotherapy in the ambulatory treatment of spinal tuberculosis. Results at three years of a study in Korea. J Bone Joint Surg (Br). 1993;75:240–8.
18. Leong JC. Tuberculosis of the spine. J Bone Joint Surg Br Vol. 1993;75(2):173–5.
19. Wang X, Pang X, Wu P, Luo C, Shen X. One-stage anterior debridement, bone grafting and posterior instrumentation vs. single posterior debridement, bone grafting, and instrumentation for the treatment of thoracic and lumbar spinal tuberculosis. Eur Spine J. 2014;23(4):830–7.
20. Rajasekaran S. The natural history of post-tubercular kyphosis in children: radiological signs which predict late increase in deformity. J Bone Joint Surg Br Vol. 2001;83(7):954–62.
21. Tuli SM. Severe kyphotic deformity in tuberculosis of the spine. Int Orthop. 1995;19(5):327–31.
22. Huang Z, Liu J, Ma K. Posterior versus anterior approach surgery for thoracolumbar spinal tuberculosis. J Coll Physicians Surg Pak. 2019;29(2):187–8.
23. Cui X, Ma YZ, Chen X, Cai XJ, Li HW, Bai YB. Outcomes of different surgical procedures in the treatment of spinal tuberculosis in adults. Med Princ Pract. 2013;22(4):346–50.
24. Rajasekaran S, Vijay K, Shetty AP. Single-stage closing–opening wedge osteotomy of spine to correct severe post-tubercular kyphotic deformities of the spine: a 3-year follow-up of 17 patients. Eur Spine J. 2010;19(4):583–92.
25. Hsu LC, Cheng CL, Leong JC. Pott's paraplegia of late onset. The cause of compression and results after anterior decompression. J Bone Joint Surg Br Vol. 1988;70(4):534–8.
26. World Health Organization, Stop TB Initiative (World Health Organization). Treatment of tuberculosis: guidelines. World Health Organization; 2010.
27. Ramachandran G, Swaminathan S. Safety and tolerability profile of second-line anti-tuberculosis medications. Drug Saf. 2015;38(3):253–69.
28. Forget EJ, Menzies D. Adverse reactions to first-line antituberculosis drugs. Expert Opin Drug Saf. 2006;5(2):231–49.
29. Leibold JE. The ocular toxicity of ethambutol and its relation to dose. Ann N Y Acad Sci. 1966;135(2):904–9.
30. Lubing HN. Peripheral neuropathy in tuberculosis patients treated with isoniazid. Am Rev Tuberc. 1953;68(3):458–61.
31. Addington WW. The side effects and interactions of antituberculosis drugs. Chest. 1979;76(6):782–4.
32. Branley HM. Tuberculosis: clinical management and medicolegal pitfalls. Clinical Risk. 2009;15(6):247–52.
33. Foy MA. Missed spinal infection: a source of litigation in the orthopaedic community? Bone Joint 360. 2014;3(3):44–5.
34. Quraishi NA, Hammett TC, Todd DB, Bhutta MA, Kapoor V. Malpractice litigation and the spine: the NHS perspective on 235 successful claims in England. Eur Spine J. 2012;21(2):196–9.
35. World Health Organization. WHO guidelines on tuberculosis infection prevention and control: 2019 update. World Health Organization; 2019.

Chapter 16
Surgical Management of TB Spine: Indications and Overview with Postoperative Protocols

Benny T. Dahl, Deepak Neradi, and Balwinder Sherry

Abstract Though the majority of spine tuberculosis is managed with antitubercular therapy, surgery is sometimes necessary to control infection, obtaining tissue samples, preventing neural damage and deformity. There is no definitive evidence on duration of antitubercular therapy for spine tuberculosis. But surgery not only helps in prevention of damage, but also it cuts down the duration of chemotherapy treatment. This chapter deals with surgical management of tuberculosis, indications, and various techniques.

Keywords Tuberculosis · Surgery · Spine · Postoperative protocols

16.1 Introduction

Tuberculosis of spine is treated primarily with chemotherapy. Long duration antitubercular chemotherapy is the essential part of treatment of spinal tuberculosis. Surgery in tuberculosis of the spine is a controversial topic, and there is no clear-cut consensus on the indications for surgical treatment. Surgical intervention may be required to prevent and treat complication of spinal tuberculosis like cold abscess, deformity, and neurological deficit. Studies comparing excisional therapy and antitubercular therapy demonstrated no differences between both. In fact, excisional therapy alone results in anterior column deficit and can result in deformity and delayed neurological deficit [1].

The Hong Kong operation first described by Ito, and made famous by Hodgson and Stock [2], consisted of thorough debridement of tuberculous focus till healthy

B. T. Dahl (✉)
Texas Children's Hospital and Baylor College of Medicine, Houston, TX, USA

Spine Unit, Department of Orthopaedic Surgery, Rigshospitalet and University of Copenhagen, Copenhagen, Denmark

D. Neradi · B. Sherry
Department of Orthopedics, PGIMER, Chandigarh, India

S. S. Dhatt, V. Kumar (eds.), *Tuberculosis of the Spine*,
https://doi.org/10.1007/978-981-16-9495-0_16

bleeding cancellous bone and dura matter, and filling of the created defect with a strut graft taken from the rib or a tricortical iliac crest bone graft. Clearance of paravertebral abscess by anterior approach allows a surgeon to clear the infection site and is usually very effective to reduce the infectious load on the patient. Observations in this study were early recovery, easiness in debridement, prevention of delayed kyphosis, prevention of relapse, and decreased hospital stay.

Earlier there were differences in the opinions regarding choice of treatment with some like Hodgson favoring surgical management while Konstam chose only medical therapy in Pott spine cases. Later studies emphasized complementary role of surgery in cases where medical therapy alone would have been ineffective. Surgery allows for removal of tuberculous focus and improves effectiveness of antitubercular drugs. Tuli's middle path regimen (proposed for low resource centers) was antitubercular drug therapy-based management supplemented by surgical intervention in selected cases [3]. According to him surgery should be performed in following scenarios:

1. Decompression for neurological complications not responding to conservative management
2. Posterior spinal lesions
3. Failure of response after 3–6 months of non-operative treatment
4. Doubtful diagnosis
5. Instability after healing
6. Recurrence of disease or neurological complication

There has been little change in the indications for surgery provided by Tuli's middle path regimen, and presently objectives of surgery include decompression of spinal cord, correction of deformity, removal of diseased focus, and providing stability to spine.

In a systematic review of case series of spinal tuberculosis from 1980 to 2011 by Ferrer et al. [4], more than 56% of the patients underwent surgery in the majority of 37 studies.

Prospective multicenter studies were conducted in multiple countries by Medical Research Council (MRC) working party on spinal tuberculosis to compare the outcome of different treatment modalities [5] (Table 16.1). They found that the *Hong Kong strategy* (Radical debridement + Strut grafting) provided better bony union, resolution of the abscess, and better spine alignment.

Table 16.1 Showing outcomes of various surgical strategies for tuberculosis of spine

Treatment group	Patients (%) achieving bony fusion after 18 months	Angle of kyphosis: At presentation	Angle of kyphosis: After 5 years
Radical debridement + Strut grafting	85	26	23
Radical debridement	52	25	33
Ambulatory chemotherapy	50	24	31
Conservative management	15	35	56

Based on the findings of the MRC study, in 2012 Mak et al. [5] recommended the following indications for surgery:

1. Progressive neurological deficit
   Early surgical decompression helps in rapid resolution of deficit leading to reduced morbidity and improvement in quality of life.
2. Progressive spinal deformity
   In the thoracic spine more kyphosis could be tolerated by compensatory lordosis in the lumbar spine, but excessive loss of lordosis in the lumbar spine is not acceptable. Sixty degrees of kyphosis can lead to paraplegia and cardiopulmonary compromise and should be surgically treated. There was no progression of kyphosis in patients undergoing the Hong Kong procedure.
3. Failure of conservative treatment
   Progression in pain or neurological deficit after 3–4 weeks of chemotherapy with/without brace/bedrest should be considered as treatment failure and managed with surgical intervention.
4. Uncertain diagnosis
   Isolation of *Mycobacterium* from lesions is the gold standard for diagnosis of spinal tuberculosis. When there is a lack of superficial abscess or samples are unobtainable/insufficient from percutaneous biopsy, it can be difficult to make a diagnosis or determine drug sensitivity. In such cases surgery should be performed to obtain sufficient tissue samples.

   In children younger than 10 years of age, there is a risk of gradual progression of the kyphosis with age due to bone growth leading to late deformity. Rajasekaran described a scoring system based on findings on X-rays [6]. One point was given to each of the following variables:

   a. Facet joint separation at apex of curve
   b. Posterior retropulsion of diseased vertebral segment
   c. Lateral translation on AP view
   d. Tilt or toppling

A score greater than two predicted an increase in kyphosis >30° and a final kyphosis >60°. These children should be operated at earlier stage to prevent late deformity.

Oguz [7] developed the GATA (**G**ulhane **A**skeri **T**ip **A**kademisi) classification system based on clinical signs and radiology to help decide on the management of spinal tuberculosis. (Table 16.2).

16.1.1 Techniques

Only posterior laminectomies were used to be done in earlier days, but they didn't result in good outcomes. In 1911, Hibbs performed in situ fusion with posterior grafting, but it was not effective in preventing delayed kyphosis. Later in 1920s,

Table 16.2 GATA classification

	Lesion	Treatment
Type IA	Limited to vertebra One level disc degeneration No abscess No collapse No neurological deficit	Antitubercular drugs Needs periodic monitoring
Type IB	Abscess formation not limited to the vertebra, No collapse/instability No neurological deficit	Debridement and drainage of abscess Anterior/posterior/endoscopic
Type II	Vertebral collapse Mild kyphosis Abscess No instability Sagittal index (SI) is <20° Neurological deficit may be there	Anterior debridement and strut cortical Graft fusion If neurological deficit – anterior decompression
Type III	Vertebral collapse Severe kyphosis Abscess Instability Sagittal index (SI) is >20° Neurological deficit may be there	Anterior debridement and strut cortical Graft fusion If neurological deficit – decompression Correction of deformity and fixation by anterolateral/posterior approaches/both

Capener and Menard introduced lateral rachiotomy using postero-lateral approach. With this approach they tried to address ventral pathology but it led to instability. Ito et al.'s anterior approach was opposed by many surgeons due to high mortality. The surgical mortality rate has come down after the introduction of chemotherapy. Drainage of cold abscess used to be done and it was also recommended by Sir Percival Pott, but studies demonstrated that it has no benefit over chemotherapy alone. Aspiration is advised only to obtain tissue for diagnosis. Aspiration can also be done in patients with large abscess with poor general condition.

Various surgical techniques include anterior decompression and grafting, staged anterior and posterior approaches, and combined anterior and posterior approaches. Surgical approaches vary depending on the site of tuberculous infection. Studies also suggested good results with aspiration of abscess under CT guidance and followed by posterior fixation which eliminates the need for laminectomy.

16.1.2 Cervical Spine

For lesions in C1 and C2, a transoral approach is preferred as it gives the surgeon direct access to the diseased vertebrae. This approach requires additional stabilization with posterior fixation. In the subaxial spine, lesions can be approached without difficulty using anterior (Smith-Robinson approach). This approach is familiar to many spine surgeons and provides access to the anterior vertebral bodies. Corpectomy and stabilization with cage and plate is essential after debridement of the lesion. Additional posterior fixation in this region depends on the extent of the disease.

16.1.3 Thoraco-lumbar Spine

Direct anterior approach for the upper thoracic vertebrae were described in the past using transsternal, right thoracic or left thoracic approaches. These approaches are technically challenging and associated with a relatively high risk of complications, since manipulation of large vessels and viscera is often necessary. Anterolateral approach using thoracotomy provides excellent visualization of anterior vertebral body. For the upper thoracic spine (T2-T9), a right thoracotomy is used, and for T10-L2 a left side approach is better. The fifth intercostal space is used for lesions above T10, and sixth intercostal space is used for lesions from T10 and below. This approach involves resection of the rib, and the same rib is utilized as a strut graft after debridement. Though a rib graft provides some structural support, it becomes weak if used as long segment graft in a multilevel decompression case. Using this approach one can clear the pathology and place a graft or cage anteriorly to maintain vertebral height and prevent kyphosis. This technique is good, but it is associated with complications, like injury to lungs, great vessels, and esophagus. It is reported that, though this approach is good it has drawbacks like development of delayed kyphosis and subsequent deficit. Surgeons started adding posterior fixation for this approach, but it was a staged procedure and left the graft unstable until fixation was achieved and resulted in failure [8]. To prevent this, some authors started operating using posterior only approach, where they perform laminectomy and debride the pus and then fix posteriorly using pedicle screws and fuse the posterior elements with the use of bone graft. This approach is good in achieving stability, but removing pathology from ventral region is difficult. This approach is criticized by many surgeons since only the healthy posterior elements of the spine were violated. Surgeons then started to approach pathology using simultaneous anterior and posterior approach, postero-lateral approach (transforaminal).

16.1.4 Simultaneous Anterior and Posterior Approach

In multilevel involvement, anterior decompression with grafting may lead to instability requiring posterior fixation which can be done in one or two stages. Jain et al. [9] recommended simultaneous anterior decompression, posterior fixation, and circumferential bone grafting using extra pleural anterolateral approach for the following indications:

1. Pan-vertebral disease
2. >3 vertebrae involvement or >1.5 vertebrae loss with neurological defect
3. Kyphosis requiring correction

With the patient in the lateral decubitus position, a T-shaped posterior incision was used. In thoracic spine three ribs at apex of kyphosis were resected posteriorly. The involved vertebral bodies were excised to achieve anterior decompression. Posteriorly, the spine was exposed up to two adjacent healthy vertebrae on either side in short segment disease and till one adjacent healthy vertebra each in long segment pathology. Posterior fixation was achieved using a pre-bent Hartshill loop. Tricortical iliac crest graft or resected ribs were used to graft the anterior defect after debridement of bodies of diseased vertebrae. With this technique a final kyphosis correction of 25° was obtained. The extra-pleural approach in lateral position has decreased risk of spinal cord injury, prevents uncontrolled correction of kyphosis, and spares respiratory function. Moon et al. had recommended a two stage surgery with posterior stabilization done first and later anterior decompression with bone grafting done at second stage.

16.1.5 Postero-lateral Approach (Transforaminal)

Multilevel non-contiguous thoracic spine involvement is an atypical presentation of Pott spine and has been primarily managed conservatively with antitubercular chemotherapy and immobilization. Zhang et al. [10] described single stage transforaminal thoracic debridement, decompression, fusion, and fixation (modified TIFF) using posterolateral approach for multilevel non-contiguous pathology. Surgical intervention should be done in patients with instability, progressive neurological deficit, severe deformity, resistance to drugs, and paravertebral abscess. In the prone position, two longitudinal skin incisions were made 5–7 cm lateral to spinous processes. The posterior elements were exposed, and facetectomy and laminectomy were performed to achieve limited decompression and debridement. The exposed diseased vertebral bodies were removed with curettes. The adjacent rib was cut 1–1.5 cm. Fixation was achieved at two levels superior and inferior to level of decompression. The defect created was filled with duplex cortical bone graft. Zhang's method allows 270° decompression and anterior reconstruction by interbody fusion. They achieved significant improvement in deformity in postoperative period and arrest of progression of kyphosis.

Earlier single staged debridement and bone grafting by anterior approach was the surgical method of choice in spinal tuberculosis. But it had a limited role in correction of kyphosis and preventing its progression. Using anterior debridement and posterior fixation, it was possible to address this issue but resulted in a significant surgical trauma and a high frequency of perioperative complications. Single segment tuberculosis can be managed effectively by a posterior approach only. In a retrospective study by Tang et al. [11], they compared anterior approach only, anterior combined with posterior approach, and posterior approach only in patients with thoracolumbar tuberculosis. They found that all patients achieved bony fusion between 6 and 12 months after surgery. Patients who had fixation through a posterior approach had better correction of the deformity, better maintenance of correction, and better stability of fixation. A combined approach was associated with significant surgical trauma leading to longest surgery time, highest blood loss, and most perioperative complications. Isolated posterior approach had fewest complications related to surgical procedure and allows for effective debridement, correction of deformity, and stable fixation. But the posterior only approach is technically difficult, provides narrow field of vision, and can cause dura injury. They concluded that the posterior approach is superior to the anterior only or combined approach when indications for it are favorable (Table 16.3).

16.1.6 Approaches Lumbo-sacral Spine

Tuberculous lesions in lumbo-sacral spine can be approached through anterior only, posterior only, or a combined approach. For the anterior approach, an oblique hypogastric incision is made with the patient in lateral decubitus position or a left paramedian incision with the patient in the supine position. After the exposure, the spine is stabilized using distractor screws on adjacent normal vertebrae. After thorough debridement of the tuberculous focus, internal fixation and bone grafting is done. Using the posterior approach, a mid spinal incision is made with the patient in position. The posterior elements are exposed, and shorter segmental fixation is achieved using transpedicular screws and rods. After removal of diseased vertebrae, defect was filled with bone graft. The deformity is corrected by manipulation of the instrumentation. In the combined approach, anterior debridement is done first, and subsequently the patient is repositioned for the posterior fixation [12–14].

In a retrospective study by Zheng et al. [12], they found that the posterior approach had significantly lower surgery time and blood loss compared to the anterior approach. All patients achieved bony fusion, and there were no significant differences in pain relief, neurological improvement, or ODI scores. Also, the posterior

Table 16.3 Comparing outcomes of different surgical approaches by Tang et al.

	Anterior approach	Combined anterior and posterior	Posterior approach
Surgery time (min)	324 ± 44	422 ± 70	257 ± 84
Blood loss (ml)	895 ± 395	1187 ± 504	805 ± 769
Cobb angle Preoperative	20.23 ± 7.62	18.74 ± 7.3	23.2 ± 9.7
Cobb angle Postoperative	10.0 ± 4.99	9.11 ± 3.63	9.8 ± 5.4
Cobb angle final follow-up	15.54 ± 6.06	10.94 ± 4.0	12.0 ± 6.2
Loss of angle	5.45 ± 3.13	1.82 ± 1.76	2.2 ± 2.6

Table 16.4 Bhoraj and Mehta classification system

	MRI findings	Treatment
Group A	Anterior lesions Stable with no kyphosis	Anterior debridement and strut grafting
Group B	Global lesions Instability with kyphosis	Anterior decompression and strut grafting posterior fixation
Group C	Anterior or global lesions High risk for transthoracic surgery	Decompression through posterior transpedicular route and posterior fixation
Group D	Posterior lesions No deformity Stable	Posterior decompression No fixation

approach achieved significantly better correction of the lumbosacral lordosis, 27° vs. 22° with anterior approach at the last follow-up. Sun et al. [13] found that the combined approach had higher surgery time, blood loss, and duration of hospitalization compared to anterior approach with ARCH plate. There was no significant difference in ESR, CRP, pain relief, neurological improvement, and ODI score between anterior and combined approach. A retrospective study by Liu et al. [14], comparing posterior approach with combined approach, found significantly lower intraoperative time, bleeding, and hospital stay in the posterior approach group. Both groups achieved bony fusion and normalization of ESR and CRP. There was no significant difference in pain relief, neurological improvement, deformity correction, ODI score, and long-term complications in both groups.

The anterior approach provides direct access to lesion allowing for complete removal of the tuberculous focus and spares the posterior elements of spine. But the anterior approach is more challenging and includes the complications related to a thoracotomy, a high risk of neurovascular injury in lumbosacral region due to complicated anatomy, and may additionally require stable fixation by posterior approach. The posterior approach is technically easier, provides access to the spinal canal for decompression of cord, allows for more stable fixation via pedicle screws, and is associated with fewer surgery-related complications.

Bhoraj et al. [15] described a classification system to help decide the surgical approach based on the site of lesion and degree of spinal deformity (Table 16.4).

16.2 Postoperative Protocol

- The drain is to be removed after the flow is less than 50 ml/day.
- The patient should be maintained in supine position for a minimum of 2 weeks and a TLSO brace support to be used when patient made to sit or stand.
- Brace treatment should be continued for a minimum period of 6–8 weeks after surgery.
- ATT should be continued till 12 months depending on the disease condition.

- Patients should be followed every 3 months for the first year, every 6 months for the second year, and then annually.
- At each follow-up, clinical symptoms, neural status, radiological signs of bony fusion, ESR, CRP, and LFT must be checked.

References

1. Neville CH. Is surgical fusion still desirable in spinal tuberculosis? Clin Orthop. 1971;75:179–84.
2. Hodgson AR, Stock FE. Anterior spinal fusion a preliminary communication on the radical treatment of Pott's disease and Pott's paraplegia. Br J Surg. 1956;44(185):266–75.
3. Tuli S. Results of treatment of spinal tuberculosis by "Midddle-Path" regime. J Bone Joint Surg. 1975;57:1301–620.
4. Ferrer MF, Torres LG, Ramirez OA, et al. Tuberculosis of the spine. A systematic review of case series. Int Orthop. 2012;36:221–31.
5. Mak KC, Cheung KMC. Surgical treatment of acute TB spondylitis: indications and outcomes. Eur Spine J. 2013;22(Suppl 4):603–11.
6. Rajasekaran S. The natural history of post-tubercularkyphosis in children: radiological signs which predict late increase in deformity. J Bone Joint Surg. 2001;83B:954–62.
7. Oguz E, Sehirlioglu A, Altinmakas M, Ozturk C, Komurcu M, Solakoglu C. A new classification and guide for surgical treatment of spinal tuberculosis. Int Orthop. 2008;32(1):127–33.
8. Cheng Z, Wang J, Zheng Q, Wu Y, Guo X. Anterolateral radical debridement and interbody bone grafting combined with transpedicle fixation in the treatment of thoracolumbar spinal tuberculosis. Medicine (Baltimore). 2015;94(14):e721. https://doi.org/10.1097/MD.0000000000000721.
9. Jain A, Dhammi I, Prashad B, Sinha S, Mishra P. Simultaneous anterior decompression and posterior instrumentation of the tuberculous spine using an anterolateral extrapleural approach. J Bone Joint Surg. 2008;90-B:1477–81.
10. Zhang H, Lin M, Shen K, Ge L, Li J, et al. Surgical management for multilevel noncontiguous thoracic spinal tuberculosis by single-stage posterior transforaminal thoracic debridement, limited decompression, interbody fusion, and posterior instrumentation (modified TTIF). Arch Orthop Trauma Surg. 2012;132:751–7.
11. Tang Y, Wu W, Yang S, Wang D, Zhang Q, et al. Surgical treatment of thoracolumbar spinal tuberculosis – a multicentre, retrospective, case-control study. J Orthop Surg Res. 2019;14:233.
12. Zheng B, Hao D, Guo H, He B. Anterior versus posterior surgical approach for lumbosacral tuberculosis. J Int Med Res. 2018;46:2569–77.
13. Sun D, Zhang Z, Mei G, Hou T, Li Y, et al. Comparison of anterior only and combined anterior and posterior approach in treating lumbosacral tuberculosis. Sci Rep. 2019;9:18475.
14. Liu Z, Zhang P, Li W, Xu Z, Wang X. Posterior- only vs. combined posterior- anterior approaches in treating lumbar and lumbosacral spinal tuberculosis: a retrospective study with minimum 7-year follow-up. J Orthop Surg Res. 2020;15:99.
15. Mehta J, Bhojraj S. Tuberculosis of the thoracic spine. A classification based on the selection of surgical strategies. J Bone Joint Surg Br. 2001;83(6):859–63.

Chapter 17
Surgical Management of Cervical Spine Tuberculosis

Ryan P. McLynn, Vibhu Krishnan Viswanathan, and Sakthivel Rajan Rajaram Manoharan

Abstract While the spine is the most common site of extrapulmonary tuberculosis (TB), cervical spine represents a small portion of cases, only roughly 3–5% [Teka et al., Pan Afr Med J 37(7):1–5, 2020; Hu and Liu, Spine J 16:e227–e229, 2016; Khanna and Sabharwal, Spine J 19:1858–1870, 2019]. Consequently, tuberculosis of the cervical spine has received substantially less attention compared to thoracolumbar disease, resulting in lower volume and poorer quality of evidence to guide physicians [Yuan B, Zhao Y, Zhou S, et al. Arch Orthop Trauma Surg, 2020].

The goals of treatment for cervical spinal tuberculosis include disease eradication, pain control, neurologic improvement, and restoration of spinal stability. As with other forms of tuberculosis, the mainstay of treatment is multidrug antitubercular chemotherapy. Appropriate chemotherapy, in conjunction with immobilization, has demonstrated remarkable efficacy in treating spinal tuberculosis. As the body heals diseased tissues, there is usually substantial improvement in neurologic deficits as well as robust healing with bony or fibrous tissues, restoring spinal stability.

Despite the success of antimicrobial treatment, there are many cases in which medical management alone fails. In these cases, surgical debridement and reconstruction may be essential to restore spinal stability, decompress neural elements, or eliminate disabling pain. In light of the rarity of cervical tuberculosis and the paucity of high-quality studies, surgical indications have not been entirely clarified. In this chapter, we have comprehensively discussed the options for surgical management of cervical TB.

Keywords Cervical spine · Tuberculosis · Cervical TB

R. P. McLynn · S. R. R. Manoharan (✉)
Department of Orthopaedics, UAB, Birmingham, AL, USA
e-mail: srajaram@uabmc.edu

V. K. Viswanathan
Department of Orthopaedics, University of Calgary, CA, USA

S. S. Dhatt, V. Kumar (eds.), *Tuberculosis of the Spine*,
https://doi.org/10.1007/978-981-16-9495-0_17

17.1 Introduction

While spinal TB accounts for 1% of all TB cases, cervical TB (CTB) constitutes just 3–5% of all spinal disease [1–3]. The literature classifies CTB into cranio-vertebral (CVJ) and sub-axial cervical disease (SACTB). Additionally, lesions involving junctional levels of the cervico-thoracic (CT) region need special consideration, owing to peculiar biomechanical properties of this transitional zone. The smaller dimension of spinal canal, proximity to vital structures (including vertebral arteries), unique facetal orientation, high mobility, and lordotic profile make cervical spine more vulnerable to malalignment, instability, and neuro-deterioration [4–9]. The management of these lesions therefore requires careful consideration of all such factors.

In accordance with the popular adage, "Uncomplicated tuberculosis is primarily a medical disease," chemotherapy remains the mainstay in the treatment of spinal TB [4, 10, 11]. Nevertheless, surgical interventions can be extremely valuable in specific circumstances. The principal objectives of surgical interventions in spinal TB include procurement of tissue samples, debridement neural decompression, and stabilization [12–14]. The usual indications for surgical intervention have been listed in Table 17.1.

17.2 Indications for Surgery

As with other infectious and infiltrative diseases of the spine, the goals of treatment for cervical spinal tuberculosis include curing disease, improving neurologic deficits, controlling pain, and preserving spinal stability. Due to the remarkable efficacy

Table 17.1 Indications for surgery in spinal TB

Absolute indications
1. Significant neuro-deficit (including bladder/bowel incontinence)
2. Progressive neurological deficits, despite 3 or 4 weeks of medical therapy
3. Spine at risk signs (in pediatric patients)
4. Multi-level or extensive disease
5. Failed or inadequate percutaneous biopsy
6. Doubtful diagnosis
7. Large or un-resolving abscess
8. Failure of medical management
9. Multidrug resistant tuberculosis
Relative indications
1. Kyphosis $\geq 30°$
2. Significant vertebral loss
3. Significant spinal canal compromise with normal neurology

of medical management, the majority of patients with cervical tuberculosis can be successfully treated with multidrug antibiotics and judicious immobilization. Many trials have demonstrated impressive success of medical management, even in patients with profound neurologic deficits or gross spinal instability. As spinal tuberculosis resolves, there is a high rate of resorption of infectious foci and replacement with bone and/or fibrous tissue. Several studies have demonstrated excellent spinal stability following treatment, even in patients who presented with frank dislocations [15–17]. Additionally, patients with advanced tuberculosis have poor physiologic reserve, making them poor candidates for major spine surgery and susceptible to high complication rates [18, 19].

Given the efficacy of antitubercular chemotherapy, surgery has become an adjunct treatment for patients who fail medical management or present with unique features unlikely to resolve with medical management alone. The challenge for physicians is to identify this minority of patients who will ultimately require surgical treatment.

The efficacy of medical management means there are few absolute indications for surgery, but there are many circumstances in which surgery should be considered. In considering the goals of treatment, the following are potential indications for surgery. Of note, even with surgical management, it is essential to promptly initiate appropriate antimicrobial chemotherapy and complete the entire course according to local protocols.

17.2.1 Failure of Medical Management

Surgery should be offered to patients who demonstrate persistent infection despite appropriate chemotherapy, based on clinical and laboratory monitoring. Assuming correct antibiotic therapy, refractory cases can be offered surgery. Similarly, patients who continue to experience severe or intolerable pain despite optimal medical management should be offered surgery [20].

17.2.2 Extent of Disease

Many experts recommend surgery for patients with massive abscesses, though no objective measurements exist to guide that decision. Disease involving both the anterior and posterior elements of a vertebra may be considered for surgery, as there may be a higher risk for neurologic injury or progressive deformity [21]. Patients with large, symptomatic retropharyngeal abscesses should be offered decompression by open or minimally invasive means [2, 16, 21–23].

17.2.3 Neurologic Deficits

Patients with major neurologic deficits such as significant weakness, inability to ambulate, or incontinence despite medical management should be offered surgery. This includes patients who demonstrate neurologic decline despite medical management or who fail to improve after 3–4 weeks of medical management [18, 22–24]. There are no absolute neurologic indications for surgery prior to trialing conservative management, but patients with >50% cord compression, severe deficits, or obvious myelomalacia or myelitis should be considered for surgery [21–23]. There are case series of successful medical management even with advanced deficits though, so treatment ultimately should be a decision made together by the patient and surgeon [17, 19, 22].

17.2.4 Instability and Deformity

Surgical indications in the setting of spinal instability remain controversial and lacking consensus guidelines. Some degree of spinal instability is not an absolute indication for surgery, as there is an excellent record of bony healing and restored stability with medical management [15–17]. In the cervical spine, this requires appropriate immobilization. While some physicians use a hard cervical collar in milder cases, many favor a halo vest for greater stability and patient compliance [15, 19]. Given the complications and discomfort, versus earlier return to ambulation and activity with surgery, physicians should discuss both options with patients. Following conservative treatment, patients who continue to experience instability or increased displacement on flexion/extension radiographs should be offered surgery.

Similarly, optimal treatment cervical kyphosis remains controversial. Nonoperative treatment tends to be associated with a small increase in kyphosis, normally within 5° but up to 15° [17, 25]. Surgery, in contrast, offers excellent restoration of cervical lordosis, and modern instrumentation has made loss of correction rare [17, 26, 27]. The challenge is identifying what degree of kyphosis leads to disability or progressive deformity. Though some surgeons treat kyphosis aggressively, one study found sagittal alignment was not associated with pain, function, or neurologic status as long as final kyphosis was <30° [28]. Kyphosis of 60° or greater faces unacceptable risk of progressing, while others have proposed 30° or 40° as thresholds due to patient discomfort and potential risk of progression [21, 28]. Accounting for limited evidence, cervical kyphosis of 60° represents a strong indication for surgery, while patients with 30°–60° should consider surgery. Surgeons should have a lower threshold to offer surgery at the cervicothoracic junction, given the increased risk for progression [29].

17.3 Craniovertebral Junctional Tuberculosis

Patients frequently present more with neuro deficits in atlantoaxial tuberculosis (AATB) than other spinal TB (including SACTB). Patients with AATB complicated by neuro deficit often have associated posterior pharyngeal wall and paravertebral abscesses, destruction of lateral mass of atlas, odontoid, or vertebral body of axis, significant atlanto-axial instability, and serious intraspinal compression of spinal cord secondary to abscess.

17.3.1 Management of AATB

While medical management is the foundation of AATB, the literature features a divide in managing patients with extensive spinal destruction or neurologic deficit. One camp strongly favors conservative measures including prolonged external immobilization [19, 30, 31], while the other more liberally advocates for surgical fixation at earlier stages [32–34]. Despite these contrasting approaches, all authors have emphasized the need to balance surgical risks with the difficulties associated with long-term external orthoses. Only one study concluded that ideal line of management in all patients with AATB is surgical, reporting superior prevention of neuro-deterioration and early mobilization [35].

17.3.2 Classification Systems

Radiographic criteria: The classic classification by Lifeso includes three stages, namely, stage 1 where ligamentous and bony architecture are preserved, stage 2 where ligamentous architecture is compromised, and stage 3 where significant osseous destruction and gross malalignment are observed [15]. Goel classified AATB into 3 stages based on extent of disease involvement [6]. Stage 1 includes lesions with unilateral involvement of cancellous portions of atlas, axis, and odontoid. Stage 2 is characterized by disease extension onto unilateral AA joint. In stage 3, disease involves bilateral AA joints. Stage 3 lesions have high prevalence of associated deficits.

Clinical criteria: Behari and Arora classified AATB into four grades (Di-Lorenzo grading), based on clinical presentation: Grade 1 includes patients with neck pain alone, grade 2 includes independent patients with minor disabilities, grade 3 and 4 include patients who are partially and totally dependent on others for activities of daily living [19, 32, 33].

Combined criteria: Teegala combined clinical and radiological parameters and developed a grading system based on neck movement, motor, and radiological scores [5].

17.3.3 Classification of Disease and Decision-Making

Goel's classification favored conservative treatment alone following tissue diagnosis for stage 1 and stable stage 2 disease [6]. Teegala recommended conservative treatment for scores 3–4 and surgical treatment for scores 7–8, while scores 5–6 were considered intermediate and required case-specific decision-making [5]. This grading was further simplified by Molliqaj, who advocated surgery for score ≥6 [7].

17.3.4 Surgical Intervention

17.3.4.1 Indications

The role of surgery is usually confined to confirming diagnosis through tissue sampling, decompression in patients with significant neurologic deficit, stabilization in stage 3 or advanced stage 2 cases to prevent deformity, or in patients who fail medical management. Similarly, Behari recommended surgery for grade 3/4 disease, presence of AAD, retropharyngeal abscess, significant osseous destruction, and poor response to ATM after 3 months [32, 33].

The role of surgery is usually confined to one of the following scenarios: (1) confirmation of diagnosis through tissue sampling, (2) debridement and decompression in patients with gross neuro-deficit, (3) stabilization in some stage 2 and all stage 3 cases to prevent deformity progression, (4) drug-resistant infection, and (5) patients' inability to tolerate ATM. Behari described five criteria for considering surgical intervention, namely, preoperative grades 3/4, presence of mobile or fixed AAD, retropharyngeal abscess, degree of osseous destruction, and poor response following 3 months of ATM [32, 33].

17.3.4.2 Need for Tissue Sampling for Confirmation

The need for histopathological diagnosis prior to starting ATM remains debated. General treatment principles favor tissue sampling before chemotherapy, but the deep location of CVJ and resulting difficulty obtaining tissue should be considered. Some investigators have highlighted paucibilliary nature and low yield of these infections, suggesting initiating ATM without prior tissue sampling unless drug-resistant infection is suspected [8, 9]. Nevertheless, the current consensus favors universal tissue sampling.

17.3.4.3 Surgical Approaches

The ideal surgical approach in AATB remains controversial. Studies have described anterior-alone, posterior-alone, and combined approaches. In general, while anterior approach gives direct access to lesion to facilitate decompression and tissue sampling, posterior approach provides biomechanically superior options for stabilization.

Molloqaj described a protocol for deciding the surgical approach, recommending posterior fusion only in individuals with clear evidence of AAD and ligamentous disruption [7]. In patients with grade ≥6 and no AAD, trans-oral decompression was advocated. In those with reducible AAD, posterior fixation of only the involved segments is necessary. In all patients with fixed AAD, combined anterior (trans-nasal/trans-oral odontoid resection) and posterior approach (C1-2 or OC fusion, as necessary) is ideal.

Anterior-only approach: While anterior-only approach has the major benefit of providing a direct window for debridement and decompression, this approach is complicated by distorted anatomy from disease, inadequate fixation options, and difficulty achieving fusion. Consequently, Fang reported 50% graft failure after anterior-only surgeries [36].

The AA joint can be exposed by trans-oral (TOA), lateral upper cervical (LUCA), anterior retropharyngeal (ARPA), or traditional anterior cervical approaches (TACA). Although TOA is the most direct approach, its limitations include poor surgical window, exposure to oral flora, possible cerebrospinal fluid fistula, and glossal/pharyngeal edema. This approach does have the unique advantage of simultaneous access to bilateral joints.

LUCA may involve ligation of external jugular vein, dissection of carotid sheath, and may place vertebral artery at risk during dissection. Although ARPA avoids contamination with oral flora and provides excellent exposure from clivus to C2 body, dissection involving the submandibular gland, hypoglossal nerve, facial artery, and other vital structures is technically challenging [37]. Wang has published a recent 12-patient series that demonstrated good healing through this approach, augmented with posterior instrumentation [38]. Although traditional anterior (Smith-Robinson) approach is familiar to most spine surgeons, it may not be feasible to eradicate disease with this approach alone.

Adjuvants to surgery: Several authors have recommended either preoperative halo traction [15] or intraoperative cervical traction [37] to reduce dislocated atlantoaxial joints.

Posterior and combined antero-posterior approaches: Although posterior-only approaches provide excellent options for stabilization, meticulous debridement and decompression are not always possible [39]. A combined approach (single- or multi-staged) integrates the benefits of both approaches and has been commonly described [32, 33, 39]. Posterior stabilization techniques include atlanto-axial and occipito-cervical fixation (OCF). Wang advocated for choosing the most conservative possible technique for AATB, routinely favoring C1-2 stabilization alone (versus OCF) to achieve adequate stability while preserving motion [38]. Goel reported the effectiveness of contralateral-only C1-2 stabilization in unilateral C1-2 involvement [6]. OCF needs to be considered only with extensive, bilateral joint destruction.

Concept of unilateral lateral mass stabilization in stage 2 lesions: Goel conceptualized that following unilateral destruction of C1/2 facets (stage 2), ipsilateral alar and transverse ligaments become incompetent [6]. This results in increased obliquity of C1 facet and leads to lateral subluxation. They described a technique of unilateral inter-facetal distraction, reduction, and unilateral stabilization.

17.3.5 Authors' Preferred Approach

The surgical approaches in AATB include anterior-alone, posterior-alone, and combined approaches. Currently, posterior approach (AA fusion or occipito-cervical fusion (OCF)) is the most preferred globally [7, 32, 33].

In patients with isolated atlanto-axial disease, AA fusion may suffice. In the presence of anterior abscess, anterior debridement is imperative to reduce recurrence and achieve good fusion rates. Preoperatively assessing reducibility of AA dislocation (AAD) is essential. Patients with reducible AAD benefit from posterior fusion alone. However, those with irreducible or rotatory AAD require posterior distraction, reduction, and stabilization or combined anteroposterior approaches. Additionally, pre- or intraoperative halo traction should be considered for irreducible AAD. In cases with extensive, bilateral AA joint destruction or basilar invagination, OCF offers superior stability. A case example is shown in Figs. 17.1, 17.2, 17.3, and 17.4.

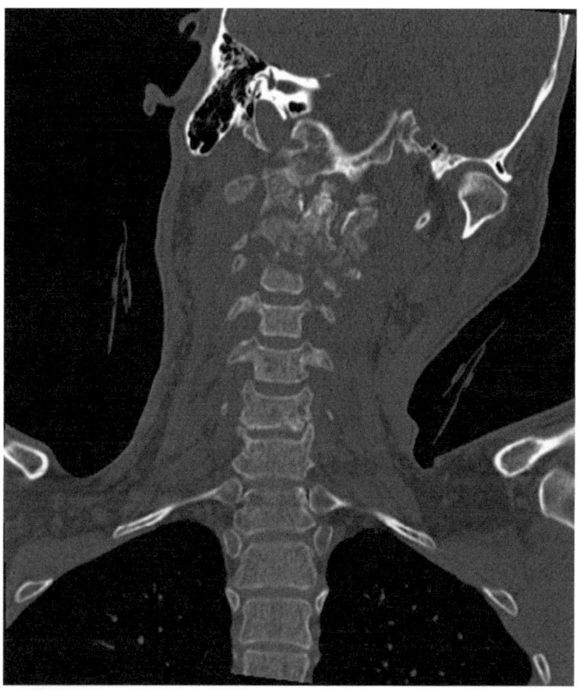

Fig. 17.1 Coronal CT showing destruction of C2-3 segment with erosive changes at C1-2 joints

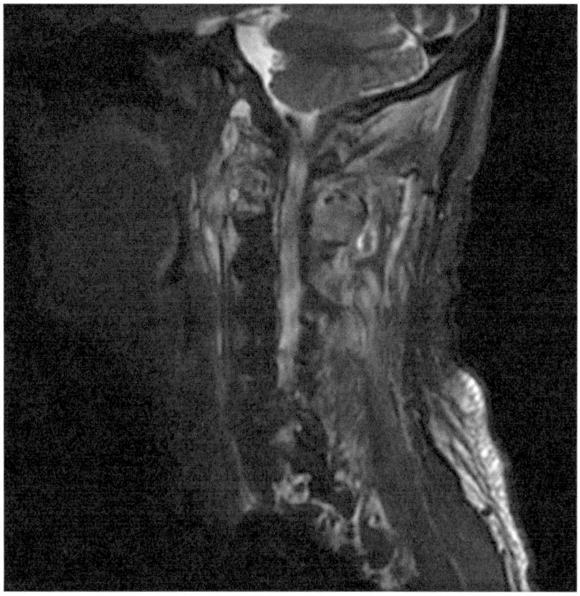

Fig. 17.2 Sagittal MRI cut shows significant prevertebral abscess and involvement of the occiput to C3 joints

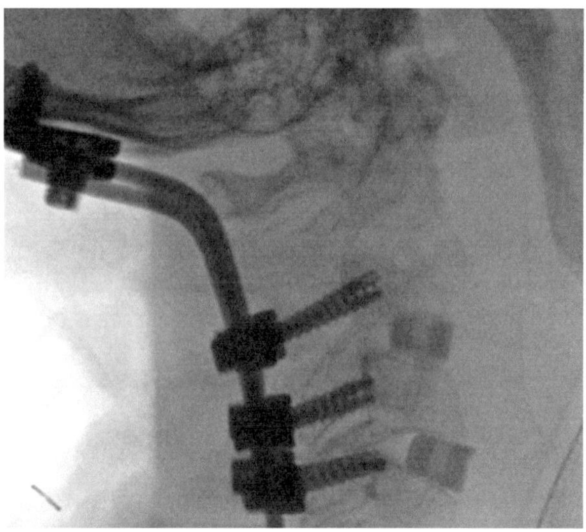

Fig. 17.3 Immediate post op films after debridement with 360°. reconstruction of the cranio-cervical and upper cervical region

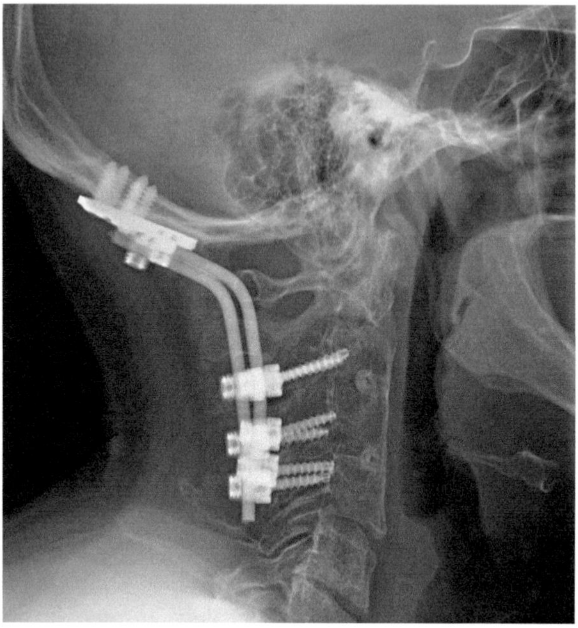

Fig. 17.4 Two-year follow-up cervical X-ray showing fusion mass across the reconstruction

17.4 Sub-axial Tuberculosis (SACTB)

17.4.1 Principles of Imaging

Plain standing radiographs provide the essential information regarding cervical alignment (C2-C7 lordosis and C2-C7 sagittal vertical axis (SVA)). Whole spine radiographs can be beneficial in identifying compensatory changes in spinal or pelvic alignment with major cervical sagittal deformities. Two-level disease is the commonest pattern, followed by single-level and then multi-level disease [40]. C5 was the most commonly involved level, followed by C6.

17.4.2 Classification Systems

Wang described a grading system that includes neck movement restriction, motor power, and radiological features (paravertebral abscess, bone destruction, and cord compression) [41]. A score of 3–4 was classified as grade 1, 5–6 as grade 2, and 7–8 as grade 3.

17.4.3 Surgical Indications

The surgical indications in SACTB are similar to general recommendations for TB involving other spinal levels [14, 24]. Indications include (1) progressive neurologic deterioration, (2) severe kyphosis at presentation, and (3) patient preference after informed decision-making. Additionally, patients with pan-vertebral disease and long-segment involvement fare better with surgical management, secondary to high propensity for progressive kyphosis and late neuro-deterioration [24]. All patients with SACTB must be offered chemotherapy initially, even in patients with neurologic deficits [24]. The patient is followed with re-evaluation of Japanese Orthopedic Association (JOA) score after 1 and 2 weeks. If JOA score is stable or improved, chemotherapy is continued. Any deterioration necessitates surgery. Recently, the importance of cervical sagittal balance has been highlighted. Patients with C2-C7 kyphosis or C2-C7 SVA >4 cm have poorer neck disability index (NDI) and higher risk of kyphosis progression. Such patients benefit from anterior debridement and reconstruction [42, 43].

17.4.4 Approaches and Surgical Techniques

Anterior approaches to cervical spine offers the best approach for direct access to the disease focus, thorough debridement, spinal decompression, robust stabilization, fusion, and restoration of lordosis. Most current studies have supported the role of anterior approach. The most commonly reported complications following anterior cervical approach include dysphagia, hematoma, and recurrent laryngeal nerve palsy.

Hsu reported 100% recovery after radical debridement and reconstruction (Hong Kong procedure) through Southwick-Robinson approach combined with ATM [40]. Similarly, Wu reported excellent outcomes following anterior debridement, decompression, and instrumented fusion with titanium mesh cage, including significant improvements in kyphosis angle and visual analog scale pain scores [26]. Similar reports demonstrated 100% fusion and neurological stabilization in 25 patients who underwent anterior debridement and reconstruction with bone graft (He). Koptan found superior alignment and reduced complications reconstructing with titanium mesh cage compared to structural iliac crest graft in a non-randomized trial [44]. A recent systematic review corroborated superior debridement via anterior approaches [45].

However, posterior approach may be necessary in patients with pan vertebral or posterior-only involvement, significant kyphosis or sagittal imbalance, long-segment disease requiring corpectomies at 3+ levels, junctional involvement, and those with significant posterior compression. Based on their clinico-radiological grading, Wang proposed a treatment protocol for SACTB: conservative treatment for grade 1, anterior debridement and fusion for grade 2; and combined anterior-posterior approach for grade 3 lesions [41].

Yin found that anterior, posterior, and combined (anterior decompression and posterior stabilization) approaches all resulted in successful neurological recovery, pain improvement, and restored alignment, concluding all are reasonable options [46]. They purported that therapeutic strategies need to be individualized, depending upon patient's condition, focal disease characteristics, and surgeon's expertise.

Special considerations in children: The pediatric cervical spine is peculiar given its continued growth until skeletal maturity. Radical debridement may damage ring apophyses and end plates, leading to growth disturbance and progressive kyphosis. Therefore, gentle, instead of radical, debridement is recommended in growing spines [25, 47].

The "spine at risk" signs (SARS), which identify posterior column failure in thoracolumbar post-tubercular kyphosis, are important indicators for deformity progression in immature spines [25, 47]. Prophylactic stabilization should be considered in all children with positive SARS, and all children managed conservatively need to be followed until skeletal maturity.

17.5 Cervicothoracic Tuberculosis

Disease involving C7-T2 carries certain unique anatomic and biomechanical features. The cervicothoracic junction constitutes a major transitional zone between kyphotic and lordotic, as well as rigid and mobile, spinal segments [48]. These factors result in increased biomechanical stresses, which may lead to severe kyphosis and instability. Therefore, surgeons should have a lower threshold to stabilize these lesions [49]. Surgical approaches are done through traditional anterior cervical or posterior approaches [50–52]. The literature has favored anterior approaches as a safe and direct approach to diseased vertebrae [48, 51, 53, 54]. The depth of vertebrae; extent of kyphosis; proximity to vital neck structures; and presence of the sternum, clavicles, mediastinum, and scapulae make exposure of this region challenging [54].

Extended anterior approaches have been described to access CT region. Various approaches involving manubriotomy, manubriectomy, and/or medial clavicle excision have been reported with good results [48–51]. Exposure to T2-T3 disc space and distally is challenging and may require manubriotomy in up to 85% of cases [53, 55, 56].

Although supplemental posterior fixation is biomechanically advantageous [57], a majority of studies report a good outcome with anterior interventions alone [50, 51, 56]. Zhu recommends adding posterior stabilization when disease focus is distal to the sternal notch based on preoperative computed tomography [54]. Wang and

Rajasekaran have favored combined anteroposterior approaches in pediatric CTTB, especially with "spine-at-risk" signs [25, 29, 47, 58, 59].

17.5.1 Clinical Outcome of CTB

Typically, the effectiveness of ATM is evident within 3 weeks, with continued subsequent improvement. Eventually, all lesions heal by fibrous union and late ossification, restoring spinal stability [6]. Overall, outcomes in both conservatively and surgically managed CTB patients have been reported to be favorable [15, 22, 24, 27, 32, 33].

17.5.2 Long-Term Outcome in AATB

In Lifeso's series, 11/12 patients (five conservative, six surgical) recovered completely [15]. Similarly, Behari reported excellent cure rates and neurologic improvement in a series of both conservatively and operatively treated patients [32, 33]. Sinha reported excellent recovery in 17/18 patients (one mortality due to meningitis) treated with combined anteroposterior surgery and ATM [37].

17.5.3 Long-Term Outcome in SACTB

Hassan demonstrated excellent neurological and radiological (improvement of kyphosis from 21.5° to 2.6°) outcome following anterior debridement, iliac crest autograft, and plating [60]. Preoperative JOA scores and number of levels involved are important predictors of recovery [24]. Both Qu and Bhandari found similar final outcomes with conservative versus surgical treatment, though recovery was much faster in patients treated surgically [22, 24].

17.6 Conclusion

The general principles of management of CTB are similar to spinal TB elsewhere. Medical therapy remains the cornerstone. When surgery is chosen, it should never delay or shorten antitubercular chemotherapy. Surgery is advocated in specific scenarios involving gross neurologic deficit, significant instability, altered sagittal balance, and unacceptable response to ATM. Surgical approaches for AATB include anterior, posterior, and combined approaches, although posterior approach is preferred. Most studies on SACTB favor anterior approaches. Posterior augmentation is necessary in long-segment or pan-vertebral disease, significant kyphosis, and junctional involvement. The overall long-term outcome in surgically-treated CTB is favorable. The craniocervical and cervicothoracic junctions frequently require more technically demanding approaches and circumferential procedures to achieve a favorable result. Patient-reported outcomes and cost-effectiveness research are absent in the literature and deserve greater attention moving forward. As many of the surgical indications are relative or equivocally evidence-based, physicians should discuss the benefits, risks, and patient's goals to jointly select a treatment.

References

1. Teka M, Ghozlen HB, Zaier AY, et al. Cervical spine tuberculosis. Pan African Medical Journal. 2020;37(7):1–5.
2. Hu X, Liu L. A huge retropharyngeal abscess causing airway and esophageal obstruction associated with cervical spine tuberculosis. Spine J. 2016;16:e227–9.
3. Khanna K, Sabharwal S. Spinal tuberculosis: a comprehensive review for the modern spine surgeon. Spine J. 2019;19:1858–70.
4. Rajasekaran S, Kanna RM, Shetty AP. Pathophysiology and treatment of spinal tuberculosis. JBJS Rev. 2014;2:e4.
5. Teegala R, Kumar P, Kale SS, et al. Craniovertebral junction tuberculosis: a new comprehensive therapeutic strategy. Neurosurgery. 2008;63:946–55.
6. Goel A. Tuberculosis of craniovertebral junction: role of facets in pathogenesis and treatment. J Craniovertebr Junction Spine. 2016;7:129–30.
7. Molliqaj G, Dammann P, Schaller K, et al. Management of craniovertebral junction tuberculosis presenting with atlantoaxial dislocation. Acta Neurochir Suppl. 2019;125:337–44.
8. Qureshi MA, Afzal W, Khalique AB, et al. Tuberculosis of the craniovertebral junction. Eur Spine J. 2013;22(Suppl 4):612–7.
9. Appaduray SP, Lo P. Nonoperative management of craniovertebral junction and cutaneous tuberculosis. Surg Neurol Int. 2015;6:157.
10. Padda IS, Reddy KM. Antitubercular medications. 2020.; https://www.ncbi.nlm.nih.gov/books/NBK557666/. Accessed 27 Dec 2020.
11. Tiberi S, Scardigli A, Centis R, et al. Classifying new anti-tuberculosis drugs: rationale and future perspectives. Int J Infect Dis. 2017;56:181–4.
12. Shetty A, Kanna RM, Rajasekaran S. TB spine—current aspects on clinical presentation, diagnosis, and management options. Semin Spine Surg. 2016;28:150–62.
13. Kothari A, Khurjekar KS, Hadgaonkar S, et al. Ultrasound-guided aspiration of psoas abscess in a 28 year-old male: a case report, literature review, and the relevance of this technique in the developing world. Asian Pacific J Health Sci. 2014;1:307–11.
14. Viswanathan VK, Subramanian S. Pott's disease. 2020. https://www.ncbi.nlm.nih.gov/books/NBK538331/. Accessed 27 Dec 2020.
15. Lifeso R. Atlanto-axial tuberculosis in adults. J Bone Joint Surg Br. 1987;69-B(2):183–7.
16. Hou K, Yang H, Zhang L, et al. Stepwise therapy for treating tuberculosis of the upper cervical spine: a retrospective study of 11 patients. Eur Neurol. 2015;74:100–6.
17. Moon M-S, Moon J-L, Kim S-S, Moon Y-W. Treatment of tuberculosis of the cervical spine: operative versus nonoperative. Clin Orthop Relat Res. 2007;460:67–77.
18. Megaloikonomos PD, Igoumenou V, Antoniadou T, et al. Tuberculous spondylitis of the craniovertebral junction. J Bone Joint Infection. 2016;1:31–3.

19. Arora S, Sabat D, Maini L, et al. The results of nonoperative treatment of craniovertebral junction tuberculosis: a review of twenty-six cases. J Bone Joint Surg Am. 2011;93-A(6):540–7.
20. Fisahn C, Alonso F, Hasan GA, Tubbs RS, Dettori JR, Schildhauer TA, Rustagi T. Trends in spinal surgery for Pott's disease (2000–2016): an overview and bibliometric study. Global Spine J. 2017;7(8):821–8.
21. Chandra SP, Singh A, Goyal N, et al. Analysis of changing paradigms of management in 179 patients with spinal tuberculosis over a 12-year period and proposal of a new management algorithm. World Neurosurg. 2013;80(1/2):190–203.
22. Bhandari A, Garg RK, Malhotra HS, et al. Outcome assessment in conservatively managed patients with cervical spine tuberculosis. Spinal Cord. 2014;52:489–93.
23. Jain AK. Treatment of tuberculosis of the spine with neurologic complications. Clin Orthop Relat Res. 2003;398:75–84.
24. Qu J-T, Jiang Y-Q, Xu G-H, et al. Clinical characteristics and neurologic recovery of patients with cervical spinal tuberculosis: should conservative treatment be preferred? a retrospective follow-up study of 115 cases. World Neurosurg. 2015;83(5):700–7.
25. Rajasekaran S, Shanmugasundaram T. Prediction of the angle of gibbus deformity in tuberculosis of the spine. J Bone Joint Surg Am. 1987;69(4):503–9.
26. Wu W, Li Z, Lin R, et al. Anterior debridement, decompression, fusion, and instrumentation for lower cervical spine tuberculosis. J Orthop Sci. 2020;25:400–4.
27. Pan Z, Luo J, Yu L, et al. Debridement and reconstruction improve postoperative sagittal alignment in kyphotic cervical spinal tuberculosis. Clin Orthop Relat Res. 2017;475:2084–91.
28. Srivastava S, Raj A, Bhosale S, et al. Does kyphosis in healed subaxial cervical spine tuberculosis equate to a poor functional outcome? J Craniovertebr Junction Spine. 2020;11(2):86–92.
29. Rajasekaran S. Natural history of Pott's kyphosis. Eur Spine J. 2013;22(Suppl 4):S634–40.
30. Gupta SK, Mohindra S, Sharma BS, et al. Tuberculosis of the craniovertebral junction: is surgery necessary? Neurosurgery. 2006;58(6):1144–50.
31. Chadha M, Agarwal A, Singh AP. Craniovertebral tuberculosis: A retrospective review of 13 cases managed conservatively. Spine (Phila Pa 1976). 2007;32:1629–34.
32. Behari S, Mehrotra A, Sharma P, et al. Tuberculosis of the Craniovertebral Junction. Craniovertebral Junction. Thieme. 2011:167–77.
33. Behari S, Nayak SR, Bhargava V, et al. Craniocervical tuberculosis: protocol of surgical management. Neurosurgery. 2003;52(1):72–80. discussion 80–81
34. Shukla D, Mongia S, Devi BI, et al. Management of craniovertebral junction tuberculosis. Surg Neurol. 2005;63:101–6.
35. Arunkumar MJ, Rajshekhar V. Outcome in neurologicaly impaired patients with craniovertebral junction tuberculosis: results of combined anteroposterior surgery. J Neurosurg. 2002;97:166–71.
36. Fang D, Leong JC, Fang HSY. Tuberculosis of the upper cervical spine. J Bone Joint Surg Br. 1983;65-B:47–50.
37. Sinha S, Singh AK, Gupta V, et al. Surgical management and outcome of tuberculous atlantoaxial dislocation: a 15-year experience. Neurosurgery. 2003;52:331–9.
38. Wang B, Shang R, Yang T, et al. Evaluation of clinical outcomes of one-stage anterior and posterior surgical treatment for atlantoaxial tuberculosis complicated with neurological damage. BMC Musculoskelet Disord. 2019;20(1):148–57.
39. Kumar A, Singh S, Dikshit P, et al. Occipital condyle syndrome in a case of rotatory atlantoaxial subluxation (type II) with craniovertebral junction tuberculosis: should we operate on "active tuberculosis"? J Craniovertebr Junction Spine. 2020;11:143–7.
40. Hsu LC, Leong JC. Tuberculosis of the lower cervical spine (C2 to C7). A report on 40 cases. J Bone Joint Surg Br. 1984;66(1):1–5.
41. Wang X-Y, Wang XY, Luo CK, Li WW, et al. A practical therapeutic protocol for cervical tuberculosis. Eur J Trauma Emerg Surg. 2013;39:93–9.
42. Sardar ZM. CORR Insights: debridement and reconstruction improve postoperative sagittal alignment in kyphotic cervical spinal tuberculosis. Clin Orthop Relat Res. 2017;475:2092–4.

43. Ba Z, Pan F, Huang Y, et al. One-stage anterior radical debridement and reconstruction with titanium mesh combined with anti-tuberculosis for cervical spinal tuberculosis: 5–13 years follow up. Int J Clin Exp Med. 2016;9(3):6368–72.
44. Koptan W, ElMiligui Y, ElSharkawi M. Single stage anterior reconstruction using titanium mesh cages in neglected kyphotic tuberculous spondylodiscitis of the cervical spine. Eur Spine J. 2011;20:308–13.
45. Narayan V, Mohammed N, Savardekar AR, et al. Tuberculous spondylolisthesis: a reappraisal of the clinicradiologic spectrum and surgical treatment paradigm. World Neurosurg. 2018;114:361–7.
46. Yin XH, He BR, Liu ZK, et al. The clinical outcomes and surgical strategy for cervical spine tuberculosis: A retrospective study of 78 cases. Medicine (Baltimore). 2018;97:e11401.
47. Rajasekaran S. The natural history of post-tubercular kyphosis in children. Radiological signs which predict late increase in deformity. J Bone Joint Surg Br. 2001;83:954–62.
48. Wang VY, Chou D. The cervicothoracic junction. Neurosurg Clin N Am. 2007;18:365–71.
49. Ramani PS, Sharma A, Jituri S, et al. Anterior instrumentation for cervical spine tuberculosis: an analysis of surgical experience with 61 cases. Neurol India. 2005;53:83–9.
50. Sundaresan N, Shah J, Foley KM, et al. An anterior surgical approach to the upper thoracic vertebrae. J Neurosurg. 1984;61:686–90.
51. Sar C, Hamzaoglu A, Talu U, et al. An anterior approach to the cervicothoracic junction of the spine (modified osteotomy of manubrium sterni and clavicle). J Spinal Disord. 1999;12:102–6.
52. Chatterjee S, Basu S. Trans-sternal decompression of postlaminectomy caries of the upper dorsal spine. Br J Neurosurg. 2003;17:270–1.
53. Kurz LT, Pursel SE, Herkowitz HN. Modified anterior approach to the cervicothoracic junction. Spine (Phila Pa 1976). 1991;16:S542–7.
54. Zhu Z, Hao D, Wang B, et al. Selection of surgical treatment approaches for cervicothoracic spinal tuberculosis: a 10-year case review. PLoS One. 2018;13(2):1–12.
55. Sharan AD, Przybylski G, Tartaglino L. Approaching the upper thoracic vertebrae without sternotomy or thoracotomy: A radiographic analysis with clinical application. Spine (Phila Pa 1976). 2000;25:910–6.
56. Mihir B, Vinod L, Umesh M, Chaudhari K. Anterior instrumentation of the cervicothoracic vertebrae. Spine (Phila Pa 1976). 2006;31(9):E244–9.
57. Singh K, Vaccaro A, Kim J, et al. Biomechanical comparison of cervical spine reconstructive techniques after a multilevel corpectomy of the cervical spine. Spine (Phila Pa 1976). 2003;28(20):2352–8.
58. Rajasekaran S. Kyphotic deformity in spinal tuberculosis and its management. Int Orthop. 2012;36:359–65.
59. Wang X, Zhou C, Xi C, et al. Surgical treatment of cervicothoracic junction spinal tuberculosis via combined anterior and posterior approaches in children. Chin Med J (Engl). 2012;125:1443–7.
60. Hassan MG. Anterior plating for lower cervical spine tuberculosis. Int Orthop. 2003;27:73–7.

Chapter 18
Anterior Surgical Approaches: TB Spine

Sashin Ahuja, Pranav Shah, and Zainab Hussain

Abstract The surgical strategy for treating spinal tuberculosis is thorough debridement of the infected tissue, effective anti-tuberculosis treatment, neural decompression, and spinal column reconstruction to achieve spinal stability. This provides a sound foundation for effective anti-tuberculosis treatment. There has been widespread debate regarding optimal surgical approach to achieve these goals.

The use of single-stage anterior spine surgical approach has been found to effectively achieve adequate debridement, decompression, and internal fixation to stabilise the spine. Generally, the disease process starts and/or is mainly localised to the anterior column, and hence the anterior approach helps address the diseased area directly. It also prevents damage to the posterior column which may not be affected by the disease, shortens the operative time, and allows sound reconstruction of the anterior spinal column and satisfactory wound healing. Thus, it is an important surgical treatment for spinal tuberculosis (Jain AK et al., Indian J Orthopaedic. 2010;44(4):409–16; Rawall et al., Musculoskelet Surg 97(1):67–75, 2013).

The anterior approach has demonstrated that often the disease frequently is found to be more extensive than suspected allowing for more effective debridement reducing the risk of subsequent relapse (Hodgson et al., Br J Surg. 48:172–8, 1960).

We shall discuss the surgical technique of anterior spinal approach for tuberculosis of the spine at different levels and also consider the recent advances in dealing with the pathology effectively while reducing the ensuing post-surgical morbidity.

Keywords Tuberculosis · Anterior approach · Spine surgery

S. Ahuja (✉) · P. Shah
Welsh Centre for Spinal Surgery & Trauma, University Hospital of Wales, Cardiff, UK
e-mail: Sashin.Ahuja@wales.nhs.uk; Pranav.Shah@wales.nhs.uk

Z. Hussain
Trent Vale Medical Practice, Trent Vale, Stoke on Trent, UK
e-mail: Zainab.Hussain@stoke.nhs.uk

S. S. Dhatt, V. Kumar (eds.), *Tuberculosis of the Spine*,
https://doi.org/10.1007/978-981-16-9495-0_18

18.1 Background

Tuberculosis of the spine commonly affects the thoracic spine. The anterior approach is utilised to surgically debride, acquire material for culture histopathology, decompress the spinal cord, and reconstruct and stabilise the spinal column. This then allows appropriate and effective medical management which is the mainstay of treatment.

The anterolateral extra-pleural spinal approach was developed by Griffiths (1956), Seddon (1956), and Roaf (1959). This approach has been slightly modified for use in tuberculous conditions for adequate debridement of diseased tissue, and for facilitating decompression of the cord with or without bone grafting to achieve anterior spinal fusion for lesions in the thoracic spine. Trans-pleural anterior approach was popularised by Hodgson and Stock (1956, 1960) and is used for tuberculous lesions of the dorsal spine [4].

We describe the common anterior approaches and recent advances below starting with the commonest, i.e., anterior trans-thoracic approach used to access the mid thoracic spine.

18.2 Surgical Technique

18.2.1 Mid Thoracic

18.2.1.1 Anterior Trans-thoracic [5]

The patient is usually positioned in a left semi-lateral position, i.e., right side is up by 45° with the help of pillow or a bean bag and the patient securely strapped. Some surgeons may prefer to seek help from a thoracic surgeon for the thoracotomy and exposure. The incision usually is based on the level of the disease, and the rule of thumb would be to gain access through the rib bed two levels above the diseased level due to anatomical alignment of the ribs. The rib level can also be gauged on a plain x-ray by subtending a horizontal line from the diseased level to the outermost rib at the lateral edge of the thoracic cage. The incision extends from anterior axillary line to about 3 cm off midline posteriorly in line with the rib (Fig. 18.1a). In multi-level spinal involvement, the fifth intercostal space is used for pathology from upper thoracic spine up to T10, and the sixth intercostal space is used for pathology from T10 and lower. The latissimus dorsi is divided in the line of the incision and so is the serratus anterior. The rib is exposed using the periosteum elevator and the rib dissectors. Take adequate care to protect the intercostal nerve and vessels which lie along the inferior aspect of the rib (Fig. 18.1b). The pleura is opened (Fig. 18.1c). A rib spreader is inserted to widen the access. Rib resection is usually avoided and reserved only for extensive exposure. Once the thorax is opened, the right lung is deflated (preoperatively you may request the anaesthetist to insert a double lumen ,

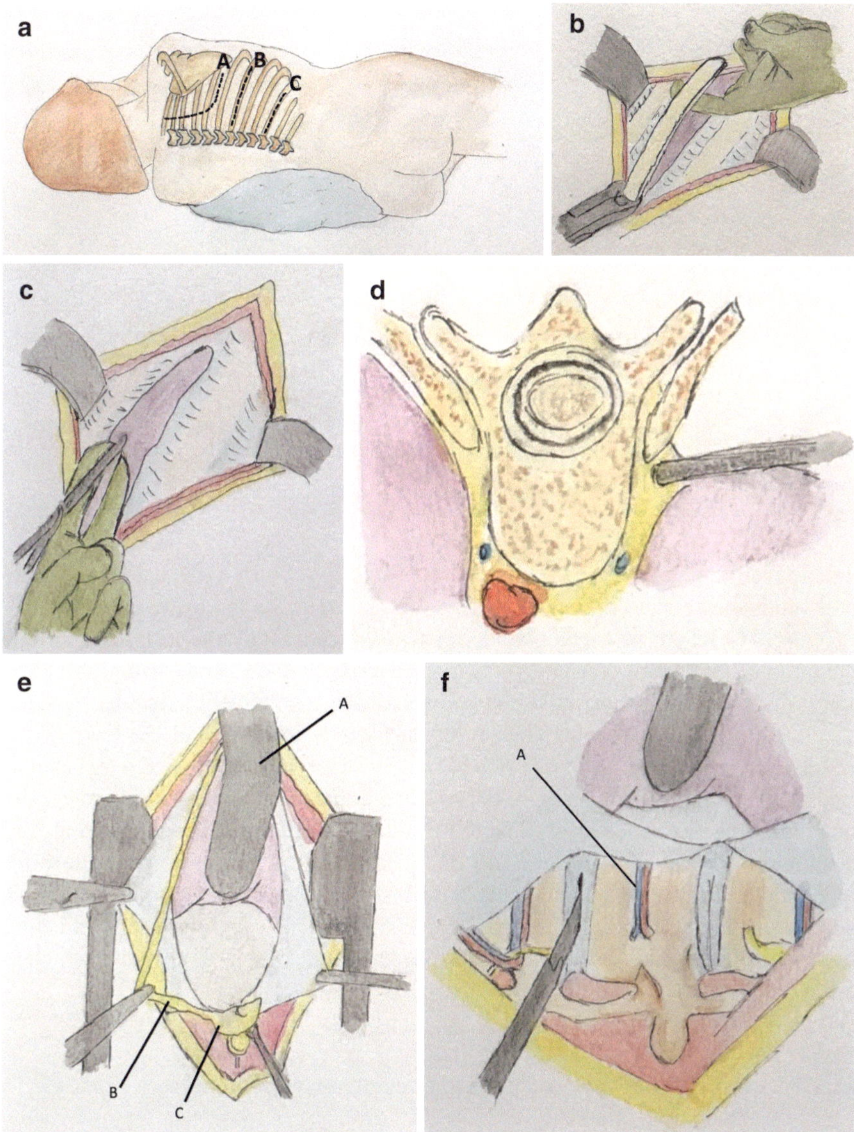

Fig. 18.1 Trans-thoracic approach (**a**)–(**h**). (**a**) Incision markings: A, upper thoracic spine up to T10; B and C: exposure below T10. (**b**) Subperiosteal dissection of the rib. (**c**) Chest cavity opened by cutting the parietal pleura using a scissors with the lung protected with finger dissection under the parietalpleura. (**d**) plane of dissection. (**e**): A-retracted deflated lung; B-segmental intercostal NV bundle; C-posterior edge of resected rib. (**f**) A-segmental vertebral vessel. (**g**, **h**) excision of the diseased vertebrae and affected discs and decompression of the spinal cord

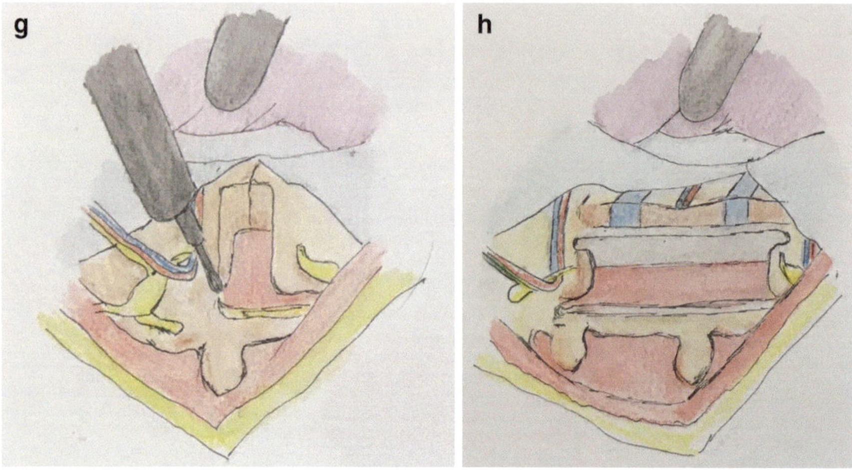

Fig. 18.1 (continued)

tube to facilitate this step) and the spine exposed (Fig. 18.1d–f). The affected vertebrae are identified and the level confirmed both clinically and using intraoperative imaging. The lung is protected with a wet swab and retracted anteriorly. The parietal pleura over the lateral oesophagus is incised and retracted gently using blunt and sharp dissection usually over the disc level which is relatively avascular to allow access to the spinal column. The segmental vessels which are at the level of the waist or the middle part of the vertebral body may need to be dissected and cauterised or ligated. The periosteum over the spine is reflected with elevators to expose involved vertebrae. The diseased vertebra and disc are debrided and the spinal cord decompressed. The pus (if any) and the debrided material is sent for culture for tuberculosis and bacteria. The spine is reconstructed as per the surgeon's choice, i.e., using rib graft/tricortical iliac crest graft/expandable cage/mesh cage and anterior stabilisation. The closure is performed in layers over a chest drain which is anchored with drain stitches (Fig. 18.1g–h).

18.2.1.2 Anterolateral Extra-pleural (Costotransversectomy) Decompression [6]

With the patient positioned in either the right lateral or prone decubitus, a semicircular incision is made starting about 7 cm proximal to the apex of the kyphus in the midline. The incision is gently curved distally and laterally to a point approximately 7 cm away from the midline to the left at the apex of the kyphus and also extending 7 cm distal to the apex.

The skin, subcutaneous tissue, and deep fascia are incised in line to create a full thickness fascio-cutaneous flap. The trapezius, peri-scapular muscles and latissimus dorsi are divided in a T-shaped manner.

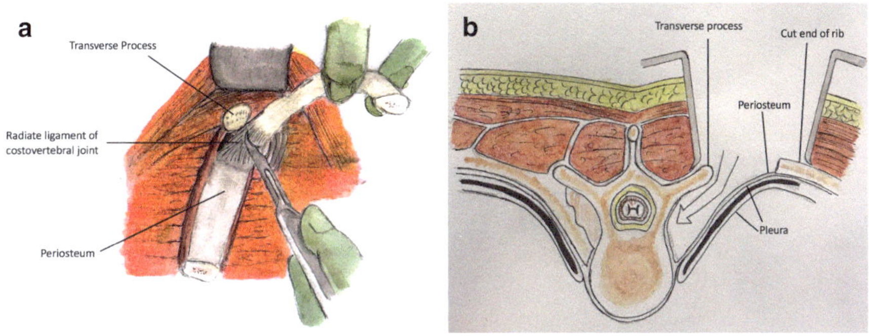

Fig. 18.2 Anterolateral extra-pleural approach (**a**, **b**)

The ribs to be removed are identified and the periosteum of each rib incised and elevated along the long axis. The rib is divided lateral to its angle at a distance of about 8 cm away from the tip of transverse process using bone cutting forceps. The paraspinal muscles are divided transversely in the line of the rib, and a cleavage is created between the transverse process and rib-head dividing the costo-transverse ligaments (Fig. 18.2a). The transverse process is removed from its base and rib including its head is detached.

After having removed the middle rib, adjacent ribs can be removed in a similar manner. At this point, the intercostal neurovascular bundle are ligated and divided 5 cm away from the spinal foramina, sparing the lowermost intercostal nerve. Subsequently, one may encounter the pre- or paravertebral abscess. The antero-lateral surface of the vertebral body is exposed, and a blunt spatula is inserted anterior to the vertebral body (Fig. 18.2b). The affected vertebrae are identified and the level confirmed both clinically and using intra-operative imaging. The diseased vertebrae and discs are debrided. The pus (if any) and the debrided material is sent for culture for tuberculosis and bacteria. The spinal cord is exposed spanning three vertebrae (i.e., 5 cm × 1 cm). Patency of the spinal canal is confirmed by inserting an infant feeding tube proximally and distally. The spinal column is reconstructed using local rib graft or reconstruction cage and the kyphosis corrected. The segment is stabilised as per the surgeon's choice of implants. The lungs are inflated to rule-out any inadvertent pleural tear before closing the wound. Chest drain is not routinely inserted.

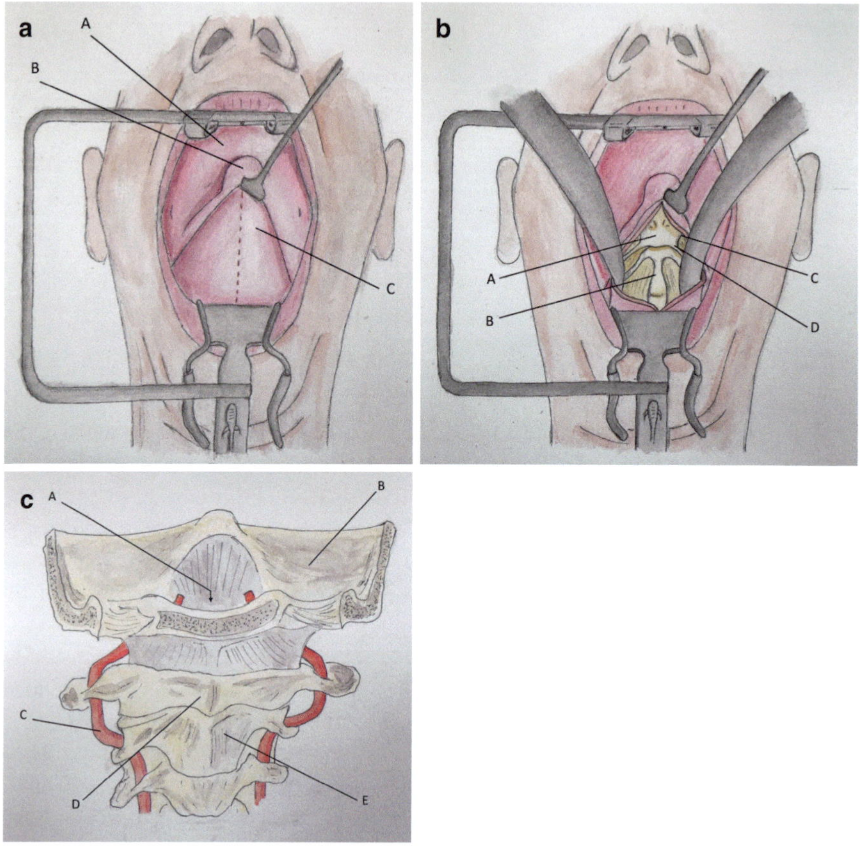

Fig. 18.3 Trans-oral upper cervical approach (**a**–**c**). (**a**) A, soft palate; B, uvula; C, posterior pharyngeal wall. (**b**) A, anterior tubercle of atlas; B, body of axis; C, longus capitis; D, longus colli. (**c**) A, foramen magnum; B, occipital bone; C, vertebral artery; D, anterior tubercle of atlas; E, body of axis

18.2.2 Upper Cervical [7]

After taking a throat swab to identify any microorganism in the pharynx and administering intravenous antibiotics at induction, which are continued for a week postoperatively, skull callipers are applied, if not already in place. 5 kg traction weight is applied. With the patient supine on the operating table, iliac crest auto-graft is harvested.

The patient is then placed in a beach-chair position and a tracheostomy is performed, anaesthesia being continued through the tube. The mouth is opened and held with a Boyle-Davis mouth gag (Fig. 18.3a). Care is taken to avoid any damage to the posterior pharyngeal wall or to the tongue. The soft palate is divided in the midline with the incision passing through either side of the uvula. The soft palate is retracted anteriorly, and the level of the spine is checked with an image intensifier.

Subsequently, the posterior pharyngeal wall is divided in the midline starting at the level of the anterior tubercle of the atlas and extending to the C2-3 disc space (Fig. 18.3b). Sharp and blunt dissection to clear the soft tissue laterally from the front of the vertebral bodies. In cases where dens is involved, it becomes imperative to clear the lower part of the inferior surface of the basi-occiput, and in some cases, the front of the spine has to be cleared below the disc at C2–C3. The atlas and axis can be exposed laterally to visualise the joints between these bones, but it is important to bear in mind that the vertebral artery is in very close proximity at this level (Fig. 18.3c). The affected vertebrae are identified and the level confirmed both clinically and using intraoperative imaging. The diseased tissue is excised and the level reconstructed as deemed appropriate.

When either there is basilar invagination, i.e., proximal migration of the dens into the foramen magnum, or if there is irreducible displacement, then the dens can be removed carefully using a high-speed burr, to the depth of posterior longitudinal ligament and the dura.

The operative field can be sprayed with antibiotic powder and the posterior pharyngeal wall closed in layers using absorbable interrupted sutures for muscle and mucosa and repairing the soft palate in layers using interrupted sutures.

18.2.2.1 Lower Cervical [8]

Lower cervical spine can be approached by the standard Smith Robinson approach whereby the operation is performed in a supine position, with a sand-bag between the shoulder blade to extend the neck. The approach could be from the right

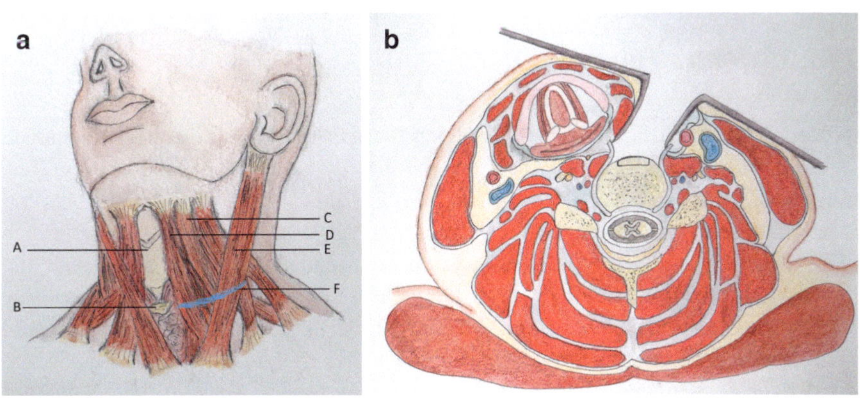

Fig. 18.4 Lower cervical approach: (i) Approach, (ii) anatomic dissection, (iii) schematic dissection. (**a**) A, thyroid cartilage; B, cricoid cartilage; C, omohyoid; D, sternohyoid; E, sternocleidomastoid; F, skin incision. (**b**) Plane of dissection between the sternomastoid and the strap muscles and in the deeper layers between the carotid sheath and the trachea and oesophangus

(preferred by most surgeons as most are right-handed) or left (due to consistent course of the recurrent laryngeal nerve and the reduced risk of its injury). The landmarks for the incision include the hyoid at C3, the thyroid cartilage at C4, and the cricoid at C6. Alternatively, image intensifier can be used with a metal marker to identify the level. A transverse incision is used, preferably in a skin crease for cosmesis. A 5–6-cm-long incision extending from midline to the medial border of the sternocleidomastoid is made (Fig. 18.4a). Dissection is carried down to platysma, which is cut transversely across the length of the skin incision. The anterior border of sternocleidomastoid (SCM) is identified, and cervical fascia is opened vertically anterior to it. With blunt dissection, the soft-tissue plane is developed between lateral aspect of the laryngeal strap muscles and medial aspect of the SCM. The carotid artery is palpated for, behind the sternocleidomastoid. Close attention should be paid to avoid dividing any structure crossing from the carotid sheath medially. Dissection is carried down to the vertebral body by retracting the trachea and oesophagus medially and the carotid sheath laterally. The prevertebral fascia is opened in the midline (Fig. 18.4b). A spinal needle is placed for level check. Once the correct level is confirmed the longus colli muscles dissected usually using a monopolar or bipolar diathermy and retracted laterally using self-retaining retractors placed beneath its medial edges to prevent retraction force directly on the oesophagus and trachea (Fig. 18.4c). These retractors should not be displaced for the remainder of the surgery.

Threaded pins are then placed in the vertebrae above and below the diseased area for distraction. The diseased tissues, i.e. vertebrae and discs, are excised with resection extending to the posterior longitudinal ligament and visualising the dura to achieve adequate decompression. The spinal column is reconstructed either using tricortical iliac crest graft or reconstruction cages and stabilised using a cervical plate.

18.2.3 Upper Thoracic [9]

Access to the upper thoracic and the cervico-thoracic region could either be achieved by extending the anterior cervical approach distally as per Fig. 18.5a or via a sternotomy approach as per Fig. 18.5b.

For the extensile anterior cervical approach, the steps for the cervical approach are as described above. The skin incision is extended vertically down over the sterno-clavicular joint and the manubrium (Fig. 18.5a). Alternatively, a sternotomy is performed, i.e. via a midline vertical sternal incision (Fig. 18.5b). The platysma is divided in the line with the skin incision. The external jugular vein is ligated and divided, and the medial supraclavicular nerve may require division. The clavicular head of the sterno-mastoid muscle is dissected and reflected upwards. Medially, the strap muscles are similarly released and reflected. The areolar tissue in the suprasternal space is excised.

The medial clavicle and the manubrium sterni are visualised with subperiosteal dissection. The medial one-third of the clavicle is resected using a Gigli saw, thus

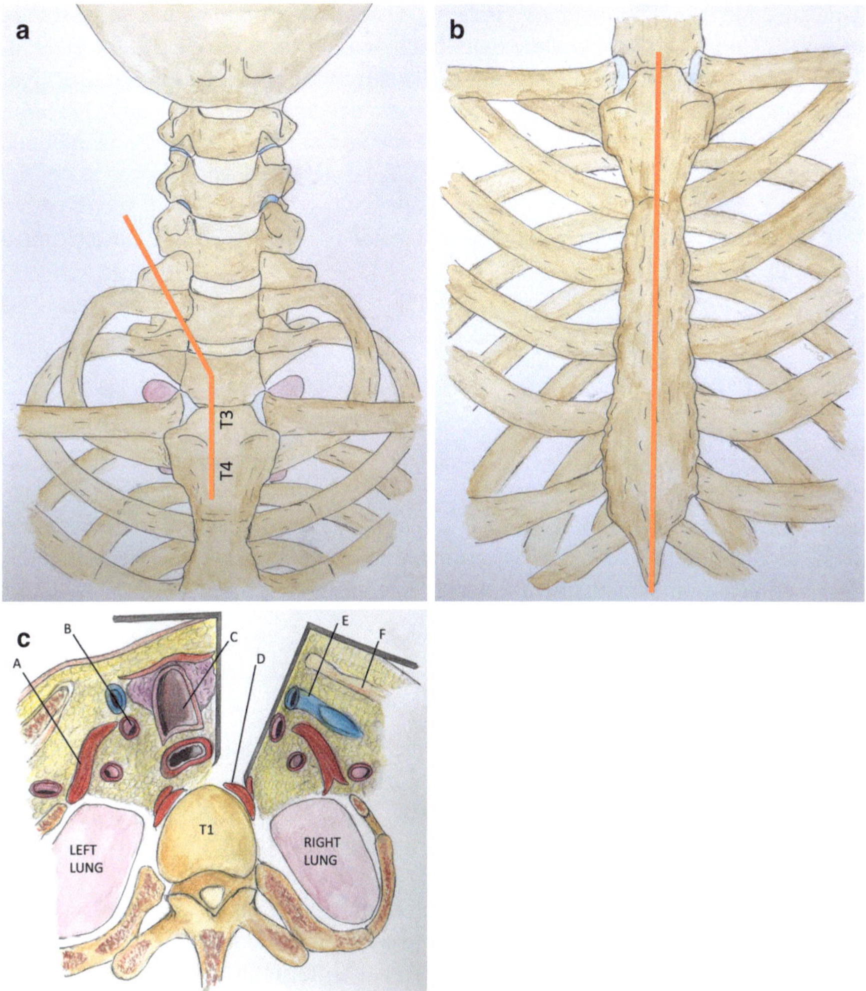

Fig. 18.5 Upper thoracic approach (**a–c**). (**c**) Schematic dissection: A, anterior scalene muscle; B, internal jugular vein and carotid artery; C, trachea; D, longus colli; E, subclavian vein; F, clavicle

disconnecting the clavicle from the sternum after curettage of the sternoclavicular joint. Often a rectangular block of sternum is removed by using a high-speed drill to thin the bone peripherally and then making the final cut using a Kerrison rongeur. Underneath the manubrium sterni lie the subclavian vein and the thymus. The subclavian vein is carefully dissected free. The thymus may be removed, if needed for additional exposure. The tissue plane, which lies between carotid sheath laterally and the trachea and oesophagus medially, is developed to approach the prevertebral space (Fig. 18.5c). The recurrent laryngeal nerve lies across the operative field and must be protected. The prevertebral fascia is opened in the midline and the breach extended laterally. The affected vertebrae are identified and the level confirmed both clinically and using intraoperative imaging. Diseased vertebral bodies and discs are resected. The pus (if any) and the debrided material is sent for culture for tuberculosis and bacteria. Resection is continued down to the posterior longitudinal ligament, and dura is visualised to ensure adequate decompression. The spinal column can be reconstructed using the excised clavicle as a strut graft or using an alternate graft or reconstruction cage. The vertebrae can be stabilised using a plate as per the surgeon's choice of implant. The wound is then closed in layers with suction drain left in situ. A collar with a thoracic extension is often used for postoperative immobilisation.

18.2.4 Lumbo-sacral

Anterior approach to lumbo-sacral spine can be accomplished by using an extra-peritoneal approach or trans-peritoneal (trans-abdominal) approach (Fig. 18.6). Some surgeons may opt for a vascular surgeon to help with access, but the recommendation would be to at least have pathways in place for easy access to a vascular surgeon in case of an inadvertent vascular emergency.

18.2.4.1 Extra-peritoneal [10, 11]

The patient is placed in supine position with a pillow under the knees to flex the hips and knees. The foot end of the table may be elevated slightly higher than the head. A para-median vertical incision is made extending from the symphysis pubis to the umbilicus. The skin and subcutaneous tissue dissected off the rectus sheath. The peritoneum is gently retracted manually or with a swab from lateral to medial to expose the psoas muscle where the genitofemoral nerve can be identified and protected. The ureter is retracted medially along with the peritoneum. The sacral promontory is located. Subsequently, the abdominal aorta, inferior vena cava, and its bifurcations are identified (it is usually helpful to identify the level of the bifurcation based on the pre-operative imaging, i.e. coronal and axial MRI to plan access to the disc levels). The major blood vessels are retracted and protected throughout the procedure. The median sacral artery and vein either can be dissected and retracted or cauterised. The hypogastric plexus is identified and protected. The prevertebral fascia is cut in the midline and dissected laterally. A level check is performed using x-rays. The lesion is isolated with wet gauze to prevent adjacent tissue contamination. The abscess is opened to drain the pus. The diseased tissue is debrided, and the spinal column is reconstructed using tricortical iliac crest graft or alternate

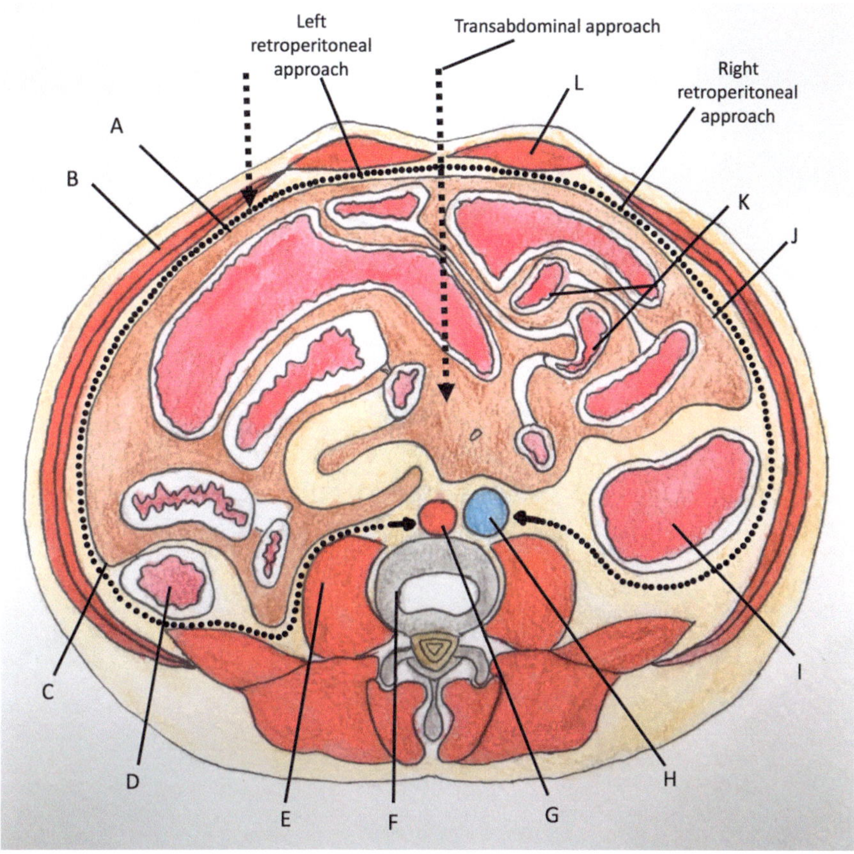

Fig. 18.6 Anterior lumbar approach schematic diagram; A, C, peritoneum; B, lateral abdominal muscles; D, left colon; E, left psoas; F, lumbar intervertebral disc; G, abdominal aorta; H, vena cava; I, right colon

reconstruction cage and stabilised anteriorly. The pus (if any) and the debrided material is sent for culture for tuberculosis and bacteria. The incision is sutured in layers.

For treatment of multi-level lumbosacral tuberculosis posterior pedicle screw instrumentation in combination with anterior debridement and fusion can be achieved with modified inverted L- or T-shaped incision using the extraperitoneal approach with the patient in a lateral position to allow additional posterior access.

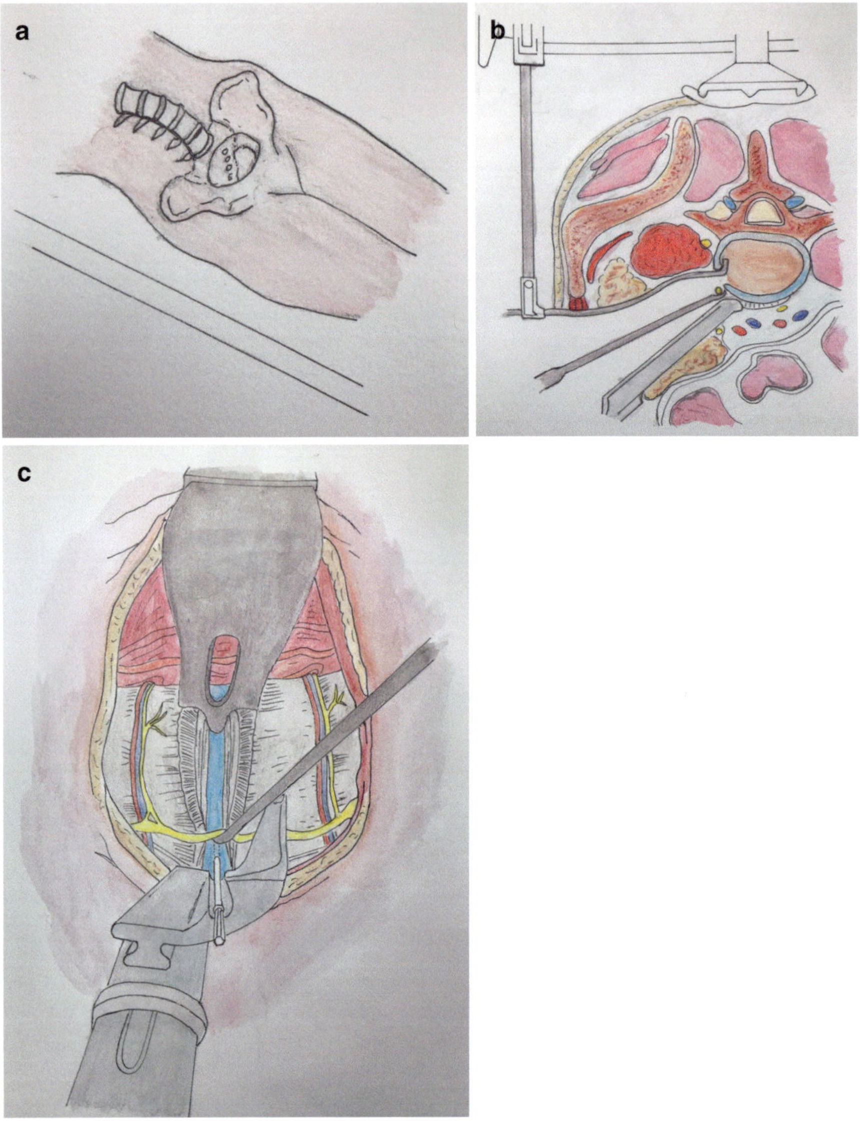

Fig. 18.7 Anterior lumbar trans-peritoneal approach (**a–c**)

18.2.4.2 Transperitoneal Hypogastric Approach [12]

The transperitoneal approach begins with patient in supine position using a Pfannenstiel incision (preferably) about 5 cm above the pubis and with vertical dissection through the linea alba (Fig. 18.7a). The pre-peritoneal fat is dissected until the peritoneal membrane can be identified (Fig. 18.6). The peritoneum is opened carefully to avoid any inadvertent injury to the bowel. The bowel is protected with swabs with the cecum retracted to the right, the sigmoid colon retracted to the left, and the small bowel superiorly (Fig. 18.7b). The L5–S1 inter-vertebral space is palpable deep in the wound. The posterior peritoneum is opened carefully to prevent causing any injury to major blood vessels underneath it. The disc space is exposed with blunt dissection to avoid injuring the superior hypogastric plexus. The remainder of the procedure comprising of level-check, discectomy, endplate preparation, and instrumentation is standard as described previously (Fig. 18.7c).

18.2.5 Minimal Invasive

18.2.5.1 Navigation-Assisted Minimally Invasive Direct Lateral Interbody Fusion in Lumbar Tuberculosis [13]

The patient is placed in a lateral position with the side with more severe bone destruction up using front and back table support and reinforcement with tape to prevent movement. The patient's hips and knees are flexed, and a cushion is kept between the legs to prevent pressure sore. The lumbar bridge (considered the centre) is aligned with the affected segment. The navigation reference frame is anchored to the postero-superior iliac spine. Navigated surgical instruments with trackers are registered to the workstation, while the O-arm is connected with the navigator and the spinal segment scanned. The navigation probe is used to locate the skin surface projection corresponding to the antero-posterior median position of the lateral side of the lesion, and the transverse incision is made about 5 cm long. After opening the skin and subcutaneous tissues, the external and internal oblique is split in the line of the incision with the index finger. The transversalis fascia is opened but be mindful of the peritoneum underneath it. The peritoneum is reflected from posterior to anterior to expose the psoas. Under navigation guidance, the position-guide needle is inserted into the intervertebral space of the lesion through the retroperitoneal space and psoas. The needle-tip position has to be in the middle of the intervertebral space on the lateral view. Expansion cannulas are inserted along the needle to widen the channel, and the tubular sheath is fixed into place with table mounted free arms. The annulus is opened and the diseased tissue is debrided. The pus (if any) and the debrided material is sent for culture for tuberculosis and bacteria. Navigation probes are used to identify the extent of lesion guiding debridement and decompression. The defect is reconstructed either using a tricortical iliac crest graft or a cage as per the surgeon's preference. The spinal column is stabilised. Computer navigation guides the optimal entrance points and angles for screws that are inserted into the posterior one-third of the vertebral body under real-time guidance in order to avoid neural injury. C-arm fluoroscopy is performed to confirm the positions of implants. The wound is closed in layers.

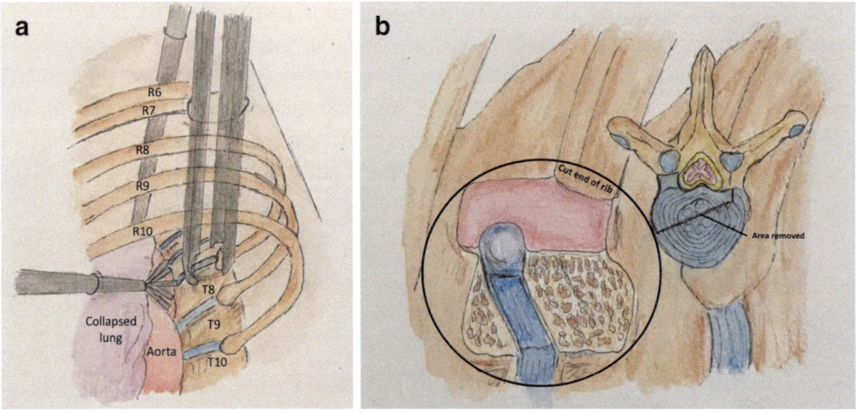

Fig. 18.8 Minimal access approach (**a**, **b**)

18.2.6 Video-Assisted Thoracoscopic Surgery [14]

Under a general anaesthetic with a double-lumen endotracheal tube in place, the patient is positioned in the left lateral decubitus on a beanbag and secured with tapes. The skin is prepared and draped for a standard posterolateral thoracotomy so that the procedure could be converted smoothly to an open one, if required. After selective collapse of the right lung, a stab incision is made to enter the chest. The initial trocar incision is made at the T6-T7 intercostal space along the anterior axillary line. Using an 11-mm metal trocar, the thoracoscope is introduced. The lesion site is identified on the video monitor, and the other two manipulating channels are made under scope-guidance and positioned at or slightly posterior to the posterior axillary line at the T5-T6 and T7-T8 intercostal spaces (Fig. 18.8a). Locating the correct lesion site could occasionally be difficult if covered by inflammatory tissue and may need appropriate dissection. Using monopolar diathermy, the mediastinal pleura overlying the lesion is divided longitudinally. Specimens are collected for culture for tuberculosis and bacteria. The intercostal arteries and veins are ligated and divided. The abscess is drained, and the diseased vertebrae and discs are debrided using curettes (Fig. 18.8b). The pus (if any) and the debrided material is sent for culture for tuberculosis and bacteria. Decompression is performed down to the epidural space and guided with video assistance. The tissue retrieval portal is protected by a flexible thoracic port. The spinal column is reconstructed either using a bone graft or reconstruction cage or stabilised with implants as per the surgeon's preference. A chest tube is inserted through one incision wound and directed to the apex of the chest.

The portals are closed in layers. A chest radiograph is performed after the operation to ensure a fully inflated lung.

18.3 Complications

Apart from the known complications for most spinal surgical procedures, some of the access specific complications are enumerated below:

18.3.1 Anterior Cervical

- Injury to recurrent laryngeal nerve leading to hoarseness of voice
- Oesophageal injury and dysphagia
- Horner's syndrome following damage to sympathetic chain
- Injury to thoracic duct (exposure from left side)
- Vertebral artery injury

18.3.2 Anterior Thoracic

- Atelectasis, pneumonia, pleural effusion, chest wall discomfort (post-thoracotomy pain syndrome) and intercostal neuralgia
- Pneumothorax and broncho-pulmonary fistula
- Injury to superior mediastinal structures (aorta, trachea, oesophagus, thoracic duct)
- Post-operative thrombi-embolic complications

18.3.3 Anterior Lumbar

- Injury to ilio-lumbar vein or segmental lumbar vessels
- Laceration of vena cava/common iliac veins
- Bowel/ureteric injury
- Sexual dysfunction due to injury to inter-mesenteric nerve plexus and superior hypogastric plexus
- Paralytic ileus
- Deep vein thrombosis

18.4 Conclusion

Anterior approaches to the spine, although less frequently employed, allow better access to the pathology and facilitate more anatomic spinal reconstruction. They are an important technique in spine surgeons' armamentarium. Good knowledge of anatomy and sound surgical skills form the foundation to perform these approaches safely.

References

1. Jain AK, Dhammi IK, Jain S, Kumar J. Simultaneously anterior decompression and posterior instrumentation by extra-pleural retroperitoneal approach in thoracolumbar lesions. Indian J Orthop. 2010;44(4):409–16.
2. Rawall S, Mohan K, Nene A. Posterior approach in thoracolumbar tuberculosis: a clinical and radiological review of 67 operated cases. Musculoskelet Surg. 2013;97(1):67–75.
3. Hodgson AR, Stock FE, Fang HS, Ong GB. Anterior spinal fusion. The operative approach and pathological findings in 412 patients with Pott's disease of the spine. Br J Surg. 1960 Sep;48:172–8. https://doi.org/10.1002/bjs.18004820819.
4. Tuli SM. Tuberculosis of the skeletal system (bones, joints, spine and bursal sheaths). 3rd ed. Jaypee Brothers: Bangalore; 2004.
5. Balasubramaniam S, Tyagi DK, Zafar SH, Savant HV. Transthoracic approach for lesions involving the anterior dorsal spine: a multidisciplinary approach with good outcomes. J Craniovertebr Junction Spine. 2016;7(4):236–42. https://doi.org/10.4103/0974-8237.193254.
6. Jain AK, Aggarwal A, Dhammi IK, Aggarwal PK, Singh S. Extra-pleural anterolateral decompression in tuberculosis of the dorsal spine. J Bone Joint Surg Br. 2004 Sep;86(7):1027–31. https://doi.org/10.1302/0301-620x.86b7.14546.
7. Fang D, Leong JC, Fang HS. Tuberculosis of the upper cervical spine. J Bone Joint Surg Br. 1983;65(1):47–50. https://doi.org/10.1302/0301-620X.65B1.6822601.
8. Smith GW, Robinson RA. The treatment of certain cervical-spine disorders by anterior removal of the intervertebral disc and interbody fusion. J Bone Joint Surg Ser A. 1958;40:607–24.
9. Sundaresan N, Shah J, Foley KM, Rosen G. An anterior surgical approach to the upper thoracic vertebrae. J Neurosurg. 1984;61(4):686–90. https://doi.org/10.3171/jns.1984.61.4.0686.
10. Shi SY, Hu SP, Fei J, Lai Z, Hang GH. Clinical application of modified inverted L-shape incision by extraperitoneal approach to lumbosacral tuberculosis. Zhongguo Gu Shang. 2017;30(9):799–804. Chinese. https://doi.org/10.3969/j.issn.1003-0034.2017.09.004.
11. Li JH, Zhang ZH, Shi T, et al. Surgical treatment of lumbosacral tuberculosis by one-stage debridement and anterior instrumentation with allograft through an extraperitoneal anterior approach. J Orthop Surg Res. 2015;10:62. https://doi.org/10.1186/s13018-015-0204-x
12. Laratta JL, Davis EG, Glassman SD, Dimar JR. The transperitoneal approach for anterior lumbar interbody fusion at L5-S1: a technical note. J Spine Surg. 2018;4(2):459–60. https://doi.org/10.21037/jss.2018.05.18.
13. Jiang J, Gan F, Tan H, Xie Z, Luo X, Huang G, Li Y, Huang S. Effect of computer navigation-assisted minimally invasive direct lateral interbody fusion in the treatment of patients with lumbar tuberculosis: a retrospective study. Medicine (Baltimore). 2018;97(48):e13484. https://doi.org/10.1097/MD.0000000000013484.
14. Huang TJ, Hsu RW, Chen SH, Liu HP. Video-assisted thoracoscopic surgery in managing tuberculous spondylitis. Clin Orthop Relat Res. 2000;379:143–53. https://doi.org/10.1097/00003086-200010000-00017.

Chapter 19
Posterior Approach for TB Spine

Abduljabbar Alhammoud and Ravinder Bains

Abstract Surgical management of the TB spine is the cornerstone to restore the spine alignment and stability, especially in failed medical management and advance disease. Surgery can be done from the front or the back.

We present in this chapter a literature review of the posterior approach for TB spine, looking for the indications, contraindications, reported outcome, and step by step, our preferred surgical approach.

Keywords TB · Spine · Posterior · Approach

19.1 Introduction

Anti-TB chemotherapy alone is not sufficient in restoring the vertebral height as well as correcting the deformity; therefore adjacent surgical treatment has become the trend aiming for the correction of the deformity caused by the destruction of the vertebral body. Also other advantages of adjacent surgical correction include decreasing the period of treatment, removal of the destructive lesion with reliving of the spinal compression, and restoration of the vertebral height which reduces disability and improves the quality of life [1].

In recent years various surgical methods have been described in the literature for treating spinal TB, and the choice of the surgical approach is still controversial; however radical debridement remains the key in surgical treatment. In cases of incomplete focal excision, sinuses may appear, and there is the likelihood of failure of both bone grafting and internal fixation [2].

Anterior only approach (Hong Kong operation) was reported first by Hodgson and Stock in 1960 [3], and it is advocated by many surgeons due to its advantages in direct access of the focal lesion and adequate debridement under direct vision

A. Alhammoud · R. Bains (✉)
Kaiser Permanente Oakland Medical Center, Oakland, CA, USA
e-mail: abduljabbar.x.alhammoud@kp.org; ravi.s.bains@kp.org

S. S. Dhatt, V. Kumar (eds.), *Tuberculosis of the Spine*,
https://doi.org/10.1007/978-981-16-9495-0_19

with decompression of the spinal cord [4–8]. When utilizing anterior only approach, there is insufficient correction of the kyphosis deformity accompanied by great loss of correction post-operatively; internal fixation and instrumentation is difficult to perform due to special anatomic characteristics and position as there is higher risk injury to the great blood vessels specially in the lumbar and lumbosacral region [8–10].

Recently many surgeons have reported the superiority of posterior only approach over the anterior only approach and combined anterior with posterior approach [4, 6, 10–12]. Adequate lesion debridement, bone grafting and three columns internal fixation, stabilization, and deformity correction can be accomplished at one less invasive incision without the need to change the patient's position when utilizing the posterior only approach. Controversy remains whether posterior approach can thoroughly remove the lesion from the TB lesion mainly concentrated in the anterior column; however in experienced hand removal of the lamina and facet joint along with moderate stretching of the nerve root and dura can provide adequate surgical space in which 360° lesion debridement, removal of dead tissues, and darning of the abscess under direct vision can be achieved [10–12].

19.2 Indications

- **Why posterior**:
  - Few affected bony segments
  - Mild vertebral destruction
  - Destruction located in posterior part of the body or near endplate
  - Disease located in paraspinal muscle without gravitation abscess
  - Medical or surgical contraindication for anterior approach
- **Why not anterior**:
  - High-grade kyphosis, which may need osteotomy
  - Poor fixation points due to anatomical consideration
  - Higher rate of catastrophic complications and longer hospital and ICU stay

19.3 Literature Review

19.3.1 Reported Surgical Techniques

Different surgical techniques were reported in the literature to address the spinal TB in posterior only approach. Those techniques extended from simple laminectomy to radical corpectomy. Posterior laminectomy, PLIF/TLIF type approach, transpedicular approach, through removing the rib head and the transverse process, transcapular inferolateral approach, lateral extrapleural approach, and extensile posterior approach with a combination of all above techniques.

The type and the extent of the approach depended on the location of the lesion and the surgeon's skills and experience.

To overcome the inadequate direct visualization in posterior only approach and in case of residual infection, saline irrigation at the lesion site along with local implantation of anti-TB drugs and the use of postural drainage were described [10, 11, 13].

19.3.2 Reported Outcome

When comparing the posterior only approach to combined approach, multiple studies have reported significantly better medical and surgical outcomes in posterior only approach.

Zheng et al. and Garg et al. reported lower blood loss, operative time, and hospital stay in posterior only approach, whereas more ICU stay and support are needed in the anterior type approach [11, 14]. Kyphosis correction in the posterior only approach was better than the combined approach, and similar results were reported by Garg et al. On the other hand, post-operative loss of correction was less in posterior only approach with comparable fusion rate above 90% in both groups reaching till 100% in posterior only approach within 6 months from the surgery [6, 11, 14, 15].

No difference in functional outcome in most of the reported literature and a better Prolo scale was reported by Greg et al. in the posterior only group.

Ma et al. reported improvement of neurological deficit in 74% with normalizing of the ESR at 8–12 months post-operatively of the posterior cohort. Similarly, Liu et al. reported 1–3° of neurological improvement and 100% cure rate with no recurrence in the one-stage posterior only approach [6, 11, 15].

Major and minor complications were reported by Moon et al. ranging from major vessel injury, spinal cord injury, and dural tears, to ileus and intercostal neuralgia. The spinal cord injury was highest in posterior approach, whereas dural tear was higher in anterior surgery. In other series, Liu et al. reported an 8% complication rate like intercostal neurologia and infection [1, 11, 15].

19.4 Our Preferred Surgical Techniques

19.4.1 Pre-operative and Anesthesia Consideration

- General anesthesia
- Perioperative antibiotics to be administered to cover skin flora within 30 min prior to incision
- Neuromonitoring to monitor the brachial plexus and the spinal cord through transcranial motor evoked potentials and somatosensory evoked potentials

19.4.2 Position and Exposure

- Prone on a radiolucent operating room table (Fig. 19.1).
- Skin is cut sharply down to fascia. Electrocautery and Cobb elevators utilized for subperiosteal dissection.

19.4.3 Instrumentation

- Pedicle screws are placed using anatomic landmarks and confirming fluoroscopically. Approximately six Pedicle screws are placed rostral and caudal to the operative level (Fig. 19.2).

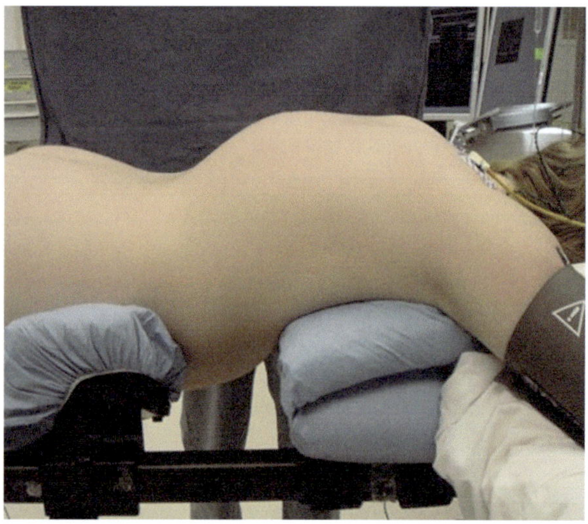

Fig. 19.1 Positioning

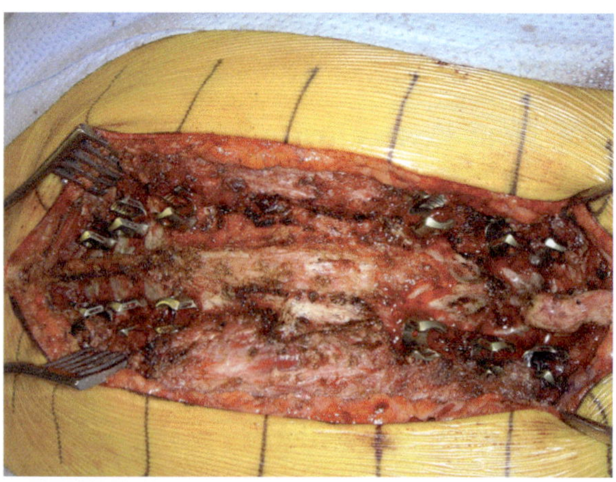

Fig. 19.2 Instrumentation

19.4.4 Debridement and Decompression

- If there is a prior laminectomy, the scar is removed from the dorsal dura.
- Normal dura plane is identified just caudal on the non-laminectomized spinal segment (Fig. 19.3).
- The dura is freed ventrally by Woodson elevator. Dissection is carried out lateral, and rib heads are removed at the VCR segment and also at the adjacent caudal segment.
- Segmental nerve can be sacrificed bilaterally or unilaterally as in this case.
- If there is no prior surgery, then the lamina, facets of the operated segment, and spinous process segment are removed.
- Discectomy was performed with the use of curettes.
- Discectomy instruments can be passed all the way across.
- On the contralateral side discectomy can also be performed.
- Corpectomy can be performed with use of a Leksell rongeur. Osteotomes were also utilized on the contralateral side.
- The PLL, posterior longitudinal ligament, is cut cranially and caudally to the vertebral column resection segment.

19.4.5 Bony Reconstruction

- Femoral ring allograft or peek or other metal composite spacers can be placed into the VCR segment (Fig. 19.4).
- The spacer can be tamped into position by using a down going curette.
- Shortening is first performed. This is usually done by approximately 5–8 mm.
- The kyphotic rod can be in situ contoured to reduce the kyphosis.
- These steps can be done repeatedly for desired correction.

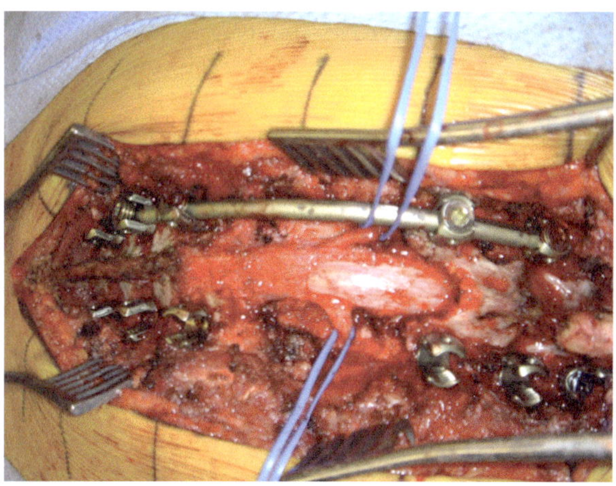

Fig. 19.3 Decompression

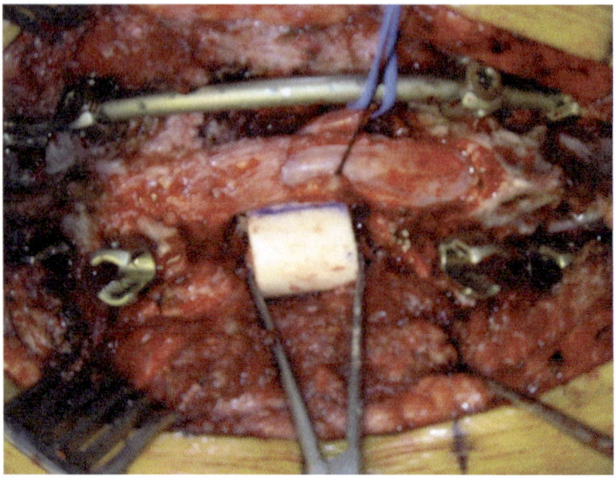

Fig. 19.4 Bony reconstruction

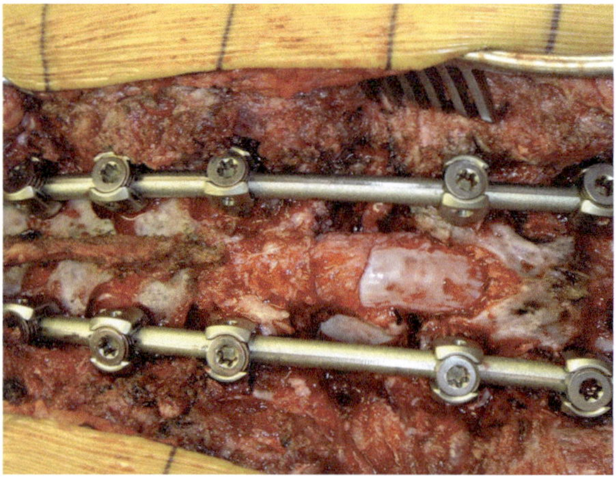

Fig. 19.5 Final construct

- The spinal cord is never shortened more than 15 mm.
- Once desired angular correction and compression has been obtained at the VCR segment, contralateral rod can be placed.
- The original rod which has been notched is removed and also replaced with a new rod (Fig. 19.5).

19.4.6 Closer and Post-operative Care

- Wound closed on layers.
- Drain usually used for 48 h.
- Decompression materials send to histopathology, culture, and sensitivity.

References

1. Moon M-S. Tuberculosis of spine: current views in diagnosis and management. Asian Spine J. 2014;8(1):97.
2. Wang Z, Ge Z, Jin W, Qiao Y, Ding H, Zhao H, et al. Treatment of spinal tuberculosis with ultrashort-course chemotherapy in conjunction with partial excision of pathologic vertebrae. Spine J. 2007;7(6):671–81.
3. Hodgson AR, Stock FE, Fang HSY, Ong GB. Anterior spinal fusion the operative approach and pathological findings in 412 patients with Pott's disease of the spine. Br J Surg. 1960;48(208):172–8.
4. Li M, Du J, Meng H, Wang Z, Luo Z. One-stage surgical management for thoracic tuberculosis by anterior debridement, decompression and autogenous rib grafts, and instrumentation. Spine J. 2011;11(8):726–33.
5. Çavuşoğlu H, Kaya RA, Türkmenoğlu ON, Tuncer C, Çolak İ, Aydin Y. A long-term follow-up study of anterior tibial allografting and instrumentation in the management of thoracolumbar tuberculous spondylitis. J Neurosurg Spine. 2008;8(1):30–8.
6. Ma YZ, Cui X, Li HW, Chen X, Cai XJ, Bai YB. Outcomes of anterior and posterior instrumentation under different surgical procedures for treating thoracic and lumbar spinal tuberculosis in adults. Int Orthop. 2012;36(2):299–305.
7. Zhao J, Lian XF, Hou TS, Ma H, Chen ZM. Anterior debridement and bone grafting of spinal tuberculosis with one-stage instrumentation anteriorly or posteriorly. Int Orthop. 2007;31(6):859–63.
8. Wang B, Lv G, Liu W, Cheng I. Anterior radical debridement and reconstruction using titanium mesh cage for the surgical treatment of thoracic and thoracolumbar spinal tuberculosis: minimum five-year follow-up. Turk Neurosurg. 2011;21(4):575–81.
9. Zaveri GR, Mehta SS. Surgical treatment of lumbar tuberculous spondylodiscitis by transforaminal lumbar interbody fusion (TLIF) and posterior instrumentation. J Spinal Disord Tech. 2009;22(4):257–62.
10. Zhang H, Lin M, Ge L, Li J, Wu J, Liu J. Surgical management by one-stage posterior transforaminal lumbar debridement, interbody fusion, and posterior instrumentation for lumbo-sacral tuberculosis in the aged. Arch Orthop Trauma Surg. 2012;132(12):1677–83.
11. Liu Z, Zhang P, Li W, Xu Z, Wang X. Posterior-only vs. combined posterior-anterior approaches in treating lumbar and lumbosacral spinal tuberculosis: a retrospective study with minimum 7-year follow-up. J Orthop Surg Res [Internet]. 2020. [cited 2021 Jan 14];15(1) https://josr-online.biomedcentral.com/articles/10.1186/s13018-020-01616-7
12. Pang X, Wu P, Shen X, Li D, Luo C, Wang X. One-stage posterior transforaminal lumbar debridement, 360° interbody fusion, and posterior instrumentation in treating lumbosacral spinal tuberculosis. Arch Orthop Trauma. 2013;133(8):1033–9.
13. Wang L, Zhang H, Tang M, Gao Q, Zhou Z, Yin X. Comparison of three surgical approaches for thoracic spinal tuberculosis in adult: minimum 5-year follow up. Spine. 2017;42(11):808–17.
14. Garg B, Upendra B, Jayaswal A, Goswami A, Kandwal P. Anterior versus posterior procedure for surgical treatment of thoracolumbar tuberculosis: a retrospective analysis. Indian J Orthop. 2012;46(2):165.
15. Liu Z, Liu J, Peng A, Long X, Yang D, Huang S. One-stage posterior debridement and transpedicular screw fixation for treating monosegmental thoracic and lumbar spinal tuberculosis in adults. Sci World J. 2014;2014:1–6.

Chapter 20
Lateral Extracavitary Approach in the Surgical Management of Tuberculosis of the Spine

Joseph Driver and Michael W. Groff

Abstract Tuberculosis of the spine, Pott's disease, presents a unique challenge for spine care professionals in general and spine surgeons in particular due to the combination of ventral compression and fixed kyphotic deformity. The indolent nature of tuberculosis has made it a persistent problem in the developing and industrial parts of the world. The Lateral Extracavitary Approach is uniquely suited to Pott's disease by virtue of the simultaneous access to both the anterior and posterior spinal columns that it affords. The LECA approach has evolved over the years to maintain its effectiveness while minimizing the morbidity.

The percepts of this approach have application to a wide range of spinal diseases.

Keywords Lateral extracavitary approach · Pott's disease · Tuberculosis

20.1 Introduction: History of LECA and Its Development for Pott's Disease

The surgical management of Pott's disease of the spine has a long history, and it has been the foundation for innovative surgical techniques that have become widespread in modern spinal surgery. Some of the early pioneers in this area, Menard and Capener, devised novel methods in the late nineteenth and early twentieth centuries for treatment of spinal TB, with the goal of accessing ventral areas of the spine. Menard, a surgeon in Paris, was one of the first to describe what is now known as the costotransversectomy for draining ventral tuberculosis abscesses. Menard described a procedure aimed at obtaining lateral access to the spine, based on a 5–7 cm incision placed laterally over the rib, with subsequent rib dissection and removal of the proximal aspect of the rib and rib head. With this bony removal,

J. Driver · M. W. Groff (✉)
Department of Neurosurgery, Brigham and Women's Hospital, Harvard Medical School, Boston, MA, USA
e-mail: mgroff@bwh.harvard.edu

S. S. Dhatt, V. Kumar (eds.), *Tuberculosis of the Spine*, https://doi.org/10.1007/978-981-16-9495-0_20

exposure of the tuberculous focus is achieved. Menard describes his experience in his landmark book published in 1900, *Etude pratique sur le mal de Pott* [1]. In 1933, Norman Capener built on the work of Menard by modifying the lateral approach and dividing the paraspinal musculature so that it could be retracted caudally and rostrally, allowing a more ventral exposure through a lateral trajectory. This approach was coined the "lateral rhachotomy" [2], and while similarly developed for Pott's disease and thoracolumbar spondylitis, Capener noted the potential utility of this approach for a wide range of thoracolumbar pathology, including tumors, trauma, and infection. While the utilization of lateral approaches for advanced Pott's disease has diminished with the advent of modern antituberculosis medications in the mid twentieth century, the refinement of this surgical technique continued. Lateral approaches to the spine were further described and popularized by Sanford Larson at Medical College of Wisconsin in 1976 when he reported his outcomes of 62 patients suffering thoracolumbar traumatic fractures [3]. Larson described the lateral extracavitary (LECA) approach for ventral decompression of the spinal canal, as well as realignment, reconstruction, and stabilization. Larson modified the procedure practiced by Capener by mobilizing the paraspinal musculature and retracting it medially, resulting in a more lateral trajectory and thus allowing true simultaneous ventral and dorsal access to the spine from a single incision.

20.2 Overview of the Lateral Extracavitary Approach

The modern day lateral extracavitary approach remains a critical technique for addressing ventral thoracolumbar spinal pathology, and while it may be more commonly applied to spinal tumor, trauma, and thoracic discs, it has an important role in management of advanced Pott's disease as well. Patients with vertebral body destruction, kyphotic deformity, with or without neurologic compromise present challenging cases requiring a "circumferential" approach. LECA is a versatile technique as it allows for ventral access to the spine from a posterior approach in the prone position and avoids entering the pleural or abdominal cavity. The lateral trajectory allows for visualization across the anterior aspect of the spinal canal, and decompression of neural elements from ventrally compressive lesions can be achieved in a safe manner. The exposure also allows for anterior column reconstruction if necessary, without spinal cord manipulation. Posterior spinal fixation can also be achieved without the need for a second incision or repositioning. This is in contrast to other ventral approaches, such as the transthoracic, transabdominal/retroperitoneal, and the thoracoabdominal approach which additionally involves diaphragmatic takedown. An important advantage of LECA is that the anterior and posterior spinal columns are exposed simultaneously allowing for an iterative operative strategy which is extremely powerful when confronting fixed kyphotic deformity. The flexibility of LECA allows a wide range of pathologies to be addressed from a single approach. Additionally, LECA can be performed without the need of a second exposure surgeon, which obviates the logistical headaches of other anterior operations. Disadvantages of LECA center on the technically demanding nature of the procedure and potential unfamiliarity with pertinent anatomy. Important anatomic landmarks include the neurovascular bundle traveling caudally to the rib, as well as the intrathoracic and intraabdominal contents. There is also risk of transgressing pulmonary structures, and it is critical to recognize when the pleural cavity has been entered as chest tube placement may be critical in the setting of a pneumothorax or pleural effusion. Given the wide exposure, there is the potential for significant blood loss. A number of retrospective studies have shown good neurologic outcomes for LECA for various pathologies, with approximately 75% of patients showing neurologic improvement [3–8]. Complication rates have been reported between 31% and 68% [9–11].

The utility of the LECA has expanded with both the refinement of surgical technique as well as the development of new technology. For example, ligation of the nerve root is now a common aspect of the procedure, something not practiced by Larson. This step allows for a wider surgical corridor and expanded access to the ventral vertebral body. Additionally, the development of expandable cage technology allows for robust anterior column reconstruction through a proportionally narrower window, further adding to the versatility. The use of posterior instrumentation, including temporary rod placement, allows for aggressive circumferential vertebrectomy while maintaining spinal stability. Lastly, the development of modern titanium-based surgical implants, cages, and pedicle screws, more resistant to biofilm formation, has allowed for safe placement of instrumentation in infected spaces [12].

Another posterolateral approach to the spine, the costotransversectomy, has also emerged as valuable approach to gain ventral access from a primarily posterior approach. The LECA when pioneered by Larson was thought of as a novel alternative procedure for lesions which otherwise would normally require a thoracotomy. The costotransversectomy achieves similar surgical goals as LECA, but can be viewed as a more incremental extension from traditional posterior surgery. The costotransversectomy improves upon the transpedicular approach for achieving ventral access by removing additional bone laterally, including the transverse process and proximal rib head. With nearly identical surgical goals, the nuances separating the costotransversectomy and the LECA today are subtle. One of the primary differences between approaches is the initial exposure and trajectory [13]. A costotransversectomy is performed under a standard midline exposure, visualizing the lamina, costovertebral joint, and proximal rib. Alternatively, the LECA involves splitting the erector spinae muscles, retracting medially, and initially exposing substantially more rib than is seen with costotransversectomy. This is followed by subperiosteal dissection medially towards the proximal rib head that will then be resected. The more lateral trajectory of the LECA allows for a more complete resection of the proximal rib head and thus improved access particularly to the ventrolateral vertebral body and the anterior aspect of the spinal canal. It should be noted that in the case of spinal column metastasis, the tumor often creates a surgical corridor that makes the medial mobilization of the multifidus muscle unnecessary.

20.3 Experiences with LECA for Spinal TB

Despite the advances in medical treatments for tuberculosis, the incidence of Pott's disease of the spine still remains significant in developing countries, and also presents a public health threat in developed countries where drug-resistant organisms have taken hold [14, 15]. Patients often present with paraplegia and kyphosis secondary to vertebral body destruction. Surgical goals may include decompression of neural elements, reestablishment of spinal alignment and correction of kyphosis, as well as debridement of abscesses and infected tissues. There have been a number of studies published evaluating the use of several anterior and posterolateral approaches, including LECA, for surgical management of Pott's disease [16–20]. Anterior decompression alone without placement of instrumentation, while attempted previously, is associated with worsening postoperative kyphosis [21]. One study evaluating 70 patients with thoracolumbar tuberculosis compared LECA to anterior approaches such as transthoracic, transpleural, and/or retroperitoneal diaphragm cutting approach. While EBL was slightly higher in the LECA group, the immediate correction of kyphosis was significantly higher, and there were fewer major complications requiring ICU care [22]. Another study evaluated 22 patients treated by LECA vs. 23 patients treated with posterior circumferential approach for thoracic/lumbar tuberculous spondylitis. Both approaches resulted in comparable high rates of deformity correction, neurologic improvement, and bony fusion, without any major complications [23]. A meta-analysis from 2019 reviewed 11 studies including 818 patients comparing anterior vs posterior approach for thoracolumbar tuberculosis [24]. The authors found equivalent operative time between anterior and posterior approaches, higher blood loss with posterior approach, no difference in hospital stay, and no difference in time to fusion. The posterior approach did however result in significantly higher rates of correction of kyphotic deformity. While this analysis is comprised of several different studies with different methodologies and surgical techniques, the concept that posterior instrumentation is important for achieving adequate kyphosis correction is affirmed. LECA, therefore, remains an excellent approach for Pott's disease as it allows ventral resection and reconstruction, but also for posterior instrumentation, which as the literature suggests, remains critical for achieving correction of kyphosis in this setting.

20.4 LECA Surgical Technique

The technical nuances of performing LECA are critical for the surgeon to understand, as the trajectory is different from traditional posterior surgery. The patient is positioned prone on the operating table with arms to the side. Neuromonitoring may be employed depending on the nature of the pathology. Once localization is achieved, the incision is planned. Historically the LECA was performed with a "hockey stick" shaped incision, as practiced by Larson, to assist in retraction of the skin laterally. This afforded a more horizontal trajectory across the anterior spinal canal. Other variations include s-shaped, and linear incisions. It is critical to extend the incision two to three levels above and below the lesion for sufficient exposure in placing posterior instrumentation and also to allow the skin to be mobilized laterally at the index level. After incision the fascia is divided and reflected, a standard subperiosteal dissected is performed, and the operative levels are identified with an intraoperative x-ray. Pedicle screws can be placed first prior to any bony resection, as this allows for placement of rods on the contralateral side to the LECA approach. Next the dissection is taken laterally, and the paraspinal muscles are mobilized and dissected to reach the desired rib. The spinal erectae muscles can be retracted medially with the aid of several penrose drains looping around the muscle when required although this step is often unnecessary. Subperiosteal dissection of the rib is performed with attention not to violate the pleural space and not to injure the neurovascular bundle running just caudal to the rib. The transverse process is removed to further expose the rib. The proximal rib can be resected with rub cutters or a rongeur, and the rib can then be disarticulated from the vertebral body using a cobb or curet. To maximize the surgical corridor, the nerve root (T2-L1) can be sacrificed. At this point the entire vertebral body is accessible from disc space above to disc space below. Depending on the goals of surgery, discectomy and/or corpectomy can now be performed. Additional exposure is achieved by resection of the facet, pedicle, and lamina. The lateral trajectory allows for direct visualization of the spinal canal while working ventrally. Anterior column reconstruction can be achieved by placement of a strut allograft or more commonly an expandable cage. Attention must be paid to ensure there is no undetected spinal fluid leak or pleural violation. A postoperative chest x-ray should be obtained to rule out a pneumothorax.

20.5 Case Example

A 24-year-old female with a history of tuberculosis presented with severe back pain and inability to ambulate for 1 month. On exam she was found to have diffuse lower extremity weakness. MRI imaging revealed Pott's disease of the spine, with thoracic vertebral body involvement and collapse, and significant ventral epidural extension of infectious phlegmon causing spinal cord compression (Fig. 20.1a). The patient was brought to the OR for a lateral extracavitary approach for ventral and dorsal decompression of the spinal canal, as well as placement of posterior instrumentation. Intraop photo (Fig. 20.1b) shows the surgical field and exposure obtained with the LECA approach. The paraspinal muscles have been dissected and are retracted medially with the assistance of several penrose drains, allowing for direct visualization of the anterior spinal canal and complete decompression of the dural tube. Postoperative plain films show good alignment of the spinal column with placement of posterior instrumentation (Fig. 20.1c).

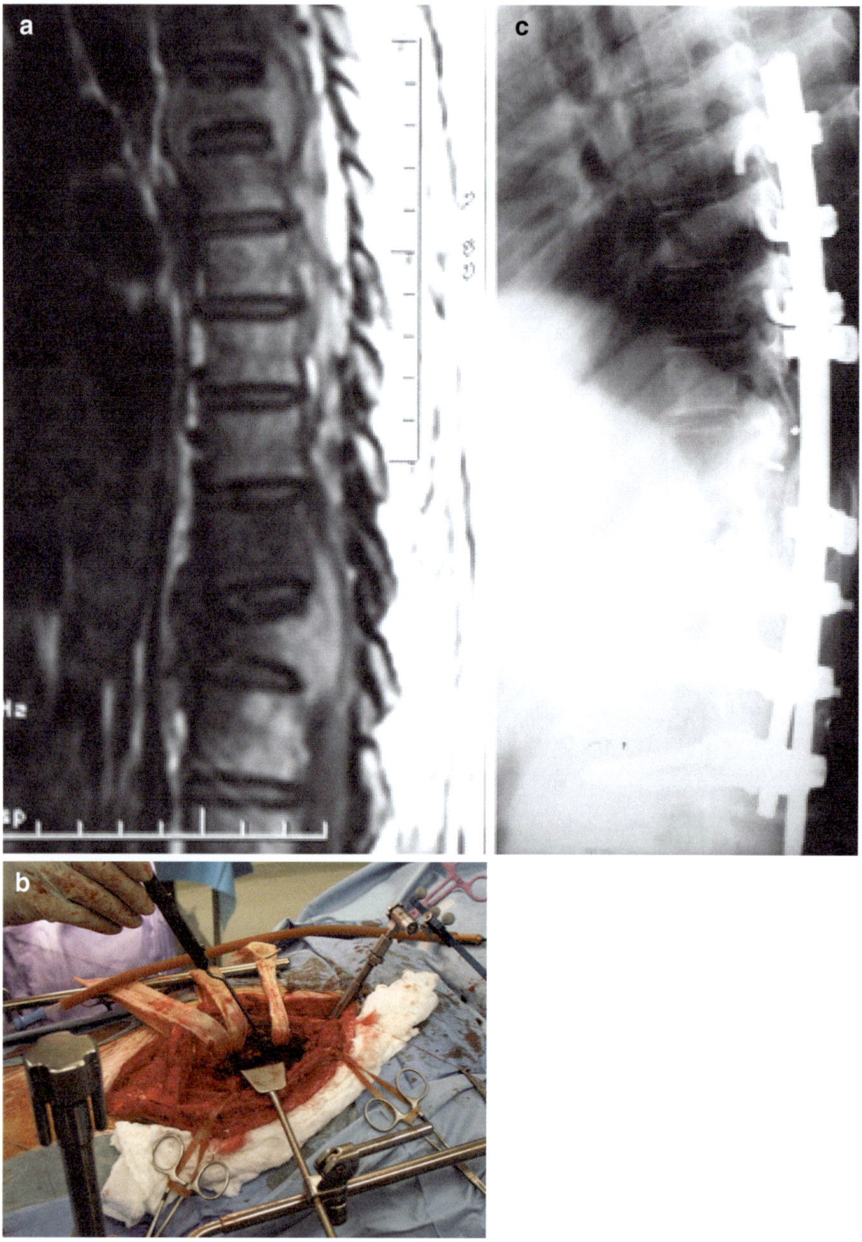

Fig. 20.1 (**a**) Preoperative image of a 24-year-old patient with Pott's disease of the spine. Image shows vertebral body involvement and collapse, as well as extension of infectious phlegmon to the ventral epidural space causing spinal cord compression. (**b**) Intraoperative photograph of the lateral extracavitary approach to the spine. (**c**) Postoperative plain films showing posterior instrumentation placement

20.6 Summary

Pott's disease of the spine remains a significant burden and challenge throughout the world. Surgical decompression and stabilization is often a critical component of the overall management of this condition. The unique aspects of Pott's disease, namely, the anterior vertebral body involvement with frequent associated collapse and kyphotic deformity, mandate an aggressive surgical strategy. The lateral extracavitary approach remains an excellent choice for achieving the surgical goals presented by these challenging cases in so far as it affords access to both the anterior and posterior spinal columns simultaneously.

References

1. Menard V. Etude Pratique sur le Mal de Pott. Paris: Masson et Cie; 1900.
2. Capener N. The evolution of lateral rhachotomy. J Bone Joint Surg Br. 1954;36-B(2):173–9. https://doi.org/10.1302/0301-620X.36B2.173.
3. Larson SJ, Holst RA, Hemmy DC, Sances A Jr. Lateral extracavitary approach to traumatic lesions of the thoracic and lumbar spine. J Neurosurg. 1976;45(6):628–37. https://doi.org/10.3171/jns.1976.45.6.0628.
4. Arnold PM, Baek PN, Bernardi RJ, Luck EA, Larson SJ. Surgical management of nontuberculous thoracic and lumbar vertebral osteomyelitis: report of 33 cases. Surg Neurol. 1997;47(6):551–61. https://doi.org/10.1016/s0090-3019(96)00242-x.
5. Delfini R, Di Lorenzo N, Ciappetta P, Bristot R, Cantore G. Surgical treatment of thoracic disc herniation: a reappraisal of Larson's lateral extracavitary approach. Surg Neurol. 1996;45(6):517–22.; discussion 522-3. https://doi.org/10.1016/0090-3019(95)00483-1.
6. Dietze DD Jr, Fessler RG. Thoracic disc herniations. Neurosurg Clin N Am. 1993;4(1):75–90.
7. Maiman DJ, Larson SJ, Benzel EC. Neurological improvement associated with late decompression of the thoracolumbar spinal cord. Neurosurgery. 1984;14(3):302–7. https://doi.org/10.1227/00006123-198403000-00007.
8. Maiman DJ, Larson SJ, Luck E, El-Ghatit A. Lateral extracavitary approach to the spine for thoracic disc herniation: report of 23 cases. Neurosurgery. 1984;14(2):178–82. https://doi.org/10.1227/00006123-198402000-00010.
9. Graham AW 3rd, Mac Millan M, Fessler RG. Lateral extracavitary approach to the thoracic and thoracolumbar spine. Orthopedics. 1997;20(7):605–10.
10. Lubelski D, Abdullah KG, Mroz TE, et al. Lateral extracavitary vs. costotransversectomy approaches to the thoracic spine: reflections on lessons learned. Neurosurgery. 2012;71(6):1096–102. https://doi.org/10.1227/NEU.0b013e3182706102.
11. Resnick DK, Benzel EC. Lateral extracavitary approach for thoracic and thoracolumbar spine trauma: operative complications. Neurosurgery. 1998;43(4):796–802.; discussion 802-3. https://doi.org/10.1097/00006123-199810000-00041.
12. Kasliwal MK, Tan LA, Traynelis VC. Infection with spinal instrumentation: review of pathogenesis, diagnosis, prevention, and management. Surg Neurol Int. 2013;4(Suppl 5):S392–403. https://doi.org/10.4103/2152-7806.120783.
13. Lubelski D, Abdullah KG, Steinmetz MP, et al. Lateral extracavitary, costotransversectomy, and transthoracic thoracotomy approaches to the thoracic spine: review of techniques and complications. J Spinal Disord Tech. 2013;26(4):222–32. https://doi.org/10.1097/BSD.0b013e31823f3139.

14. Polley P, Dunn R. Noncontiguous spinal tuberculosis: incidence and management. Eur Spine J. 2009;18(8):1096–101. https://doi.org/10.1007/s00586-009-0966-0.
15. Manjelievskaia J, Erck D, Piracha S, Schrager L. Drug-resistant TB: deadly, costly and in need of a vaccine. Trans R Soc Trop Med Hyg. 2016;110(3):186–91. https://doi.org/10.1093/trstmh/trw006.
16. Chandra SP, Ramdurg SR, Kurwale N, et al. Extended costotransversectomy to achieve circumferential fusion for pathologies causing thoracic instability. Spine J. 2014;14(9):2094–101. https://doi.org/10.1016/j.spinee.2013.12.028.
17. Ma YZ, Cui X, Li HW, Chen X, Cai XJ, Bai YB. Outcomes of anterior and posterior instrumentation under different surgical procedures for treating thoracic and lumbar spinal tuberculosis in adults. Int Orthop. 2012;36(2):299–305. https://doi.org/10.1007/s00264-011-1390-8.
18. Luo C, Wang X, Wu P, Ge L, Zhang H, Hu J. Single-stage transpedicular decompression, debridement, posterior instrumentation, and fusion for thoracic tuberculosis with kyphosis and spinal cord compression in aged individuals. Spine J. 2016;16(2):154–62. https://doi.org/10.1016/j.spinee.2013.11.014.
19. Shen X, Liu H, Wang G, Liu X. Single-stage posterior-only approach treating single-segment thoracic tubercular spondylitis. Int J Clin Exp Pathol. 2015;8(9):11051–9.
20. Zeng H, Zhang P, Shen X, et al. One-stage posterior-only approach in surgical treatment of single-segment thoracic spinal tuberculosis with neurological deficits in adults: a retrospective study of 34 cases. BMC Musculoskelet Disord. 2015;16:186. https://doi.org/10.1186/s12891-015-0640-0.
21. A 10-year assessment of a controlled trial comparing debridement and anterior spinal fusion in the management of tuberculosis of the spine in patients on standard chemotherapy in Hong Kong. Eighth Report of the Medical Research Council Working Party on Tuberculosis of the Spine. J Bone Joint Surg Br 1982;64(4):393–8. https://doi.org/10.1302/0301-620X.64B4.7047536.
22. Garg B, Kandwal P, Nagaraja UB, Goswami A, Jayaswal A. Anterior versus posterior procedure for surgical treatment of thoracolumbar tuberculosis: a retrospective analysis. Indian J Orthop. 2012;46(2):165–70. https://doi.org/10.4103/0019-5413.93682.
23. Omran K, Abdel-Fattah AS, Othman AMA, et al. Lateral extracavitary approach versus posterior extensive circumferential decompression in the treatment of complicated thoracic and lumbar tuberculous spondylitis. Clin Spine Surg. 2017;30(9):E1211–9. https://doi.org/10.1097/BSD.0000000000000485.
24. Wang K, Wang N, Wang Y, Xia Y, Song F, Liu J. Anterior versus posterior instrumentation for treatment of thoracolumbar tuberculosis: a meta-analysis. Orthopade. 2019;48(3):207–12. https://doi.org/10.1007/s00132-018-03662-w.

Chapter 21
Drug Eluting Ceramics in the Field of Spinal Infections

Venugopal Menon

Abstract Background: Synthetic ceramics have been used to expand or replace autologous bone graft in many clinical situations. The present study looks at the use of such substitutes as local drug delivery systems in bone infections. This is a retrospective observational study.

Methods: One hundred and twenty patients with infections of the spine due to pyogenic bacteria, *M. tuberculosis*, or brucellosis were included in this study. Nanoporous hydroxyapatite (HA), HA and β tricalcium phosphate (TCP), or HA and bioglass (Bg) were the ceramic compositions used. The granules were loaded with appropriate antibiotic, vancomycin, in pyogenic infection and streptomycin in Tb and placed in the debrided surgical site. Patients were followed up for infection-related complications.

Results: All the infective pathologies healed well without discharging sinus formation or persistent disability. Two cases of Tb spine in children had surgical scar breakdown and implant pullout in one that needed revision. Three patients in the adult pyogenic group also needed revision for implant failure and one case re-debridement. Radiologically all the lesions healed well but depending on the type of ceramic used it resorbed and integrated with the bone differently.

Discussion: Drug leeching ceramics have the advantage of high concentrations of local delivery of drug along with no donor site issues and immediate, large-scale availability with no storage concerns compared to biological solutions for the same condition. It is therefore our procedure of choice in infective pathology of the spine.

Keywords Bioceramics · Spinal infections · Drug delivery systems · Spinal Tb · Bioactive glass · Hydroxyapatite

V. Menon (✉)
Department of Orthopaedics, Bharati Vidyapeeth Medical College, Pune, India

S. S. Dhatt, V. Kumar (eds.), *Tuberculosis of the Spine*,
https://doi.org/10.1007/978-981-16-9495-0_21

21.1 Introduction

Autologous bone graft has been acknowledged as the "Gold Standard" for substitution or augmentation of skeletal and dental defects in mankind [1]. Their biological and mechanical properties are considered optimal for the reconstruction of normal skeletal tissues [2]. In terms of osteogenecity, osteoinductivity, and osteoconductivity, autologous bone has no parallel till date. Yet the demand for synthetic skeletal substitutes has increased exponentially in the last few decades. There are several reasons for this paradox. Optimisation of mechanical and biological properties of the ceramic to suit each individual application is but one of them. Reconstruction of ever larger defects left by trauma, tumour, and infectious disease of the bone is now possible and indeed often demanded. The availability of harvested bone is limited and the quality often suboptimal in young children and older individuals making autograft a poor option. Donor site morbidity can be a serious issue in approximately 20% cases in trauma surgery [3].

Interestingly, Albee, the pioneer of bone grafting, is also credited with the first experimental application of synthetic bone substitutes in 1920 [4]. He had earlier described spinal fusion with autologous bone in 1915 [5]. The earliest clinical application of self-setting bioactive ceramics was recorded by Koster [6]. Branemark coined the term osteointegration and is considered the father of Dental Implantology [7]. Hench is credited with the first description of silicated calcium phosphates (Bioactive Glasses) in 1969 [8, 9]. Today the discipline of tissue engineering is poised to take reconstructive surgery to newer dimensions [10] with a wide variety of bioactive (both degradable and non-degradable) ceramics and glasses available in the market. Two novel technologies that have emerged in recent years that are poised to revolutionise the bioceramic science base are Nanotechnology and 3-D printing technology [11, 12].

Targeted drug delivery to the end organ to limit the disadvantages of systemic administration and to reduce the toxicity of drugs is a relatively old concept. In skeletal tissues the currently available options are PMMA cement beads, collagen fleeces, polymers (PLA, PL-GA composites), and a host of ceramic formulations [13]. The mechanical and biological properties of an ideal ceramic substitute can be tailored to suit the needs of the local environment, at the same time deliver adequate concentrations of the drug over a prolonged period of time, and eventually allow it to disappear by integration into the surrounding bone. Wu and coworkers have used a magnesium substituted glass diopside to achieve these results while Varma's team have used nanopore technology to obtain similar results [13, 14]. CaSi composites have been extensively used in the spine as well [15]. Nagineni et al. have looked at 108 cases with 204 fusion levels with over 90% fusion rate using stand-alone ceramic graft substitute [16]. Similar results were observed by Alimi's team [17] in 234 patients. The author's experience with calcium phosphate ceramics in postero-lateral fusions of the lumbar spine have not been so encouraging, and we have recommended the product only as a graft volume expander [18]. Evidently phospho-silicates of calcium perform better than calcium ortho-phosphates with regard to radiological fusion. Salamanna's recent systematic review [19] suggests that most studies have significant bias in favour of the synthetic substitute and the evidence needs to be carefully evaluated.

Many drugs have the potential to be delivered locally into diseased bone. Antibiotics, anti-cancer drugs, anti-osteoporotic medications, anti-rheumatics, etc. are some of the potential recipients of such attention. Traditionally osteomyelitis of the extremities has been treated with PMMA beads loaded with antibiotics or intramedullary implants coated with similar drugs [20]. Others have employed continuous antibiotic infused saline irrigation systems as in septic arthritis.

In India the development of bioceramics was initiated by the SCTIMST in the late 1980s and 1990s, and the next decade saw several clinical trials of the Chitra HA and bioglass composite materials in cancellous bone fracture augmentation studies [21–25]. The HA:Bg composite was optimised for mechanical and biological properties to an 80:20 ratio and most clinical trials used this composite. The composite has had extensive applications in skeletal and spine surgery and is available in the market (B-Ostin granules). Under strict Ethics Committee approved conditions, the authors have conducted 120 surgeries in patients with spinal infections (both pyogenic and tubercular), and this report is based on the results of this case series.

21.2 Materials and Methods

One hundred and twenty patients from three different centres formed the cohort of spondylodiscitis cases studied herein. Their data was prospectively collected but analysed retrospectively. One centre in the Middle East had predominantly pyogenic infections in adults while the second from Western India had predominance of Tb cases and the third from Southern India had near equal numbers of Tb and pyogenic infections. Three different categories of ceramics were used to supplement autologous bone graft in every case—β Tri calcium phosphate (Chronos- Synthes USA), nano porous hydroxyapatite (BMT wing, SCTIMST, Trivandrum, India), and HA: Bg composite 80:20 (BMT wing, SCTIMST, Trivandrum, India). The mixture ratio was 50:50 autologous cancellous bone and ceramic by volume and approximated.

21.2.1 The Patients

Centre 1 was Khoula Hospital in Muscat, Oman. The cohort had 62 patients consisting of 4 children and 58 adults. There were 10 Tb cases and 50 pyogenic infections in this series with one Brucella and one mixed infection [26].

Centre 2 was Bharati Vidyapeeth Medical College Pune, India, where 12 cases of which only one was pyogenic and the rest were Tb.

Centre 3 was Amrita Institute of Medical Sciences, Kochi, Kerala, India, where 46 cases were treated of which 18 cases were pyogenic and 28 were Tb. There were no children in the series from Kerala, while two from Pune were children under 5 years with Tb spine.

There was a generalised male preponderance in all the regions studied. The median age group was 45–50 years. While the pyogenic infections had frequent immune-compromising co-morbid conditions, the Tb patients were otherwise generally healthy.

21.2.2 Surgical Technique

A standard surgical technique was adopted for all the spondylodiscitis in the thoracic, thoraco-lumbar, and lumbar spine. The spine was approached posteriorly and one side instrumented with Titanium pedicle screw devices. The side where the vertebral body was less affected was typically chosen, and the montage was one or two levels above to the same below. Through the lateral extra-cavitary approach, the vertebral bodies were exposed on the side opposite to the instrumentation; in the thoracic spine two ribs were sacrificed approximately 5 cm from the head. The vertebral bodies, discs and necrotic material and pus were removed piecemeal, and the resultant space filled with the augmented bone graft (rib graft in case of the thoracic spine and iliac graft in the lumbar spine) Fig. 21.1a through g. The second side instrumentation was mounted and assembly tightened.

In the cervical spine the anterior approach was chosen for the debridement and reconstruction. After excising the diseased vertebra and necrotic material reconstruction was done with tricortical iliac graft and supplemented with ceramic augmented chips on either side to fill the dead space. Anterior plates are used to stabilize the construct.

Antibiotic loading of the ceramic was done in the following manner—all Tb cases had streptomycin and all pyogenic patients had vancomycin added to the ceramic. The drug was mixed in two ml of N saline and added to the ceramic granules taken in a 50 syringe. Applying negative suction, the syringe was shaken for 2–3 min till the liquid disappeared completely into the ceramic. The ceramic was mixed with equal volumes of bone graft by volume and packed into the defect left by the vertebral body removal.

Post operatively the patients were mobilized normally without external support, and appropriate chemotherapy was started forthwith. The patients were followed up at 6 weeks, 3 months, 6 months, and 1 year.

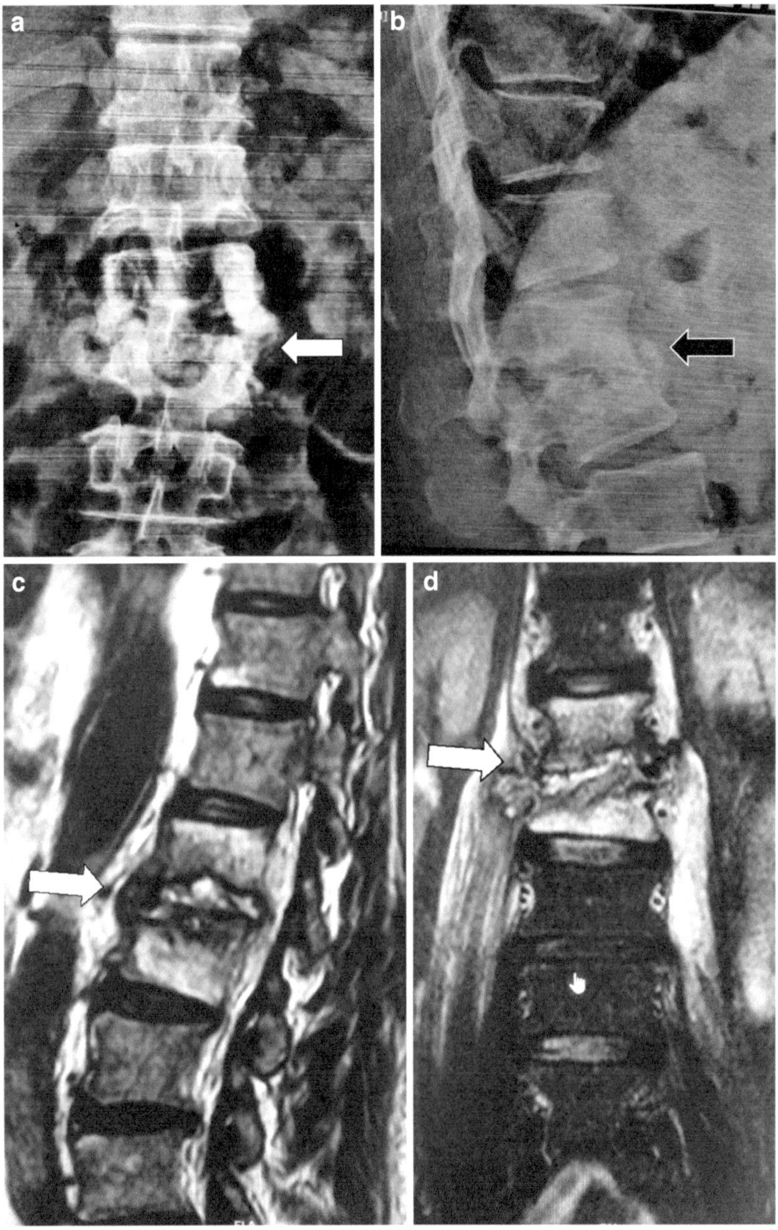

Fig. 21.1 (**a**) Antero-posterior roentgenogram of the spine depicting the L2–3 spondylodiskitis with loss of height and end plate destruction. (**b**) Lateral radiograph of the same spine where the changes of infection are visible. (**c**) MRI images of the same patient. Sagittal T2 W images show the extent of the infection and pus in the disc space very clearly. (**d**) Coronal T2 weighted image of this case. (**e**) Axial T2 weighted image through the disc space depicts the infective process. (**f**) Post operative X-rays. AP view illustrating the stabilization done through the posterior approach. (**g**) The lateral X-ray shows the instrumentation in situ and the ceramic filling of the debrided cavity within the infected bone

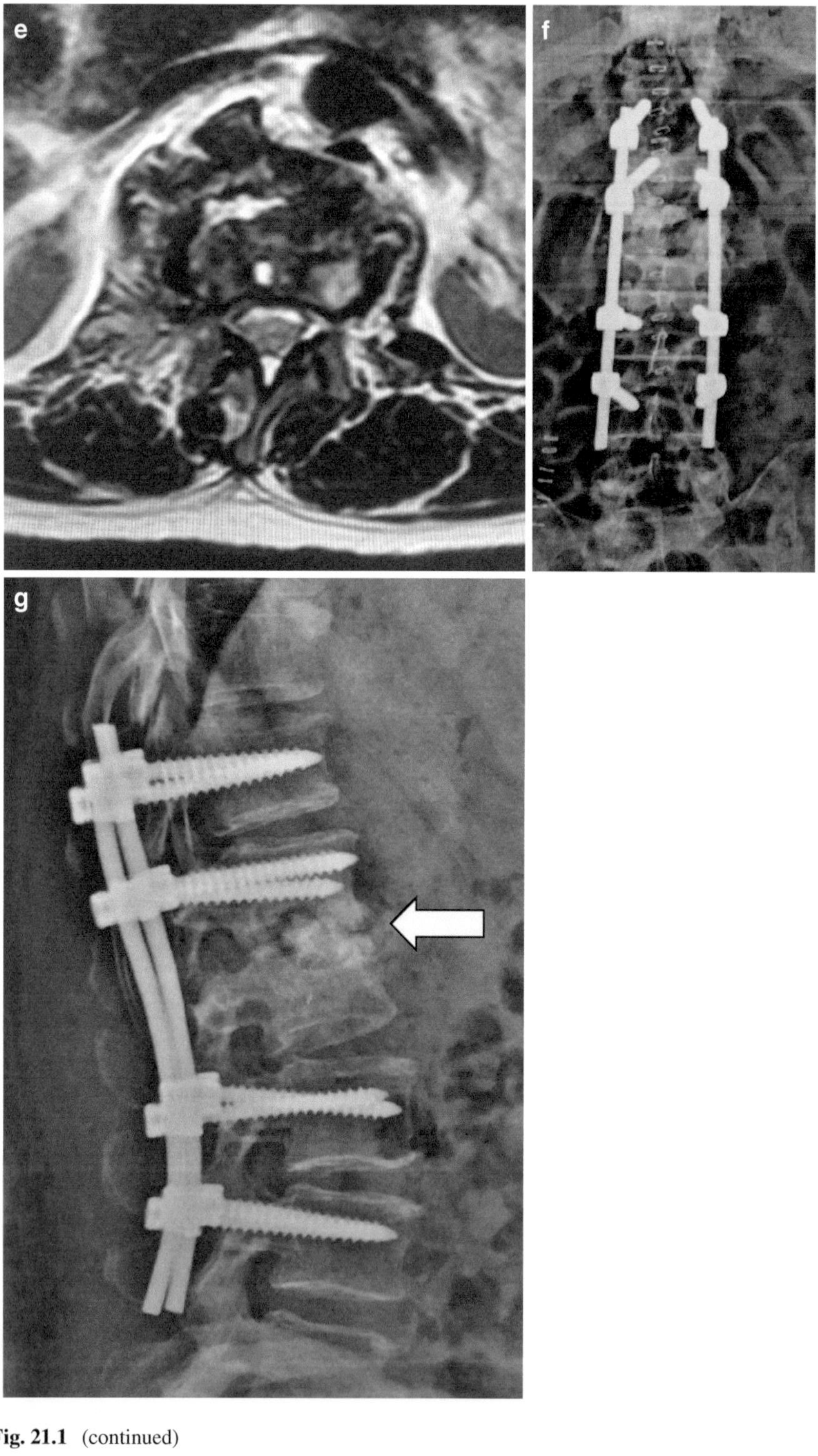

Fig. 21.1 (continued)

21.3 Results

Among the pyogenic group of patients, there was one case of wound dehiscence that needed debridement and closure without implant revision. Two cases had early implant failure and needed implant removal without revision of the vertebral procedure. One patient had implant failure with pseudoarthrosis and is awaiting revision (and is likely to need revision of the bony fusion procedure). In the tuberculosis spine group, one patient needed revision of the entire implant due to pullout (paediatric patient), while another had wound dehiscence that healed with prolonged dressing and wound care (again a paediatric age group patient). All other patients were followed up to healing of the osseous pathology by clinical, haematological, and radiological parameters. While the β TCP was fully resorbed radiologically, the HA and HA:Bg was incompletely resorbed, and radiological residue of the ceramic was visible at 1 year (Fig. 21.2). All the infective lesions healed well with no sinus formation or residual discharge. Radiological fusion was also seen in these cases at 1 year follow-up. Many cases did have minimal progression of the regional kyphosis though this did not appear symptomatic.

21.4 Discussion

Several authors have described techniques of drug delivery into infected vertebral bodies. Catheter-assisted drug delivery is the most obvious technique and has the advantage of not leaving any foreign material in after completion of procedure. It was developed as a continuum of the long bone infection protocol based on external fixation and topical antibiotic irrigation; Magerl and colleagues described the technique along with their spinal external fixator for pyogenic infections [27]. PMMA

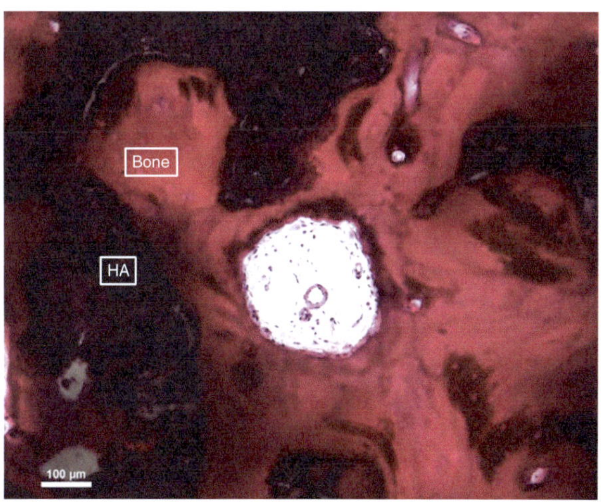

Fig. 21.2 Histological picture of the interface between the bone and the ceramic in a well-integrated specimen. H&E stain × 100 magnification. Courtesy: Dr Sabareeswaran A

cement beads came next [28, 29] and is still extensively used in prosthetic infections and traumatic bone infections. Antibiotic loaded collagen fleeces have been immensely popular [28] and are extensively used though the nature of the protein matrix lends itself to immunological reactions in a small number of cases. Biodegradable ceramics also have a potential advantage over PMMA cement beads that it doesn't need a second surgery for removal. The advantages of using ceramic as a graft substitute in the infective setting are numerous:

- Filling of the dead space created by debridement of infected tissue.
- Mechanical properties of the granules (over collagen fleece) in load bearing bones.
- They are osteoconductive, inductive, and integrative as compared to other degradables.
- Biodegradable after function is achieved. In bone this property has been described as osteo-transduction.
- Saves bone graft harvesting and all its attendant complications.
- Drug delivery at site of action for an average of 3 weeks at MIC concentration.
- Radiological visibility of the fate of the ceramic (HA) up to 2 years.
- Compared to allograft and xenograft, it is non-antigenic.
- Sensitive antibiotic can be loaded intra-operatively.
- Available in large quantities.
- Can be stocked at room temperature without special equipment.
- Can be autoclaved.

Disadvantages:

- Cannot be used as standalone graft substitutes (preferably mixed with autologous cancellous bone); this is limited to those ceramics with larger proportions of HA. TCP and bioglass predominant ceramics resorb very quickly.
- Drug leaching period is limited (3 weeks is maximum).
- HA containing ceramics resorb poorly and persist for a long time.
- Drug leeching can be erratic and often is nonlinear.
- Optimum structural support is often not provided by granules particularly as the HA content decreases.
- Ceramics can very rarely act as foreign materials in the body.

21.5 Conclusions

Based on the current series the authors recommend the use of biodegradable ceramic granules impregnated with antibiotic as an autograft augmentation and drug eluting device to be used in cases of infective spondylodiskitis (Tb, pyogenic infections, and brucellosis).

Acknowledgement Dr Sabareeswaran A, Scientist, Histopathology Lab, Dept. of Applied Biology, BMT Wing, SCTIMST, Trivandrum, Kerala, for the histology slide used in study.

References

1. Pape HC, Evans A, Kobbe P. Autologous bone graft: properties and techniques. J Orthop Trauma. 2010;24(Suppl 1):S36–40. https://doi.org/10.1097/BOT.0b013e3181cec4a1.
2. Khan SN, Cammisa FP Jr, Sandhu HS, Diwan AD, Girardi FP, Lane JM. The biology of bone grafting. J Am Acad Orthop Surg. 2005;13(1):77–86.
3. Dimitriou R, Mataliotakis GI, Angoules AG, Kanakaris NK, Giannoudis PV. Complications following autologous bone graft harvesting from the iliac crest and using the RIA: a systematic review. Injury. 2011;42(Suppl 2):S3–15. https://doi.org/10.1016/j.injury.2011.06.015. Epub 2011 Jun 25
4. Albee FH. Studies in bone growth: triple calcium phosphate as a stimulus to osteogenesis. Ann Surg. 1920;71(1):32–9. https://doi.org/10.1097/00000658-192001000-00006.
5. Albee FH. Bone graft surgery. Philadelphia PA; London, UK: WN Saunders Company; 1915.
6. Köster K, Karbe E, Kramer H, Heide H, König R. Experimenteller Knochenersatz durch resorbierbare Calciumphosphat-Keramik [Experimental bone replacement with resorbable calcium phosphate ceramic (author's transl)]. Langenbecks Arch Chir. 1976;341(2):77–86. German. https://doi.org/10.1007/BF01262779.
7. Branemark PI. Osteointegration and it's experimental background. J Prosthetic Dent. 1983;50:399–410. https://doi.org/10.1016/S0022-3913(83)80101-2.
8. Hench LL, Splinter RJ, Allen WC, Greenlee TK. Bonding mechanisms at the interface of ceramic prosthetic materials. J Biomed Mater Res. 1971;5:117–41. https://doi.org/10.1002/jbm.820050611.
9. Hench LL. The story of bioglass. J Mater Sci Mater Med. 2006;17(11):967–78. https://doi.org/10.1007/s10856-006-0432-z. Epub 2006 Nov 22
10. Baino F, Novajra G, Vitale-Brovarone C. Bioceramics and Scaffolds: a winning combination for tissue engineering. Front Bioeng Biotechnol. 2015;3:202. https://doi.org/10.3389/fbioe.2015.00202.
11. Barberi J, Baino F, Fiume E, Orlygsson G, Nommeots-Nomm A, Massera J, Verné E. Robocasting of SiO_2-based bioactive glass scaffolds with porosity gradient for bone regeneration and potential load-bearing applications. Materials (Basel). 2019;12(17):2691. https://doi.org/10.3390/ma12172691.
12. Ma H, Feng C, Chang J, Wu C. 3D-printed bioceramic scaffolds: from bone tissue engineering to tumor therapy. Acta Biomater. 2018;79:37–59. https://doi.org/10.1016/j.actbio.2018.08.026. Epub 2018 Aug 28
13. Simon D, Manuel S, Varma H. Novel nanoporous bioceramic spheres for drug delivery application: a preliminary in vitro investigation. Oral Surg Oral Med Oral Pathol Oral Radiol. 2013;115(3):e7–14. https://doi.org/10.1016/j.oooo.2011.10.021. Epub 2012 May 19
14. Wu C, Zreiqat H. Porous bioactive diopside (CaMgSi(2)O(6)) ceramic microspheres for drug delivery. Acta Biomater. 2010;6(3):820–9. https://doi.org/10.1016/j.actbio.2009.09.025. Epub 2009 Oct 1
15. Romagnoli C, D'Asta F, Brandi ML. Drug delivery using composite scaffolds in the context of bone tissue engineering. Clin Cases Miner Bone Metab. 2013;10(3):155–61.
16. Nagineni VV, James AR, Alimi M, Hofstetter C, Shin BJ, Njoku I Jr, Tsiouris AJ, Härtl R. Silicate-substituted calcium phosphate ceramic bone graft replacement for spinal fusion procedures. Spine (Phila Pa 1976). 2012;37(20):E1264–72. https://doi.org/10.1097/BRS.0b013e318265e22e.
17. Alimi M, Navarro-Ramirez R, Parikh K, Njoku I, Hofstetter CP, Tsiouris AJ, Härtl R. Radiographic and clinical outcome of silicate-substituted calcium phosphate (Si-CaP) ceramic bone graft in spinal fusion procedures. Clin Spine Surg. 2017;30(6):E845–52. https://doi.org/10.1097/BSD.0000000000000432.
18. Acharya KN, Kumar RJ, Varma HK, Menon KV. Hydroxyapatite-bioactive glass ceramic composite as stand alone graft substitute for posterolateral fusion of lumbar spine: a prospective matched and controlled study. J Spinal Disord Tech. April;21(2):106–11.

19. Salamanna F, Tschon M, Borsari V, Pagani S, Martini L, Fini M. Spinal fusion procedures in the adult and young population: a systematic review on allogenic bone and synthetic grafts when compared to autologous bone. J Mater Sci Mater Med. 2020;31(6):51. https://doi.org/10.1007/s10856-020-06389-3.
20. Inzana JA, Schwarz EM, Kates SL, Awad HA. Biomaterials approaches to treating implant-associated osteomyelitis. Biomaterials. 2016;81:58–71. https://doi.org/10.1016/j.biomaterials.2015.12.012. Epub 2015 Dec 18
21. Varma HK, Sivakumar R. Preparation and characterization of free flowing hydroxyapatite powders. Phosphorus Res Bull. 1996;6:35–8. https://doi.org/10.3363/prb1992.6.0_35.
22. Srinivasan A, Varma HK, Kumary TV, John A, et al. Preliminary in vitro and in vivo characterization of a sol–gel derived bioactive glass–ceramic system. Bull Mater Sci. 2002;25(5):419–29. https://doi.org/10.1007/BF02708021.
23. John A, Varma HK, Kumari TV, Nisha VR, Narayanan D. Cytocompatibility studies of a novel bioactive glass coated porous hydroxyapatite bioceramic for use as a bone substitute. Key Eng Mater. 2005;284–286:317–20. https://doi.org/10.4028/www.scientific.net/kem.284-286.317.
24. Easwer H, Rajeev A, Varma H, et al. Cosmetic and radiological outcome following the use of synthetic hydroxyapatite porous-dense bilayer burr-hole buttons. Acta Neurochir. 2007;149:481–6. https://doi.org/10.1007/s00701-007-1131-3.
25. Menon KV, Varma HK. Tibial plateau fractures treated with percutaneously introduced synthetic porous hydroxyapatite granules. Eur J Orthop Surg Traumatol. 2005;15(3):205–13.
26. Menon KV, MMS T. Epidemiologic and demographic attributes of primary spondylodiscitis in a Middle Eastern population sample. World Neurosurg. 2016;95:31–9. S1878-8750(16)30632-5. https://doi.org/10.1016/j.wneu.2016.07.088.
27. Jeanneret B, Magerl F. Treatment of osteomyelitis of the spine using percutaneous suction/irrigation and percutaneous external spinal fixation. J Spinal Disord. 1994;7(3):185–205. https://doi.org/10.1097/00002517-199407030-00001.
28. Seligson D, Berling S. Antibiotic-laden PMMA bead chains for the prevention of infection in compound fractures: current state of the art. Eur J Orthop Surg Traumatol. 2015;25(6):969–74. https://doi.org/10.1007/s00590-015-1652-z. Epub 2015 Jun 9
29. van Vugt TAG, Walraven JMB, Geurts JAP, Arts JJC. Antibiotic-loaded collagen sponges in clinical treatment of chronic osteomyelitis: a systematic review. J Bone Joint Surg Am. 2018;100(24):2153–61. https://doi.org/10.2106/JBJS.17.01140.

Chapter 22
Extensile Approaches to the Spine in Tuberculosis

Venugopal Menon

Difficult roads often lead to beautiful destinations—Unknown

Abstract Spinal tuberculosis surgery typically mandates adequate exposure to obtain thorough debridement of all infected material, neural decompression and reconstruction with graft or cage for immediate mobilization. Extensile approaches are often required in strategically located vertebrae to achieve these goals. This study describes four such exposures the author has used extensively:

1. The "Fallen T" approach to the dorsal spine
2. The labio-mandibulo-glossotomy approach to the cranio-cervical junction
3. The Mercedes Benz approach to the lumbosacral spine
4. The medial claviculectomy approach to the cervico-thoracic junction

The history, anatomical rationale and surgical technique are described in detail with the advantages and potential disadvantages of each. The author also appends a brief summary of his personal case series in each technique.

Keywords Tuberculosis · Extra-cavitary approach · Mercedes Benz incision · Lumbosacral spine · Upper cervical spine · Cervico-thoracic junction · Medial claviculectomy · Cranio-cervical junction

22.1 General Introduction

Surgical access is known to determine both the ease and thoroughness of any surgery. Needless to say, some targets are particularly difficult to access due to its precarious location and critical surrounding tissues. The occipito-cervical junction

V. Menon (✉)
Department of Orthopaedics, Bharati Vidyapeeth Medical College, Pune, India

S. S. Dhatt, V. Kumar (eds.), *Tuberculosis of the Spine*,
https://doi.org/10.1007/978-981-16-9495-0_22

and the cervico-thoracic junction are particularly difficult to approach anteriorly when the vertebral bodies need reconstruction as in infective pathology, tumour or trauma. Similarly, the extra-cavitary approach to the thoracic spine to access the vertebral body from the posterior approach and the lumbosacral junction to expose the L5-S1 interspace for reconstruction can be particularly challenging. This section describes the authors' experience in treating tuberculosis of the spine needing extensile exposures for reconstructive procedures utilizing four such approaches with substantial personal modifications. The author describes the following approaches:

1. "Fallen T" approach to the posterior and extra-cavitary anterior aspect of the thoracic spine
2. Mercedes Benz approach to the lumbosacral spine
3. The labio-mandibulo-glossotomy (LMG) approach to the anterior aspect of the upper cervical spine
4. Medial claviculectomy approach to the anterior aspect of the cervico-thoracic junction

22.2 The "Fallen T" Approach to the Thoracic Spine

22.2.1 Introduction

The extra-cavitary approach to the anterior aspect of the thoracic spine through the posteriorly placed incision is well known and has been used for anterior column reconstructions along with posterior instrumentation in the same sitting. The traditional incision has been a "Capner's" curved incision which allows one to dissect the rib heads and transverse processes on the convex side of the curved incision [1]. The costo-transversectomy approach described by Menard [2] and the lateral Racheotomy approach described by Capner are quite similar [3]. This approach was popularized for tuberculosis by Ito and coworkers [4]. These approaches were subsequently modified by Dott and Konstam et al. [5, 6]. In recent literature of spinal tuberculosis surgery, this approach has been favourably mentioned [7, 8].

22.2.2 Anatomy

The muscles of the back are arranged in four layers [9]. The superficial layer consists of the latissimus dorsi and the trapezius muscles (muscle fibres are largely vertically oriented). Immediately under it are the deep extrinsic muscles of the back—levator scapulae, rhomboids and the serratus posterior superior and inferior muscles (this layer is almost entirely horizontally or obliquely oriented). The next is the superficial layer of the erector spinae consisting of the iliocostalis, longissimus and spinalis muscles—again vertically oriented. The deepest layer is the short muscles of the back interspinales, intertransversales, rotatores, levator costarum and the prominent multifidus and semispinalis in the lumbar and cervical spine. The deep two layers (intrinsic spinal muscles) are innervated by the posterior primary rami of the segmental spinal nerves, and the extrinsics are supplied by nerves from the brachial plexus or the spinal accessory nerve entering the muscle at their lateral ends. Only the serratus posteriors are supplied by the intercostal nerves. This pattern is important because the hypothesis is that the horizontal limb of the incision does not denervate a large area of multiple layers of muscle but only in the peri-incisional area [10].

22.2.3 The Approach

Under general anaesthesia the patient is positioned prone on a Montreal Frame, and the spine and paraspinal areas cleaned and draped up to the posterior axillary folds. The affected vertebrae are identified by image intensification. The skin incision is marked such that the vertical limb is two to three segments above and the same below the affected segment (Fig. 22.1). The horizontal limb of the incision is marked on the left side (or in case of significant pus collection or vertebral destruction that needs direct access, on the right side) approximately 10 cm long. The skin is infiltrated with 1:500,000 adrenaline solution. The vertical limb of the incision is made

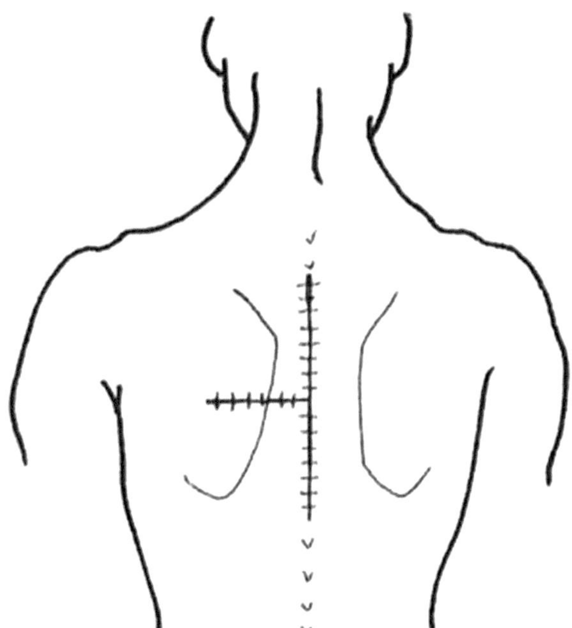

Fig. 22.1 Skin incision for the "fallen T" approach

first and carried to the bone; the muscles are reflected to either side and held with self-retaining retractors. The horizontal limb is next made en-masse without dissecting out each layer. The tissue edges are held up with tissue holders and the muscle cuts made with cutting diathermy up to the ribs. The resulting flaps are reflected back and held with self-retaining retractors (Fig. 22.2). I generally prefer to install pedicle screws on the contralateral side and hold it with a temporary rod to prevent the spinal cord being unduly manipulated. Laminectomy is usually not done unless clearance of an epidural mass under vision is indicated.

Next the ribs (typically 2) are removed from the transverse process and cut laterally about 6 cm from the edge. The intercostal vessels and the segmental nerves will usually have to be sacrificed. The parietal pleura is gently retracted exposing the lateral aspect of the vertebral body; removal of the transverse process and facetal mass often enhances the visibility. A curved malleable copper retractor or Hohman's retractor can be placed anterior to the vertebral body to help the debridement. Segmental vessels need ligation, but often in tuberculosis they are congealed and non-functional. The vertebral body is bluntly opened, and with curettes and disc rongeurs the bone, disc and necrotic materials are removed piecemeal. Once the bony endplates of the vertebrae are reached, the gap is measured, and a mesh cage, expanding cage or strut graft is planned in the defect. The rib graft is minced and (when needed augmented with synthetic ceramic loaded with streptomycin) packed

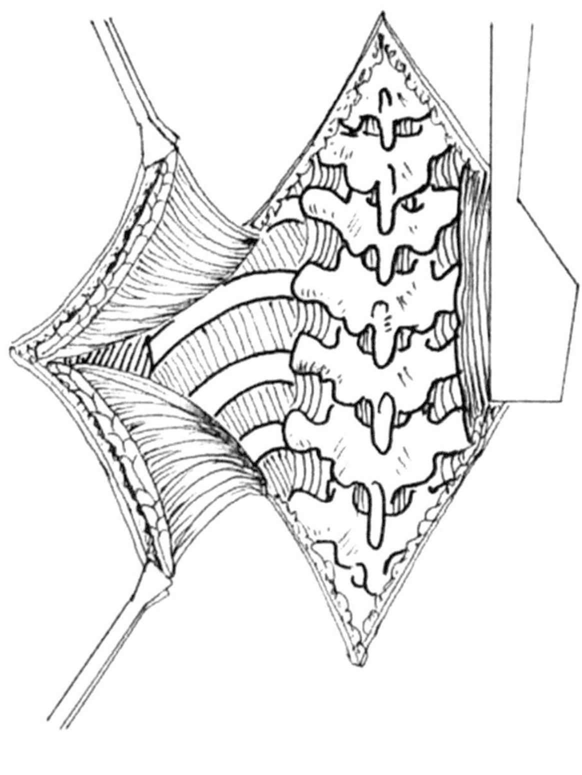

Fig. 22.2 The exposure obtained by the lateral dissection of the technique. The structures exposed are self-evident

in the defect and around the cage. The pleura is allowed to fall back. The left side montage of pedicle screws and rod is completed and tightened under compression. The vertical incision is closed as usual. The horizontal incision is closed in three layers. The muscles are approximated en-masse with No. 1 Vicryl interrupted sutures, while the subcutaneous tissue is closed with 2-0 Vicryl and the skin with staples/sutures. The junction of the horizontal and vertical limbs is first approximated with an apical subcutaneous suture.

The advantage of this approach are:

1. Procedure completed in one position through a single incision.
2. Almost the entire vertebra and discs can be removed.
3. Spinal canal can be decompressed by removing the pedicles and facets and if required the lamina at the affected segments.
4. Posterior instrumentation possible through the same approach.
5. Most surgeons familiar with the access.
6. The nerve supply to the paraspinal muscles is best preserved by this approach.
7. Bone graft harvesting is not needed separately since rib is automatically available. If the rib is also diseased, additional ribs can be removed.
8. Some authors have described less blood loss through the posterior extra-cavitary approaches [8].

Disadvantages are:

1. This is a unilateral approach; bilateral application of the horizontal limb often causes necrosis of the apical skin.
2. The skin flap viability is at risk, and meticulous handling of soft tissues is unavoidable. The tissue planes are not dissected out.
3. This is best suited for subtotal corpectomy and discectomy as in infective diseases; where curative resection is mandated as in primary tumours, this approach tends to leave some of the far cortex on the right lateral side of the vertebral body.
4. Visibility can be somewhat compromised in some cases. Tilting the table away from the surgeon can enhance the accessibility.

22.3 Mercedes Benz Incision to the L-S Junction; Posterior Approach

22.3.1 Introduction

Traditionally the lumbar spine has been approached by the vertical midline incision. It is perhaps the most familiar access to the entire length of the spine; additionally, the absence of visceral organs in the access trajectory, ease of decompression of the cord and the ease of currently available instrumentation strategies, etc. make it the gold standard. There are numerous advantages to this approach as well as many limitations. Access to the inter-transverse bed for fusion involves cumbersome, often painful muscle retraction as well as the less recognized denervation of the paraspinal muscles that inevitably occurs when exposure extends beyond the facet joints. Fixation to the pelvis and iliac graft harvesting that often accompanies posterior lumbar procedures are difficult through the vertical incision and frequently need additional exposure.

In recent years, minimal access surgery has gained considerable popularity, partly from recognizing the need to limit access-related morbidity. Nonetheless, extensile exposure is sometimes required in this region to achieve adequate decompression, debridement of the damaged tissues and stable reconstruction of the affected segment. The author has found the use of the M-B incision helpful in cases of L-S junction tuberculosis where all these requirements are met adequately.

22.3.2 History

The origins of the Mercedes Benz incision to the LS Junction is unclear. Kluger has described the approach in German literature in relation to spondylolisthesis reduction [11]. The present authors developed the technique from Dr Patrick Kluger's personal communication and subsequently modified it to suit the individual surgery requirements. The anatomic studies and technical descriptions have been personally developed by the authors. A transverse incision has been mooted by Setti Rengachari for access to sacral tumour resection, but extension of dissection to the lower lumbar spine through this approach can be cumbersome [12, 13]. A deep U-shaped incision is the standard access for the combined anterior and posterior approach to sacral tumour resection but has not been reported for other pathologies of the lumbosacral junction [13]. The authors' team has performed over 600 such cases with excellent outcomes and minimal complications. The key to the successful performance is the meticulous dissection of tissues and appreciation of the local vascular and neural anatomy.

22.3.3 Anatomy

Zhi's study of the anatomy has demonstrated that the medial branch of the posterior ramus that supplies the facets, posterior ligaments and the paraspinal muscles divides into three branches supplying the iliocostalis, longissimus and multifidus from lateral to medial and typically runs one level caudally [14]. The distal fibres of the multifidus are typically oblique and not vertical in orientation [15]. These features make it eminently suitable to dissect between the fibres and help preserve the nerve supply of the muscle [16].

The vascular anastomosis of the region is also established by several authors. The ilio-lumbar vessels, posterior segmental vessels, posterior sacral vessels, the superior and inferior gluteal vessels all form an anastomosis supplying the skin of this area. The surgical planes of the M-B incision try and preserve much of the vascular supply. It also ensures that the dissection proceeds along true anatomical planes [17].

22.3.4 Surgical Technique

Under general anaesthesia the patient is positioned prone on an appropriate device (the Montreal mattress is the author's choice). Both the PSIS are marked; the L5 spinous process is marked (if it is at or above the intercristal line). The vertical limb of the incision is from L4 to L5 spinous process but can be extended upwards as required. The two oblique limbs are next marked from the L5 to each PSIS. A Mercedes Benz sign is thus created with 120° between each limb (Fig. 22.3). The skin is infiltrated with 1:500,000 adrenaline. The vertical limb and one oblique limb is incised first. The fascia is divided in line with the skin incision. Only in the vertical limb the muscles are elevated from the midline structures with a Cobb elevator and retracted laterally up to the facet joints. The multifidus muscle is found to be

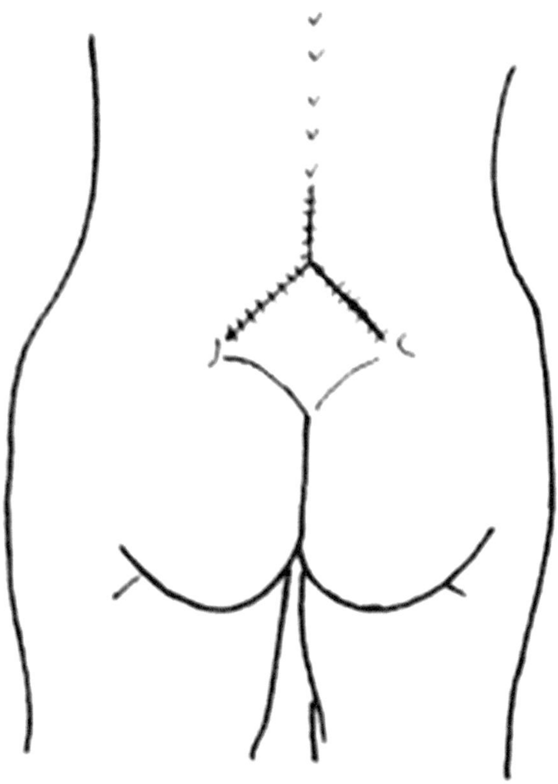

Fig. 22.3 The Mercedes Benz incision marked on the skin

obliquely oriented in the distal limbs and can be split in line with the fibres. The ilio-lumbar vessels are seen in the middle of this segment (between the L5 transverse process and Ala of the sacrum) and needs to be ligated or coagulated. Next the oblique limb of the other side is similarly opened. The L5 spinous process is vertically split with a bone shear and then cut horizontally at its base from S1 and S2 (this is a blind manoeuver done by feel). The triangular distal flap thus created is reflected distally. It is important to note that this osteo-myo-fascio-cutaneous flap is reflected in toto and at no stage should the layers be dissected separately. The Cobb's elevator is used to reflect the distal segment of the multifidus off the sacrum. The spine is now exposed from the L4 to S2 dorsal surface and both PSIS (Fig. 22.4). Further distal exposure is possible even to the extent of performing a total sacrectomy and ilio-iliac and ilio-lumbar reconstruction through the same access.

Closure proceeds from distal to proximal direction. The triangular flap is first replaced and the L5 spinous process is sutured back. The split muscle now falls back in place and need not be sutured. The fascia is sutured with No. 1 Vicryl bilaterally. The vertical limb of the incision is then closed in layers routinely. Subcutaneous and skin sutures are applied as usual.

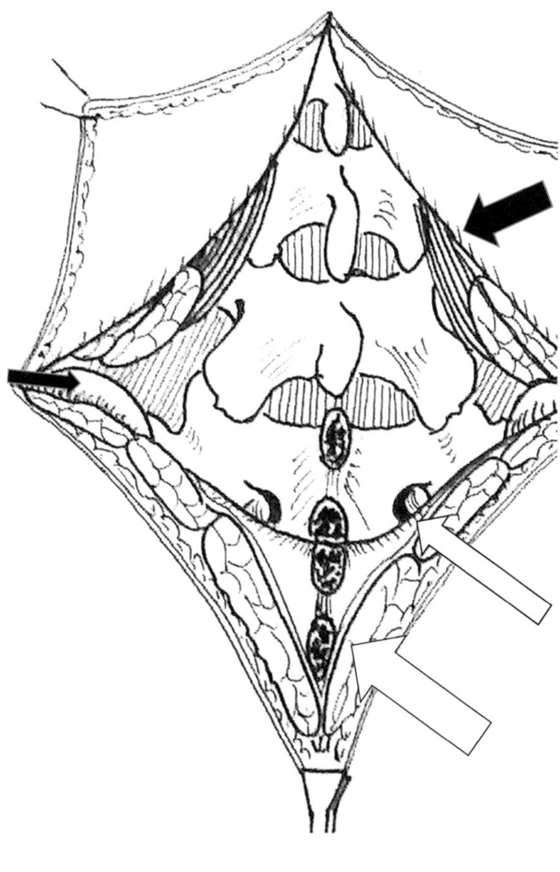

Fig. 22.4 The extent of exposure obtained by the M-B incision. Thick white arrow shows the reflected spinous processes; thin white arrow the sacral foramina. The tick black arrow points to the cut multifidus and the thin black arrow the PSIS

22.3.5 Advantages

1. Simultaneous exposure of the lumbar spine, sacrum and both iliac crests
2. Ability to extend the incision in all directions
3. Bone graft harvesting from both iliac crests
4. Anatomical planes of dissection and no vascular compromise of the flaps (provided the principles are followed)
5. Minimal denervation of the muscle despite the extensile access

22.3.6 Disadvantages

1. Potential for distal flap necrosis if the layers are dissected separately
2. Contra-indicated in post irradiation skin (as in tumours)

22.3.7 Author's Series

The author recently reviewed a series of 642 patients operated by this approach in three centres by five surgeons. The indications were lumbosacral degenerative disorders, spondylolisthesis, sacral tumours, sacro-coccygeal infective lesions and adult deformity surgeries needing fixation to the pelvis. The outcomes of this exposure were excellent. There were three patients who had major wound necrosis and needed flap coverage; all three were tumour cases who had had pre-operative radiation to the lesions. There were 11 patients who developed deep infection and needed wound debridement and secondary closure. The series has recorded 32 superficial infections that were treated with local wound management without surgical interventions.

22.4 The Labio-Mandibulo-Glossotomy (LMG) Approach to the Upper Cervical Spine

22.4.1 Introduction

Approaching the anterior aspect of the C0–C3 vertebrae can be challenging. The trans oral approach is limited by mouth opening and downward retraction of the tongue and is typically used for odontoidectomy and biopsies. Reconstructive procedures are rarely possible through the access obtained. The approach through the hypoglossal triangle is fraught with major tissues like the carotids, jugulars, salivary glands and ducts and hypoglossal and glossopharyngeal facial nerves and has limited unilateral exposure. This approach has recorded over 25% complication rate.

22.4.2 History

The LMG approach was originally described by Trotter in the 1920s for access to the tongue base [18]. Though familiar to facio-maxillary surgeons, spine surgeons rarely encounter this mode of access to the upper cervical spine. Wood [19] and Hall [20] reinvented the approach and described the technique to reach the clivus and cervical spine, respectively. Menzes has reported one of the largest personal experiences with this technique [21].

22.4.3 Anatomy

The midline of the tongue and the jaw is devoid of neurovascular structures and is the best cleavage plane for dissection to the posterior pharynx and anterior cervical spine. The median raphae of the tongue and the floor of the mouth gives attachment to the muscles of these structures that are bilaterally symmetrical. The vascular and nerve tissues do not cross the raphae making it ideal for safe approach.

22.4.4 Surgery Technique

The patient is positioned supine on a Mayfield head holder and images taken to confirm the feasibility. Tracheostomy is performed and endotracheal tube inserted through it and secured. The incision is marked from the hyoid bone to the lower lip and infiltrated with 1:500,000 adrenaline solution. The skin and lower lip are incised and reflected laterally to the mental foramina and the midline is marked (Fig. 22.5). Though a step cut osteotomy has been recommended by some authors, I prefer the straight osteotomy. The roots of the teeth are to be protected during the bone cut. The tongue is lifted out and infiltrated as before. It is split with diathermy along the median raphae till the base of the epiglottis. Crockard's or Dingman's retractors are placed to hold the cheeks, split tongue and the mandibles apart, and the floor of the mouth is retracted down against the upper teeth. The posterior pharyngeal wall is incised and the cervical spine is exposed (Fig. 22.6).

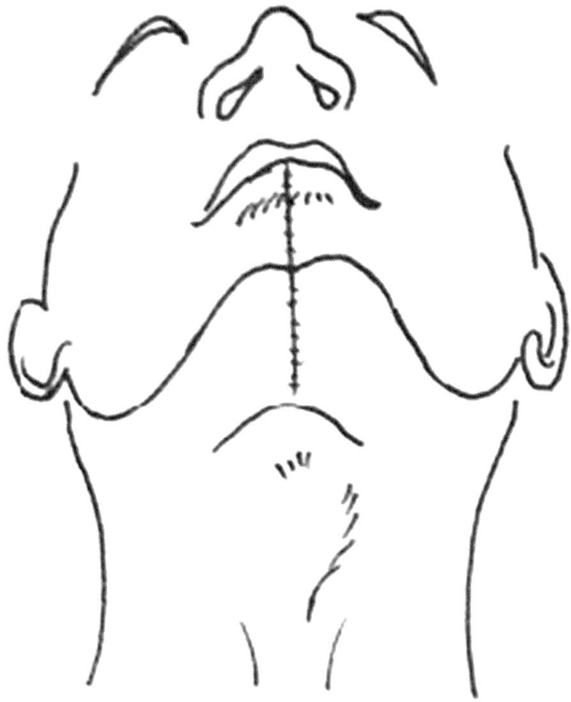

Fig. 22.5 Skin incision for the LMG approach extends from the lower lip to the hyoid bone

Closure starts from the back to the front. The posterior pharyngeal wall is repaired. The tongue is sutured from the back to the front along the dorsal surface and depth. Once the tip is reached the under surface is also sutured. The mandible is next fixed with mini plates and the buccal mucosa repaired. The skin of the mentum and neck are closed in layers.

22.4.4.1 Advantages

The LMG approach provides excellent visibility from the clivus to C4 (C0–C4). Wide retraction is possible laterally unlike the transoral approach, and when the surgeon stays in the midline, there are no neurovascular structures coming in the way. Postoperative healing is also very good, and since elective tracheostomy is performed, the concern of post operative oedema of the tongue and floor of the mouth is less.

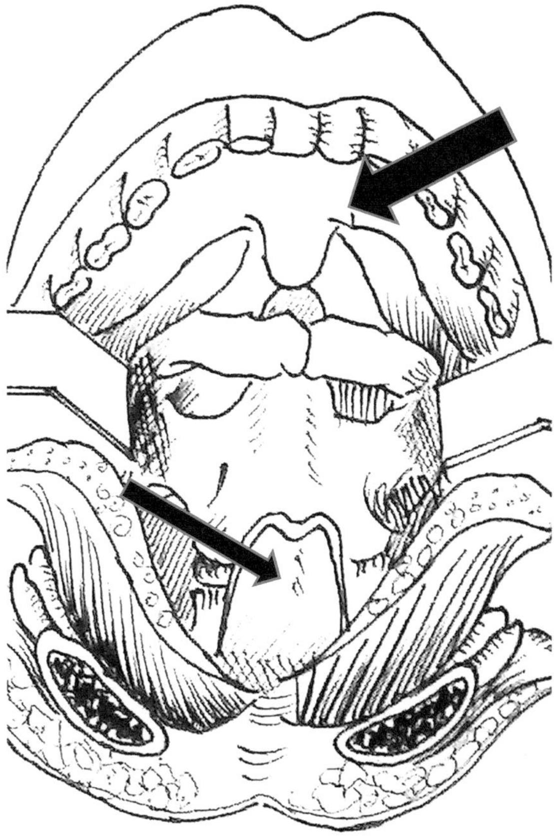

Fig. 22.6 The Ci and C2 are exposed here. The thick white arrow points to the osteotomized mandible and the thin white arrow the split tongue. The thick black arrow depicts the uvula and the thin black arrow the epiglottis

22.4.4.2 Disadvantages

It is indeed a grotesque approach with significant tissue trauma. The tracheostomy has to be maintained for 3–4 days post operatively, and the mandible takes 6 weeks to heal. The patient often needs Ryles tube feeding for a week or so. Some authors have recommended a circumglossal approach after mandibulotomy to avoid splitting the tongue. Infection is an ever-present possibility when the mouth is exposed, and the mandible can sometimes not unite or malunite. Anterior pharyngeal wall necrosis is the most dreaded complication of this approach and needs meticulous tissue dissection to prevent such complications.

22.4.5 Advantages

1. Exposure from clivus to the C3 vertebra is possible for anterior decompression and reconstruction.
2. Avascular and aneural planes of dissection.
3. No critical structure like nerves, salivary glands or vessels falls in the path of access.

22.4.6 Disadvantages

1. Grotesque appearance due to the mandible and tongue split.
2. These two organs need repair at the end and it is time consuming.
3. Tracheostomy anaesthesia is mandatory; it has to be maintained post operatively.
4. Potential increase in infection due to the opening of the posterior pharyngeal wall.
5. Needs special retractor system.

22.4.7 Case Series

The author has till date performed eight cases of the LMG approach. They are all tumour, infection or trauma of the C2 vertebrae where reconstruction was mandated; most had combined posterior fixation as well. No major complication was encountered in our series though hospitalization was prolonged in one case of tumour with neurological compromise due to rehabilitation requirements.

22.5 The Medial Claviculectomy Approach to the Anterior Aspect of the Cervico-Thoracic Junction

22.5.1 Introduction

Anterior access to the lower cervical and cervico-thoracic junction is often hampered by the thoracic cage. Most surgeons are not familiar with the sternotomy, manubriotomy, claviculotomy approaches and require the help of a thoracic surgeon for access. The medial claviculectomy access is a relatively simple procedure that gives excellent view of the upper thoracic vertebrae up to T3 in most and often T4 in thin individuals who require anterior corpectomy and reconstructive procedures.

22.5.2 History

The trans-sternal approach was first described by Cauchoix and Binet and popularized by Hodgson et al. [22, 23]. Mihir and colleagues reinvented the approach with modification in 2006 [24]. Yin and coworkers have recently described the access for Tb spine involving the junctional regions of the spine [25]. These authors had 15 cases of cervico-thoracic junction Tb approached by this technique. Though several authors have reported that posterior surgery produces excellent results (Mehta and Bhojraj) in junctional kyphotic disease often anterior plus posterior surgery is mandated to correct the biomechanics of the deformity [26]. Wu's study reported 74 cases, and they recommended anterior access as the procedure of choice [27]. Donnarumma and team recommend manubriotomy for access to the CT Jn so that they can preserve the sternoclavicular junction [28]. Kurz et al. described the medial end claviculectomy approach, and I have not found the preservation of S-C junction to be critical and tend to sacrifice the medial end of the clavicle with little cosmetic and functional consequences [29].

22.5.3 Surgical Technique

Under general anaesthesia the patient is positioned supine over a rolled towel under the shoulders to extend the neck. The left-sided approach is preferred due to the more consistent position of the recurrent laryngeal nerve [30]. The original Kurz technique involved a hockey stick incision. Though I tend to use a lazy Z incision—the vertical limb along the sternomastoid muscle, the horizontal limb along the medial 1/3rd of the clavicle and the lower vertical limb along the edge of the manubrium (Fig. 22.7). The platysma is incised and the external jugular vein is ligated as required. The sternomastoid muscle is detached from the insertions and reflected proximally. The medial third of the clavicle and the adjoining manubrium are exposed subperiosteally. The medial 1/3rd of the clavicle is excised and preserved. The proximal part of the incision is developed between the carotid sheath and the trachea/oesophagus up to the pre-vertebral fascia. The inferior thyroid vessels are sacrificed and the recurrent laryngeal nerve seen and preserved. The Rt brachiocephalic trunks are retracted laterally to the rt and the left carotid and subclavian vessels to the left and downwards using blunt retractors exposing the prevertebral fascia up to the D4. The fascia is incised exposing the vertebral bodies and the longus colli muscle (Fig. 22.8). After corpectomy the clavicle is shaped to reconstruct the space and plate is applied as indicated. Wound closure proceeds routinely, and the reflected

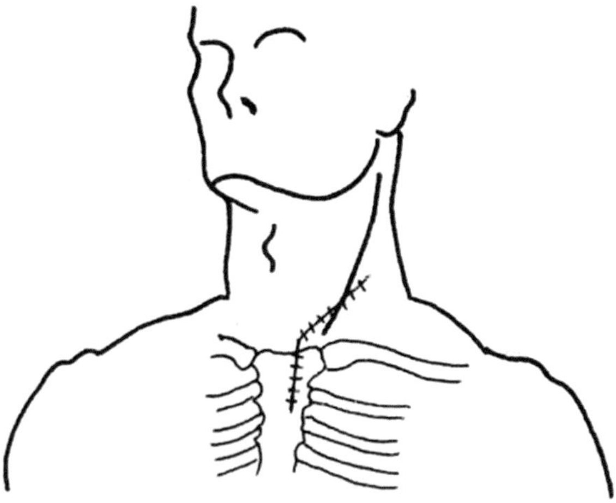

Fig. 22.7 The skin incision for medial claviculectomy approach to the cervico-dorsal spine

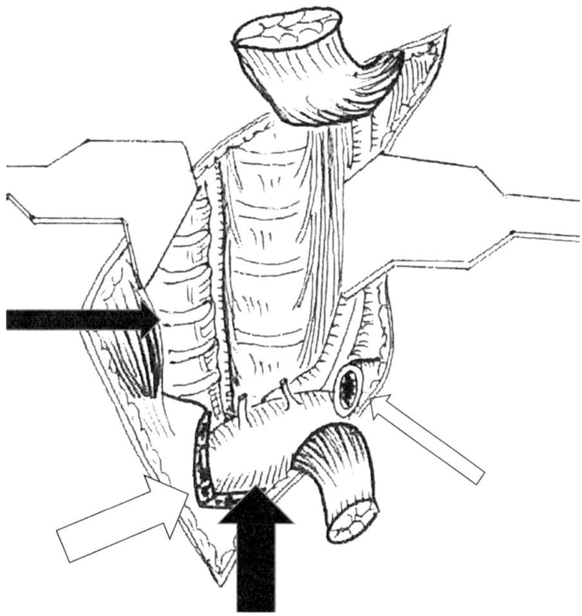

Fig. 22.8 The anterior aspect of C6–T2 exposed by the approach. Thin black arrow depicts the trachea and oesophagus; thick black arrow the left brachiocephalic trunk with ligated inferior thyroid veins. The thin white arrow shows the cut end of the clavicle and the thick white arrow the cut manubrium. The cut reflected sternomastoid muscle is also visible

strap muscles are attached back to the manubrium. Chest tube is not normally indicated. Suction drain is used routinely at our centre.

22.5.4 Advantages

1. No sternotomy or manubriotomy needed.
2. Excellent exposure from C3 to D4.
3. Little retraction of the major vessels in the base of the neck compared to other similar approaches.
4. The excised clavicle provides good structural graft for anterior reconstruction.
5. The Sundaresan's technique involves a T-shaped incision removing the clavicle and a segment of the manubrium to enhance the exposure.

22.5.5 Disadvantages

1. Excision of clavicle theoretically causes shoulder dysfunction, though we have not seen this complication in our series.
2. Potential injury to deep visceral structures. The author has had one thoracic duct injury.

22.5.6 *Author's Series*

Our experience consists of 18 cases of which 17 are for tuberculosis and 1 for tumour. None of the patients reported any shoulder dysfunction, and the only visceral injury encountered was one thoracic duct injury which was managed conservatively. The outcomes were rated as uniformly satisfactory by this approach.

References

1. Capner N. Evolution of a lateral rizotomy. J Bone Joint Surg. 1954;36B(2):173–9.
2. Menard V. Cause of paraplegia in Potts's disease. Rev Orthop. 1894;5:47–64.
3. Capener N. Vertebral tuberculosis and paraplegia. J Bone Joint Surg (Br). 1967;49(4):605–6.
4. Ito H, Tsuchiya J, Asami G. A new radical operation for Pott's disease. Report of ten cases. J Bone Joint Surg Am. 1934;16(3):499–515.
5. Dott NM. Skeletal traction and anterior decompression in the management of Pott's paraplegia. Edinburgh Med J. 1949;54:620–7.
6. Konstam P, Blesovsky A. The ambulant treatment of spinal tuberculosis. Br J Surg. 1962;50:26–38.
7. Bohlman H, Eismont F. Surgical techniques of anterior decompression and fusion for spinal cord injuries. Clin Orthop. 1981;154:57–73.
8. Lubelski D, Abdullah KG, Mroz TE, Shin JH, Alvin MD, Benzel EC, Steinmetz MP. Lateral extracavitary vs costotransversectomy approaches to the thoracic spine: reflections on lessons learned. Neurosurgery. 2012;71(6):1096–102. https://doi.org/10.1227/NEU.0b013e3182706102.
9. Hu ZJ, Fang XQ, Fan SW. Iatrogenic injury to the erector spinae during posterior lumbar spine surgery: underlying anatomical considerations, preventable root causes, and surgical tips and tricks. Eur J Orthop Surg Traumatol. 2014;24:127–35. https://doi.org/10.1007/s00590-012-1167-9.
10. Lemperle G, Tenenhaus M, Knapp D, Lemperle SM. The direction of optimal skin incisions derived from Striae distensae. Plast Reconstr Surg. 2014;134(6):1424–34. https://doi.org/10.1097/01.prs.0000438462.13840.21.
11. Kluger P, Weidt F, Puhl W. Spondylolisthesen und Pseudospondylolisthesen. Behandlung durch segmentale Reposition und interkorporelle Fusion mittels Fixateur interne [Spondylolisthesis and pseudospondylolisthesis. Treatment by segmental reposition and interbody fusion with fixateur interne]. Orthopade. 1997;26(9):790–5. German. https://doi.org/10.1007/s001320050157.
12. Zhang HY, Thongtrangan I, Balabhadra RSV, Murovic JA, Kim DH. Surgical techniques for total sacrectomy and spinopelvic reconstruction. Neurosurg Focus. 2003;15(2):E5. https://doi.org/10.3171/foc.2003.15.2.5.
13. Fourney DR, Rhines LD, Hentschel SJ, Skibber JM, Wolinsky JP, Weber KL, Suki D, Gallia GL, Garonzik I, Gokaslan ZL. En bloc resection of primary sacral tumors: classification of surgical approaches and outcome. J Neurosurg Spine. 2005;3:111–22.
14. Hu ZJ, Zhang JF, Xu WB, Zhao FD, Wang JY, Fan SW, Fang XQ. Effect of pure muscle retraction on multifidus injury and atrophy after posterior lumbar spine surgery with 24 weeks observation in a rabbit model. Eur Spine J. 2017;26(1):210–20. https://doi.org/10.1007/s00586-015-4247-9. Epub 2015 Dec 19
15. Creze M, Soubeyrand M, Gagey O. The paraspinal muscle-tendon system: its paradoxical anatomy. PLoS One. 2019;14(4):e0214812. https://doi.org/10.1371/journal.pone.0214812.

16. Watkins RG. Posterior approach to the lower lumbar spine. Surgical approaches to the spine. New York, NY: Springer; 1983. https://doi.org/10.1007/978-1-4684-0155-4_26.
17. Carmichael SW. The tangled web of Langer's lines. Clin Anat. 2014;27(2):162–8. https://doi.org/10.1002/ca.22278. Epub 2013 Aug 27
18. Shaha AR, Johnson R, Miller J, Milhorat T. Transoral-transpharyngeal approach to the upper cervical vertebrae. Am J Surg. 1993 Oct;166(4):336–40. https://doi.org/10.1016/s0002-9610(05)80327-7.
19. Wood BG, Sadar ES, Levine HL, Johnn DF, Tucker HM. Surgical approaches to the base of the skull; an interdisciplinary approach. Arch Otolaryngol. 1980;106:1–5.
20. Hall JE, Dennis F, Murray J. Exposure of the upper cervical spine for spinal decompression by the mandible and tongue splitting approach. Case report. J Bone Joint Surg Am. 1977;59:121–3.
21. Menezes AH, Foltz GD. Transoral approach to the ventral craniocervical border. Oper Tech Neurosurg. 2005;8:150–7.
22. Cauchoix J, Binet JP. Anterior surgical approaches to the spine. Ann R Coll Surg Engl. 1957;21(4):237–43.
23. Hodgson AR, Stock FE, Fang HS, Ong GB. Anterior spinal fusion: the operative approach and pathological findings in 412 patients with Pott's disease of the spine. Br J Surg. 1960;48:172–8. https://doi.org/10.1002/bjs.18004820819.
24. Mihir B, Vinod L, Umesh M, Chaudhary K. Anterior instrumentation of the cervicothoracic vertebrae: approach based on clinical and radiologic criteria. Spine (Phila Pa 1976). 2006;31(9):E244–9. https://doi.org/10.1097/01.brs.0000214883.11874.80.
25. Yin H, Wang K, Gao Y, Zhang Y, Liu W, Song Y, Li S, Yang S, Shao Z, Yang C. Surgical approach and management outcomes for junction tuberculous spondylitis: a retrospective study of 77 patients. J Orthop Surg Res. 2018;13(1):312. https://doi.org/10.1186/s13018-018-1021-9.
26. Mehta JS, Bhojraj SY. Tuberculosis of the thoracic spine: a classification based on the selection of surgical strategies. J Bone Joint Surg (Br). 2001;83(6):859–63. https://doi.org/10.1302/0301-620X.83B6.11142.
27. Wu WJ, Tang Y, Lyu JT, Yang S, Wang DG, Zhang Q, Liu X, Deng JZ, Luo F, Hou TY, Xu JZ, Zhang ZH. Clinical efficacy of three surgical approaches for the treatment of cervicothoracic tuberculosis: a multicenter retrospective study. Orthop Surg. 2020;12(6):1579–88. https://doi.org/10.1111/os.12527. Epub 2019 Sep 30
28. Donnarumma P, Nigro L, Tarantino R, De Giacomo T, Delfini R. The Manubriotomy is a safe option for the anterior approach to the cervico-thoracic junction. J Spine Surg. 2017;3(3):426–8. https://doi.org/10.21037/jss.2017.06.23.
29. Kurz LT, Fischgrund JS, Pursel SF, Herkowitz HN. The modified anterior Anterior approach to the cervicothoracic junction. In: Bridwel, Dewald, editors. Lippincott Raven; 1997. p. 237–41.
30. singh K, et al. Anterior cervico thoracic approach. In: Bradford DS, Zdeblick TA, editors. Master techniques in orthopaedic surgery – the spine. Philadelphia: Lippincott Williams Wilkins; 2004. p. 87–99.

Chapter 23
Role of Full Endoscopic Procedures in Management of Tuberculosis of Spine

Pramod V. Lokhande

Abstract The treatment of spinal tuberculosis in the present era has become more complex because of the rise in immunocompromised conditions like HIV, diabetes mellitus and presence of drug-resistant tuberculosis. Tissue biopsy is always the mainstay treatment in uncomplicated spinal TB, whereas surgery is necessary in complicated spinal TB. Minimally invasive spine surgeries (MIS) are commonly used in the management of degenerative spinal conditions. Full endoscopic surgeries, a type of MIS surgeries, are already established techniques in the management of disc herniations and spinal stenosis. In this chapter we discuss in detail the role of full endoscopy in obtaining tissue biopsy, their efficacy in debridement of the lesion and instrumented fusion when necessary in select cases. We have compared their effectiveness with current standard procedures like CT-guided biopsy and open surgical procedures like anterior debridement and fusion. We have also discussed the indications and limitations of these procedures.

Keywords Full endoscopy · FEDD · PEDD · Endoscopic debridement and drainage · Transforaminal endoscopy · Interlaminar endoscopy · Tuberculosis spine · Endoscopic fusion

23.1 Introduction

Spinal tuberculosis is a paucibacillary disease and is one of the commonest forms of extra pulmonary tuberculosis, accounting for approximately 1–3% of all tuberculosis cases [1–4]. It accounts for nearly half of skeletal tuberculosis, most commonly affecting the thoracic and thoracolumbar spine [5–7]. Developed countries have recently reported an increase in the tuberculosis (TB) cases due to diabetes mellitus (DM), HIV and other immunocompromised states which are on rise [5]. Eradicating

P. V. Lokhande (✉)
Department of Orthopedics, SKN Medical College & Hospital, Pune, India

S. S. Dhatt, V. Kumar (eds.), *Tuberculosis of the Spine*,
https://doi.org/10.1007/978-981-16-9495-0_23

infection, protecting neurologic function and maintaining structural alignment are the three main objectives in the treatment of spinal tuberculosis [8–10].

Spinal tuberculosis is said to be uncomplicated if there is no significant neurological involvement, spinal instability or kyphosis. The primary treatment approach in such cases remains conservative with antituberculous drugs, rest and bracing [1, 5, 10].

Although chemotherapy is the mainstay treatment of spinal tuberculosis, empirical treatment is not advisable for multiple reasons. Firstly spinal tuberculosis can be a great mimicker. It can be mistaken for malignancy or vice versa. Secondly resistance to first line anti-tuberculous drugs has been observed in 8–12% of tuberculosis patients [11]. Thirdly sometimes the infection can be due to atypical nontuberculous mycobacteria (NTM) like *M. chelonae*, *M. fortuitum* or fungi, or there can be mixed infections due to more than one organism, which may not respond to conventional anti-tuberculosis drugs.

Therefore biopsy is the first step in the management of uncomplicated tuberculosis to identify the causative pathogen [9].

In complicated spinal tuberculosis, there is significant neurological involvement or spinal instability. Therefore surgical intervention is necessary. Surgical intervention is also indicated when conservative treatment fails, or neurological deficit appears during treatment [1, 5, 12].

Benefits of surgery are quicker pain relief, earlier ambulation, less kyphosis deformity, immediate neurological decompression, faster bony fusion and less relapse [2, 13–19]. As the disease primarily involves the vertebral bodies adjacent to the disc space, conventional open surgical approaches focus on anterior debridement, bone grafting and posterior internal fixation [8, 20]. These approaches can be quite extensive and very morbid, particularly in the thoracic spine, therefore poorly tolerated by the patients, especially elderly patients with multiple comorbidities or immunocompromised patients [8, 9, 21–23].

Minimally invasive surgery (MIS) approaches help in reducing these access related bony and soft tissue injuries, thus reducing postoperative pain, blood loss and a reduced length of hospitalization [8, 9, 24].

CT or ultrasound guided percutaneous aspiration, drainage and continuous irrigation [25–29], thoracoscopy or laparoscopic-assisted surgery [2, 8, 12]. Tubular retractor system assisted minimally invasive surgeries [2, 30], and percutaneous endoscopic debridement and drainage (PEDD), also labelled as full endoscopic debridement and drainage (FEDD) by some surgeons ,are examples of MIS procedures [20, 31–36].

The focus of this chapter is to discuss the role of full endoscopy, also known as PELD, in the management of such tuberculous lesions in the spine. The endoscope used is a rigid working channel endoscope using normal saline as irrigation fluid. The fluid pressure not only causes haemostasis but also maintains a clear field of vision by washing away the debris and blood clots. There are two main approaches, transforaminal approach which utilizes the intervertebral foramen's Kambin triangle to access the spinal canal and the interlaminar approach which is similar to conventional interlaminar procedures like microdiscectomy (Fig. 23.1).

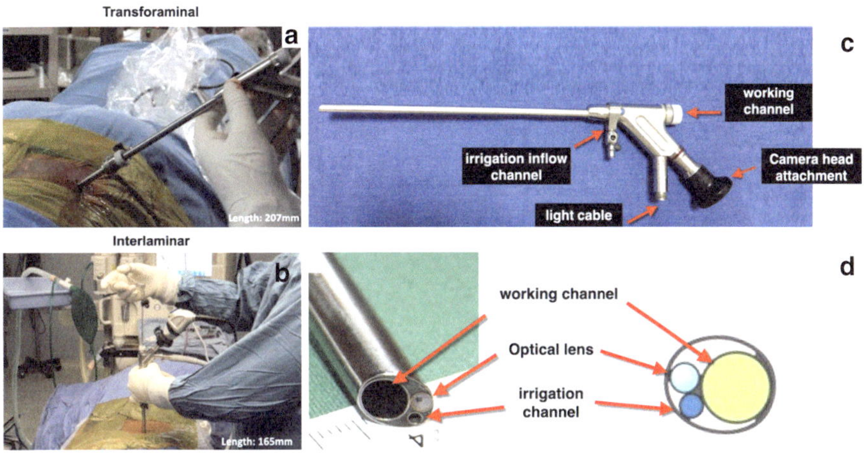

Fig. 23.1 Working channel endoscope and endoscopic approaches. (**a**) Clinical photo of transforaminal approach. (**b**) Clinical photo of interlaminar approach. (**c**) Parts of working channel endoscope. (**d**) Cross-section of working channel endoscope

23.2 Role of Endoscopy in Infective Spondylodiscitis

23.2.1 Biopsy

Biopsy is the mainstay treatment of uncomplicated tuberculosis [37]**.** Although CT-guided biopsy is a standard procedure, it has a variable success rate ranging from 36% to 91% [31, 38–42]. The commonest reason being the aspirate often is inadequate and sometimes no organism has been cultured [24].

Fouquet achieved a 36% positive rate through needle culture [31]. **Yang** obtained a positive rate of 47% for CT-guided biopsy [24]. **Staatz** obtained a positive rate of 76% for CT-guided biopsy [41].

Whereas numerous literature citations showed FEDD has higher biopsy success rate of 80–90% [24, 32–34, 43–45]**,** the positive culture rate of PEDD was comparable with traditional open surgery [24].

High biopsy success rate of endoscopy can be attributed to various factors. Compared to CT-guided biopsy which uses smaller puncture needle, endoscope has larger-diameter working portal (3-7 mm to 4.1 mm) through which large-sized material can be excised [35]. Secondly most percutaneous biopsy procedures use CT or ultrasound to localize the lesion and are relatively blind. Endoscope allows direct visualization of the lesion and helps us to remove infected material from the most affected region, thus minimising the sampling error [24, 35].

A sufficient amount of material can be obtained directly from the infected disc region for microbiologic examination, which provides a higher diagnostic accuracy. Additionally, the opportunity to debride some of the infected disc material may hasten the time of infection control and spontaneous healing [44]. Higher positive rate of culture and early identification of pathogenic strains greatly reduce the likelihood of patients needing further open surgery.

Shih-Chieh Yang compared the efficacy of CT-guided biopsy with percutaneous endoscopic biopsy and debridement. Out of 52 patients, 20 patients underwent percutaneous endoscopic discectomy and drainage by an orthopaedic surgeon, and the other 32 patients underwent CT-guided biopsies by a radiologist. Causative bacteria were identified more frequently with percutaneous endoscopy than in CT-guided biopsy (18 of 20 [90%] versus 15 of 32 [47%]).

23.2.2 Debridement and Abscess Drainage

Debridement of the lesion, decompression of the nerve root and collection of sufficient biopsy specimens are the advantages of endoscopy over previous minimally invasive surgeries [32]. With PEDD, one can directly observe the lesion, collect sufficient specimen, eradicate and debride the infected and necrotic tissue from the disc and epidural space, drain pus directly, release intradiscal pressure, irrigate inflammatory factors—and most importantly—relieve pain immediately [20, 24]. Endoscope provides real-time images that allow direct visualization of the disc space and epidural space. Studies have shown that it achieves results similar to open or other minimally invasive spine procedures in terms of clearance of the infected tissue and radical debridement [20, 33, 34].

If achieving a thorough debridement by unilateral approach was difficult, a bilateral approach can be considered [24, 33]. Psoas abscesses communicating with the disc space can easily be suctioned, drained and irrigated through the working cannula. Indwelling negative pressure Hemovac drainage can continuously drain the remaining abscess postoperatively.

For noncommunicating psoas abscesses, **Ching-Hsiao Yu** recommended a “Trocar-rotating technique” where the working cannula was withdrawn, repositioned and rotated through 180 degrees to face the psoas muscle [35].

One of the biggest advantages of full endoscopy is, being a water-mediated procedure, the continuous saline irrigation can generate hydraulic pressure which maintains a clear field of vision and also reduces intraoperative bleeding. It also helps in flushing out the abscesses and necrotic bone fragments. There is also added benefit of reduced occurrence of incision infection, keeping it as low as possible [33].

Thus, the advantages of PEDD include the removal of pathological tissues under direct visual control, guarantee of sample size and reduction of sampling errors because it is performed under direct visualization. It also avoids excessive radiographic exposure, access related trauma and potential complications caused by open surgery.

Most authors also believed that back pain is rapidly resolved after endoscopy probably by thorough debridement under vision and lavage by continuous irrigation fluid.

According to **Hsin-Chuan Chen**, the safe and minimally invasive nature of this procedure broadens the application of operative treatment for infectious spondylodiscitis, even in the thoracic and upper lumbar level [46].

Most authors recommended that the procedure is best indicated in patients with early-stage spondylodiscitis who show mild to moderate destructive changes in the vertebrae [24, 46].

Xuepeng Wang retrospectively analysed 17 patients. The three cases of failure in their study were all multi-segment infections. They concluded that endoscopy was likely inadequate for the debridement of the multilevel infections [36].

Similarly, other investigators also opined that patients with multisegment infection may not benefit from FEDD because of poor infection control and mechanical instability at the affected segments [20, 33, 44, 45, 47, 48].

Tsai-Sheng Fu retrospectively analysed the outcomes of PEDD and traditional anterior open debridement and interbody fusion. They found that the blood loss in the PEDD group was significantly less than that for the traditional anterior open surgery group (<50 mL versus 585 ± 428 mL, $p < 0.001$). The duration of hospitalization in the PEDD group was shorter than the open group. And there was statistically significant faster CRP and ESR normalization rate in the PEDD group ($p < 0.001$, $p = 0.009$, respectively). They successfully isolated the causative organism from 30 patients (81.1%) following PEDD and from 25 patients (80.6%) following the open surgery [48].

Yi Mao performed a meta-analysis and systematic review to give an objective estimate of the outcomes of PEDD. Nine single-arm PEDD articles (158 patients) were included.

The pooled event rate was 82% for positive bacteria culture, 81% for pain control satisfaction and 21% for reoperation. They concluded that PEDD not only has a high rate of causative-pathogen identification, but also provides satisfactory clinical outcome. Early PEDD intervention in spinal infection is encouraging [49].

Case Example 1

A 47-year-old female patient came with the complaints of back pain with bilateral leg pain since 6 months. Patient had minor weakness 4/5 in right quadriceps. MRI showed infective spondylodiscitis affecting L34 level with a localized ventral epidural abscess. We planned a right-sided transforaminal approach because right leg pain was more severe. Surgery was done under local anaesthesia because the patient was cooperative and not hypertensive. The main aim was to obtain adequate biopsy and to debride the disc space and decompress the nerve root. Patient had satisfactory pain relief after surgery and was mobilized immediately and discharged the next morning. Organism was rifampicin sensitive MTB. Patient received anti-tuberculous medicines for 1 year and has remained asymptomatic for the last 3 years (Fig. 23.2).

Case Example 2

A 13-year-old male was suffering from severe low back pain and right leg radicular pain. Patient had normal neurology. MRI showed significant involvement of L45 disc space with some endplate destruction. Since the intradiscal abscess was involving the anterior part of the disc space, we planned a right-sided interlaminar

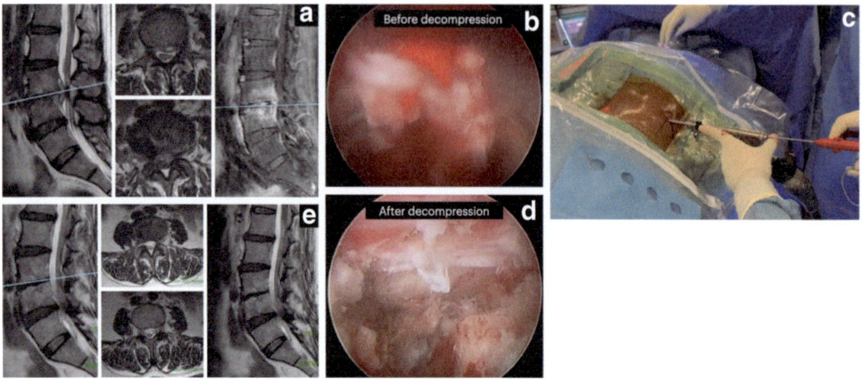

Fig. 23.2 (**a**) Preoperative MRI pictures showing L34 disc space infection with localized ventral epidural abscess. (**b**) Endoscopic picture immediately after insertion of endoscope. (**c**) Clinical picture of showing handling of transforaminal endoscope. (**d**) Endoscopic picture after completion of debridement and decompression. (**e**) Postoperative MRI pictures showing complete resolution of infection

approach for this patient. Surgery was done under GA. Disc space was debrided completely with forceps, and endoscopic drill was used to remove part of vertebral endplates to expose deep-seated abscess. Entire procedure was done under direct visualization. Patient was started with anti-tuberculous medicines and lumbar brace use was advised for 3 weeks. Postoperative MRI done after 6 months shows complete resolution of infection (Fig. 23.3).

Case Example 3: Large Epidural Abscess
A 70-year-old male had predominant back pain which was aggravated since last 15 days. Patient had a normal neurology at the time of presentation. MRI showed large ventral epidural abscess behind L5 body extending up to upper margin of L4 body. Right-sided interlaminar approach was performed under GA. Since the L5S1 disc space was minimally involved, only the epidural abscess was drained and washed out with irrigation fluid. Patient was discharged next day. Pathogen was rifampicin sensitive *Mycobacterium tuberculosis*. Patient responded well to anti-tuberculous drugs (Fig. 23.4).

Case Example 4: Extensive Ventral Epidural Abscess
A 20-year-old male patient presented with bilateral leg pain, difficulty in walking and back pain since 3 months which aggravated recently since last 7 days. Patient had mild fever.

Power in lower limbs was 4/5. There were no signs of myelopathy. MRI showed an extensive ventral epidural abscess extending from S2 body to upper border of L1 vertebra. The lower part of abscess behind L5 and sacrum looked thick, consolidated, multiloculated and caseous whereas the upper part of abscess was uniloculated and liquid. We planned a right L5S1 interlaminar approach. The thick caseous part of the abscess was manually removed with forceps under direct vision. A small silastic tube was then inserted through the endoscope and passed upwards to first

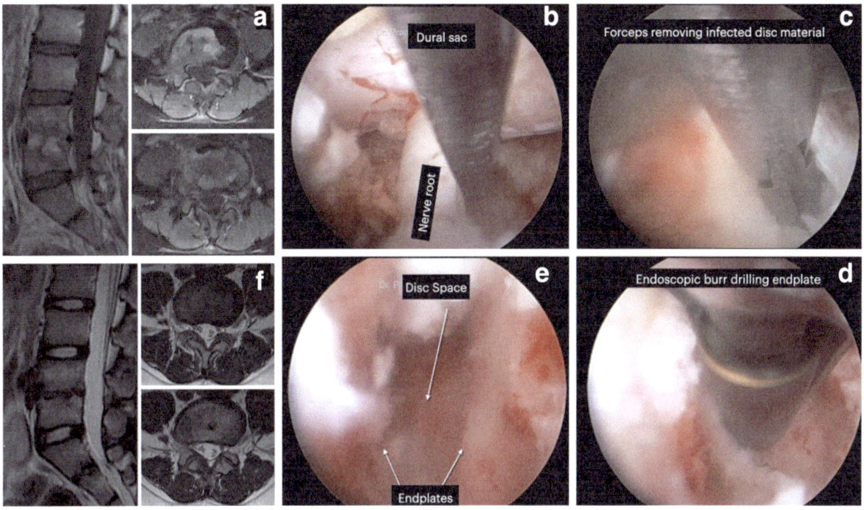

Fig. 23.3 (**a**) Preoperative MRI pictures showing L45 disc space infection reaching up to anterior part of the disc space with moderate destruction of endplate. (**b**) Endoscopic picture showing nerve root being retracted by the dura dissector. (**c**) Endoscopic picture showing forceps removing infected tissue and disc material. (**d**) Endoscopic picture showing endoscopic burr removing some part of endplates to expose the abscess cavities hidden in the middle of disc space. (**e**) Endoscopic picture showing completely removed abscess cavity and well debrided disc space. (**f**) Postoperative MRI picture after 8 months showing complete resolution of infection without any instability

aspirate the abscess and then irrigate the area with normal saline. The entire procedure was done through an 8 mm incision. No suction drain was kept. Patient responded well to anti-tuberculous drugs (Fig. 23.5).

23.2.3 Approach: Unilateral or Bilateral

Both unilateral and bilateral approaches for transforaminal technique have been described.

Li-Chen Hsu performed bilateral transforaminal approach for debridement and drainage for single-level lumbar pyogenic spondylitis with a biopsy success rate of 86.4%. Satisfactory relief of back pain was seen in 81.8% patients [50]. **Yang et al**. also performed bilateral approach to effectively treat pyogenic spondylitis with a paraspinal abscess and recurrent postoperative infection [51].

Dongying Wu performed a comparative study between unilateral and bilateral approach (PEDL). Procedures were performed under local anaesthesia [32]. Unilateral PEDL was performed in patients with obvious unilateral nerve root symptoms, and bilateral PEDL was performed if patients did not have unilateral nerve compressed symptoms. Two procedures yielded comparable and satisfactory results. Unilateral PEDL showed shorter operative time and decreased

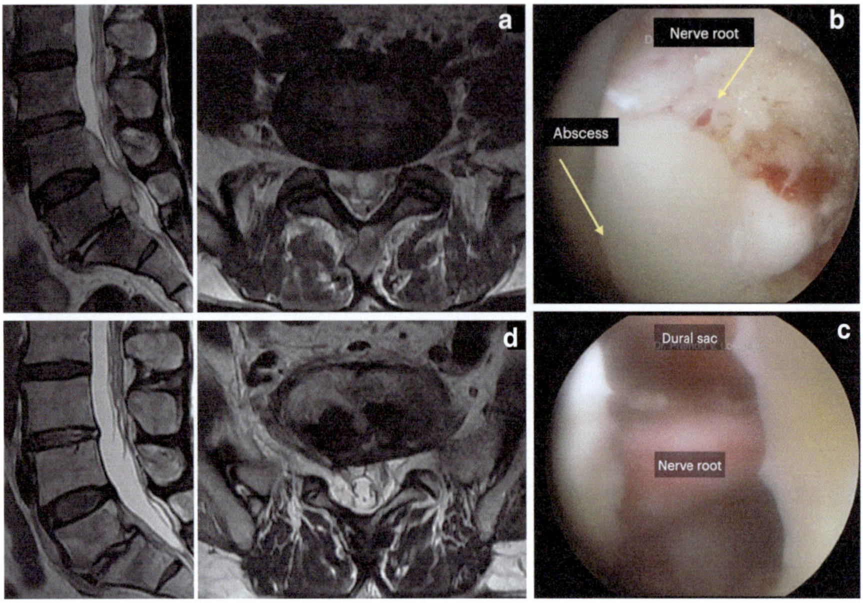

Fig. 23.4 (**a**) Preoperative MRI pictures showing large ventral epidural abscess from L5S1 disc level to upper margin of L4 body. L5S1 disc space was not significantly involved. (**b**) Endoscopic picture showing liquid abscess seen after the nerve root was retracted. Abscess was drained and irrigated with fluid. (**c**) Endoscopic picture showing dural sac and nerve root through the slit in the ligamentum flavum after complete removal of abscess. (**d**) Postoperative MRI after 3 months showing complete resolution of abscess and relatively undamaged L5S1 disc space

intraoperative fluoroscopy times compared with bilateral PEDL, whereas bilateral PEDL may acquire more specimens and perform radical debridement. In addition, the irrigation fluid flow was smoother, and the drainage tube was not easily blocked in bilateral PEDL surgery. Their results showed that the TB-positive rate in the unilateral group was similar to that in the bilateral group, indicating that bilateral PEDL had no advantage over unilateral PEDL in terms of acquisition of sample quantity. Postoperative results were similar in both groups.

23.2.4 Anaesthesia: Local or General

Regarding type of anaesthesia used, many authors preferred to perform transforaminal approach under local anaesthesia. Ito et al. evaluated the clinical results of transforaminal endoscopic debridement, abscess drainage and irrigation in patients with pyogenic spondylodiscitis under local anaesthesia and suggested that this procedure could be used in patients with multiple comorbidities who are not candidates for major spinal surgery or general anaesthesia [43].

Zhongyang Xu also emphasized that for patients with severe underlying diseases, diabetes mellitus, coronary heart disease and cerebrovascular diseases, and for patients who cannot tolerate major operations and need early mobilization, endoscopy under local anaesthesia is a very good option. It requires less time, causes less injury, with reduced effects on the heart, blood vessels and lung, and lower complication rates. The local anaesthesia adopted can achieve quick recovery after surgery without the need to enter the ICU. **Dongying Wu** believed that it is a preferred choice for patients who cannot tolerate open surgical complications or general anaesthesia [32].

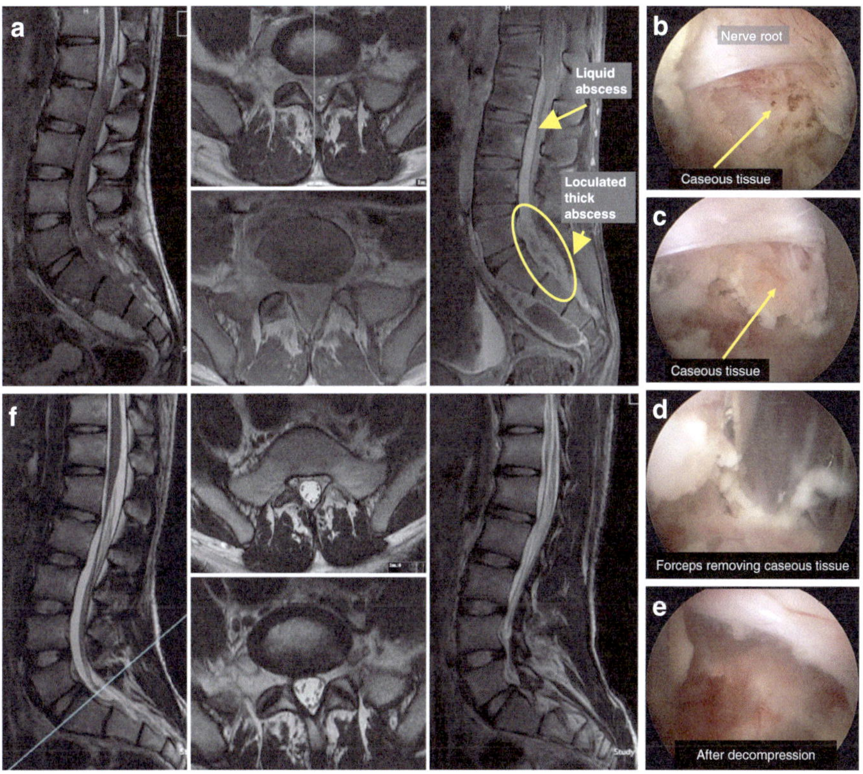

Fig. 23.5 (**a**) Preoperative MRI pictures showing extensive ventral epidural abscess from mid sacrum to T12-L1 junction. (**b**) Endoscopic picture showing caseous tissue under the nerve root. (**c**) Another Endoscopic picture of caseous tissue under nerve root. (**d**) Forceps removing the caseous tissue. (**e**) After complete removal of infected material with well decompressed nerve root. (**f**) Three months postoperative MRI showing complete resolution of abscess with undamaged disc and paraspinal structures. (**g**) Intraoperative clinical photo showing tilting of the endoscope to access the upper part of thickened abscess. (**h**) Intraoperative fluoroscopy photo showing the tip of flexible probe reaching lower border of L4 vertebra

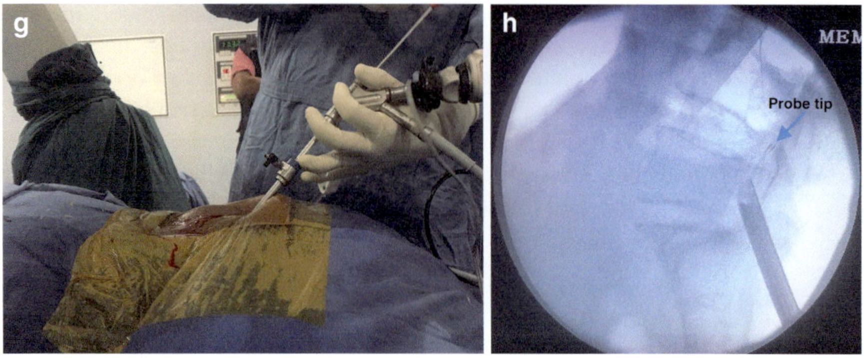

Fig. 23.5 (continued)

23.2.5 Endoscopic Fusion Surgery

Endoscopic fusion surgery for degenerative spondylolisthesis has been described in the last decade [52, 53]. **Liu** retrospectively analysed 33 patients having single segment infective spondylodiscitis who underwent percutaneous endoscopic discectomy and drainage (PEDD) and percutaneous pedicle screw fixation (PPSF) under local anaesthesia [54]. He thought that removal of the endplate during the operation can make the lesion removal more thorough and contribute to a lower recurrence rate, which can't be achieved by other minimally invasive methods except for direct vision using an endoscope. Also, when adjacent soft tissues and endplates are removed during debridement, some amount of instability remains before spontaneous fusion occurs, resulting in persistent back pain after surgery. Percutaneous posterior instrumentation provides initial spinal stability and alleviates back pain.

Duan K performed percutaneous endoscopic debridement with percutaneous pedicle screw fixation for lumbar pyogenic spondylodiscitis in 45 patients under general anaesthesia.

He believed that the lesion clearance of PEDD and the vertebral stability brought by PPSF facilitates spontaneous fusion among vertebral bodies, enabling early mobilization and reduced the incidence of perioperative complications. The incidence of postoperative back pain was also low after this procedure.

Case Example 5: Endoscopic Debridement, Abscess Drainage and Fusion
A 21-year-old male patient had severe back pain with right leg radicular pain since 3 months with recent aggravation. X-rays and MRI showed infection at L5S1 level with partial destruction of lower part of L5 body in the anterior half. There was a large abscess in the iliacus muscle which was communicating with the disc space.

We performed right-sided interlaminar approach under general anaesthesia to debride the anterior part of the disc space, drain the abscess with bone grafting and fusion. Once the working cannula entered the anterior part of the disc space, large liquid abscess started flowing out. Drainage was done as much as possible followed by suction and irrigation. Cancellous bone grafts were obtained from the posterior

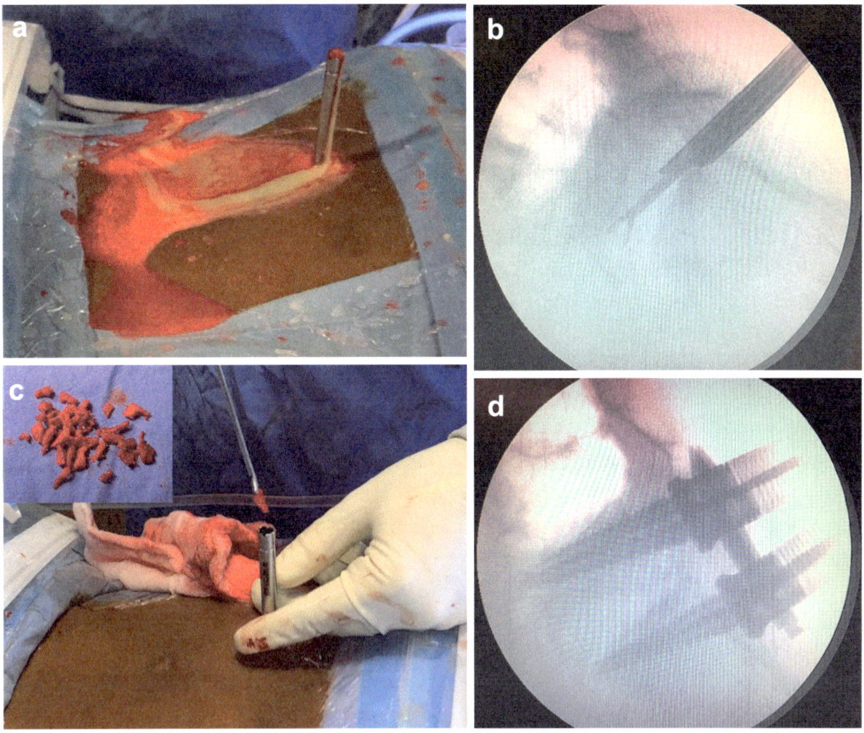

Fig. 23.6 (**a**) Interlaminar approach: Psoas abscess communicating with the disc space coming out of working channel. (**b**) Forceps reaching the anterior part of the disc space for debridement and clearance of disc space. (**c**) Bone grafts being inserted through the working channel for fusion. Bone grafts were obtained from posterior iliac crest. (**d**) Percutaneous pedicle screws fixation

part of right iliac crest and inserted through the cannula into anterior part of the disc space and packed with a punch. Percutaneous screws were inserted under fluoroscopy guidance to stabilize the segment. Patient remained asymptomatic for 3 months and was lost to follow-up during the COVID lockdown situation (Fig. 23.6).

23.3 Discussion

Endoscopy for infective spondylodiscitis is a superior procedure compared to percutaneous CT-guided biopsy in terms of better biopsy success rate and bacterial yield [24]. As the debridement is performed under direct visual control, it is very thorough and direct neural decompression is possible. Many authors believe that adequacy of debridement is comparable to open surgical procedures [48, 49]. We believe that the transforaminal approach can be considered superior to open surgical procedures in upper lumbar or thoracic spine where even midline lesions which are lying under the dural sac can be adequately debrided without neural retraction.

Although both transforaminal and interlaminar approaches have been described, in literature choice of approach has been decided as per surgeon's experience and comfort. Surgeons, who are comfortable with both approaches, chose their approach depending upon the location and extent of pathology, in such a way that there is minimal access portal related injury. This ultimately helps in reducing postoperative morbidity, hospital stay and most importantly it helps in avoiding fusion. Although some authors like **Ching-Hsiao Yu** [55] reported that transforaminal approach is better suited for anterior pathology group like discitis, spondylodiscitis, psoas abscess and "anterior" epidural abscess and interlaminar approach is advisable for "posterior" epidural abscess or paraspinal abscess, our experience has been different. We believe that if the ventral epidural abscess is multiloculated and extending beyond the margins of the disc space, interlaminar approach, by virtue of its superior mobility, can access and cover a significant area for thorough debridement and abscess removal, just by tilting the endoscope upwards and downwards. We also believe that interlaminar approach has better ability to reach the anterior part of the disc space and helps in more thorough debridement as compared to transforaminal approach. Interlaminar approach can also help introduce and pack morselized bone grafts into the anterior part of disc space during endoscopic fusion procedures.

We preferred transforaminal approach for infection which were limited to disc space. Transforaminal approach also provides better central clearance of infections at upper lumbar and thoracic spine, without excessive retraction of the dural sac and nerve root.

We always prefer a unilateral transforaminal approach. Approach is always done from the side of leg pain or more severe abscess or lesion. We do not find any added advantage of bilateral approach. We considered it mainly for bilateral nerve root decompression in patients with bilateral leg pain.

During the procedure, precaution should always be taken to ensure adequate bacterial yield and improve the biopsy success rate. The biopsy should be taken immediately after insertion of the endoscope before starting the irrigation fluid. In a transforaminal approach, biopsy was taken under fluoroscopy guidance, many times before the insertion of the endoscope. Care was to avoid injury to the neural structures by opening the forceps opposite to and away from the dura. Endoscope was then inserted to inspect and complete the procedure. For interlaminar approach the fluid was switched off on entering the epidural space after the ligamentum flavum was opened. Once the biopsy was taken, the irrigation flow was restarted.

Endoscopic debridement and drainage procedure is not recommended for all type of cases. It is a good procedure for single level disease with mild to moderate vertebral involvement. We do not recommend this procedure in patients with significant adjacent vertebral body involvement and destruction, because these cases need a good anterior column reconstruction with a strut graft or a cage, which we cannot insert through the endoscope. We can only insert morselized bone grafts through the endoscope. The procedure is also ineffective in patients with multilevel involvement and therefore not recommended.

In uncomplicated cases with stable spine segment, FEDD without instrumentation is operation of choice. However, in complicated cases with segmental instability, instrumentation is suggested to provide better stability [29, 35].

Regarding choice of anaesthesia, most authors prefer to perform the procedure under local anaesthesia for the reasons discussed previously. Choice of approach also decided the choice of anaesthesia for most surgeons. Surgeons using transforaminal approach preferred to perform the procedure under local anaesthesia, whereas surgeons using Interlaminar approach performed the procedure under general anesthesia. We prefer to perform the procedure under general anaesthesia unless the infection is in the early stages, limited to disc space, young and cooperative patients or very elderly patients where GA is contraindicated. The problems of local anaesthesia are the efficacy of local anaesthetic drugs can be reduced in the presence of active infection and patient may remain uncomfortable and noncooperative during the procedure. Usually in infection the intraoperative bleeding is also more because of severe inflammation and infected granulation tissue. General anaesthesia can provide a drug-induced hypotension which will reduce the bleeding and provide a better visual field. Another disadvantage of performing the procedure under local anesthesia is that sometimes if the surgical time exceeds, the patient can become very uncomfortable lying in prone position with the bolsters irritating the chest. Insuch cases the patient becomes restless and starts moving a lot, interfering with the surgery.

23.4 Conclusion

Full endoscopic operations are excellent procedures for management of early spinal infections without significant neurological involvement, instability or kyphosis. They are day care procedures which significantly reduce the perioperative morbidity, blood loss, hospital stay and risk of anaesthesia and surgery and allow early mobilization and return to activity. The biopsy yield and adequacy of debridement is comparable to that of open surgeries. But they are best suited for early stage infections and single level diseases and are not recommended for multilevel pathology. For more severe cases open surgical debridement and fusion, which is the gold standard, should remain the treatment of choice.

References

1. Jain AK. Tuberculosis of the spine: a fresh look at an old disease. J Bone Joint Surg Br Vol. 2010;92(7):905.
2. Gan F, Jiang J, Xie Z, Huang S, Li Y, Chen G, Tan H. Minimally invasive direct lateral interbody fusion in the treatment of the thoracic and lumbar spinal tuberculosis Mini-DLIF for the thoracic and lumbar spinal tuberculosis. BMC Musculoskelet Disord. 2018;19:283.

3. Zhang Z, Fei L, Qiang Z, Fei D, Dong S, Xu J. The outcomes of chemotherapy only treatment on mild spinal tuberculosis. J Orthop Surg Res. 2016;11(1):1–8.
4. Faciszewski T, Winter RB, Lonstein JE, Denis F, Johnson L. The surgical and medical perioperative complications of anterior spinal fusion surgery in the thoracic and lumbar spine in adults. A review of 1223 procedures. Spine. 1995;20(14):1592–9.
5. Tuli SM. Tuberculosis of the skeletal system. 4th ed. New Delhi, ND: Jaypee Brothers Medical Publishers (P) Ltd; 2010.
6. Gautam MP, Karki P, Rijal S, Singh R. Pott's spine and Pott's paraplegia. J Nep Med Assoc. 2005;44(159):106–15.
7. Turgut M. Spinal tuberculosis (Pott's disease): its clinical presentation, surgical management, and outcome. A survey study on 694 patients. Neurosurg Rev. 2001;24:8–13.
8. Garg N, Vohra R. Minimally invasive surgical approaches in the management of tuberculosis of the thoracic and lumbar spine. Clin Orthop Relat Res. 2014;472:1855–67.
9. Chen H-C, Huang T-L, Tsou Y-JCH-K, Lin W-C, Hung C-H, Tsai C-H, Hsu H-C, Chen H-T. Clinical study: a minimally invasive endoscopic surgery for infectious spondylodiscitis of the thoracic and upper lumbar spine in immunocompromised patients. Biomed Res Int. 2015;2015:780451. https://doi.org/10.1155/2015/780451. Epub 2015 Jul 26.
10. Lin C-Y, Chang C-C, Chen Y-J, Tsai C-H, Tsou H-K, Lin C-S, Ho M-W, Chen H-T, Hsu H-C. New strategy for minimally invasive endoscopic surgery to treat infectious spondylodiscitis in the thoracolumbar spine. Pain Physician. 2019;22:281–93.
11. Garg RK, Somvanshi DS. Spinal tuberculosis: a review. J Spinal Cord Med. 2011;34:440–54.
12. Jayaswal A, Upendra B, Ahmed A, Chowdhury B, Kumar A. Video-assisted thoracoscopic anterior surgery for tuberculous spondylitis. Clin Orthop Relat Res. 2007;460:100–7.
13. Xiong W, Yu B, Zhang Y, Wang C, Tang X, Cao H, Zhang X, Song Q, Tan F, Tan J. Minimally invasive far lateral debridement combined with posterior instrumentation for thoracic and lumbar tuberculosis without severe kyphosis. J Orthop Surg Res. 2020;15:221.
14. Moon MS. Tuberculosis of the spine. Controversies and a new challenge. Spine (Phila Pa 1976). 1997;22:1791–7.
15. Tuli SM. Severe kyphotic deformity in tuberculosis of the spine. Int Orthop. 1995;19:327–31.
16. Wang X, Pang X, Wu P, Luo C, Shen X. One-stage anterior debridement, bone grafting and posterior instrumentation vs. single posterior debridement, bone grafting, and instrumentation for the treatment of thoracic and lumbar spinal tuberculosis. Eur Spine J. 2014;23:830–7.
17. Ha KY, Kim YH, Seo JY, Bae SH. Percutaneous posterior instrumentation followed by direct lateral interbody fusion for lumbar infectious spondylitis. J Spinal Disord Tech. 2013;26:E95–100.
18. Wang QY, Huang MG, Ou DQ, Xu YC, Dong JW, Yin HD, Chen W, Rong LM. One-stage extreme lateral interbody fusion and percutaneous pedicle screw fixation in lumbar spine tuberculosis. J Musculoskelet Neuronal Interact. 2017;17:450–5.
19. Lü G, Wang B, Li J, Liu W, Cheng I. Anterior debridement and reconstruction via thoracoscopy-assisted mini-open approach for the treatment of thoracic spinal tuberculosis: minimum 5-year follow-up. Eur Spine J. 2012;21:463–9.
20. Duan K, Qin Y, Ye J, Zhang W, Hu X, Zhou J, Gao L, Tang Y. Percutaneous endoscopic debridement with percutaneous pedicle screw fixation for lumbar pyogenic spondylodiscitis: a preliminary study. Int Orthop. 2020;44:495–502.
21. Faciszewski T, Winter RB, Lonstein JE, Denis F, Johnson L. The surgical and medical perioperative complications of anterior spinal fusion surgery in the thoracic and lumbar spine in adults. A review of 1223 procedures. Spine (Phila Pa 1976). 1995;20:1592–9.
22. Fessler RG, Sturgill M. Review: complications of surgery for thoracic disc disease. Surg Neurol. 1998;49:609–18.
23. Graham AW III, Mac Millan M, Fessler RG. Lateral extra-cavitary approach to the thoracic and thoracolumbar spine. Orthopedics. 1997;20:605–10.
24. Yang SC, Fu TS, Chen LH, Chen WJ, Tu YK. Identifying pathogens of spondylodiscitis: percutaneous endoscopy or CT-guided biopsy. Clin Orthop Relat Res. 2008;466:3086–92.

25. Hanaoka N, Kawasaki Y, Sakai T, Nakamura T, Nanamori K, Nakamura E, et al. Percutaneous drainage and continuous irrigation in patients with severe pyogenic spondylitis, abscess formation, and marked bone destruction. J Neurosurg Spine. 2006;4:374–9.
26. Nagata K, Ohashi T, Ariyoshi M, Sonoda K, Imoto H, Inoue A. Percutaneous suction aspiration and drainage for pyogenic spondylitis. Spine. 1998;15:1600–6.
27. Onik G, Shang Y, Maroon JC. Automated percutaneous biopsy in postoperative diskitis: a new method. Am J Neuroradiol. 1990;11:391–3.
28. Tofuku K, Koga H, Yone K, Komiya S. Continuous irrigation in pyogenic spondylitis accompanied by iliopsoas abscess. Spine. 2007;15:E382–7.
29. Yu WY, Siu C, Wing PC, Schweigel JF, Jetha N. Percutaneous suction aspiration for osteomyelitis: report of two cases. Spine. 1991;16:198–202.
30. J Jiang, F Gan, H Tan, Z Xie, X Luo, G Huang, Y Li, S Huang. Effect of computer navigation-assisted minimally invasive direct lateral interbody fusion in the treatment of patients with lumbar tuberculosis A retrospective study. Medicine (Baltimore). 2018;97(48):e13484. https://doi.org/10.1097/MD.0000000000013484. PMID: 30508977; PMCID: PMC6283231.
31. Fouquet B, Goupille P, Jattiot F, Cotty P, Lapierre F, Valat JP, Amouroux J, Benatre A. Discitis after lumbar disc surgery: features of "aseptic" and "septic" forms. Spine. 1992;17:356–8.
32. Wu D, Sun J, Fan W, Yuan F. Unilateral or Bilateral Percutaneous Endoscopic Debridement and Lavage Treatment for Lumbar Spinal Tuberculosis. World Neurosurg. 2020;140:e73-e80. https://doi.org/10.1016/j.wneu.2020.04.132. Epub 2020 Apr 25. PMID: 32344133.
33. Yang JS, Chu L, Deng R, Chen CM, Wang XF, Xie PG, Yu KX, Rong LM, Hao DJ, Wei JM, Deng ZL. Treatment of Single-Level Thoracic Tuberculosis by Percutaneous Endoscopic Débridement and Allograft via the Transforaminal Approach Combined with Percutaneous Pedicle Screw Fixation: A Multicenter Study with a Median Follow-Up of 36 Months. World Neurosurg. 2019;122:e1472–e1481. https://doi.org/10.1016/j.wneu.2018.11.087. Epub 2018 Nov 19. PMID: 30465947.
34. Lin GX, Kim JS, Sharma S, Sun LW, Wu HH, Chang KS, Chen YC, Chen CM. Full endoscopic discectomy, debridement, and drainage for high-risk patients with spondylodiscitis. World Neurosurg. 2019;127:e202–11.
35. Yu CH. Full-endoscopic debridement and drainage treating spine infection and psoas muscle abscess. J Spine Surg. 2020;6(2):415–23.
36. Wang X, Zhou S, Bian Z, Li M, Wu J, Hou C, Zhu L. Unilateral percutaneous endoscopic debridement and drainage for lumbar infectious spondylitis. J Orthop Surg Res. 2018;13:306.
37. Kim BJ, Lee JW, Kim SJ, et al. Diagnostic yield of fluoroscopy-guided biopsy for infectious spondylitis. AJNR Am J Neuroradiol. 2013;34:233–8.
38. Chew FS, Kline MJ. Diagnostic yield of CT-guided percutaneous aspiration procedures in suspected spontaneous infectious disk-itis. Radiology. 2001;218:211–4.
39. Parker LM, McAfee PC, Fedder IL, Weis JC, Geis WP. Minimally invasive surgical techniques to treat spine infections. Orthop Clin North Am. 1996;27:183–99.
40. Rankine JJ, Barron DA, Robinson P, Millner PA, Dickson RA. Therapeutic impact of percutaneous spinal biopsy in spinal infection. Postgrad Med J. 2004;80:607–9.
41. Staatz G, Adam GB, Keulers P, Vorwerk D, Gunther RW. Spondylodiskitic abscesses: CT-guided percutaneous catheter drainage. Radiology. 1998;208:363–7.
42. Vinicoff PG, Gutschik E, Hansen SE, Karle A, Rieneck K. CT-guided spinal biopsy in spondylodiscitis. [in Danish]. Ugeskr Laeger. 1998;160:5931–4.
43. Ito M, Abumi K, Kotani Y, Kadoya K, Minami A. Clinical outcome of posterolateral endoscopic surgery for pyogenic spondylodiscitis: results of 15 patients with serious comorbid conditions. Spine. 2007;32:200–6.
44. Yang SC, Fu TS, Chen LH, Niu CC, Lai PL, Chen WJ. Percutaneous endoscopic discectomy and drainage for infectious spondylitis. Int Orthop. 2007;31:367–73.
45. Xu Z, Zheng Y. Percutaneous endoscopic debridement and irrigation for thoracic infections. Rev Assoc Med Bras. 2018;64(6):518–24.

46. Chen HC, Huang TL, Chen YJ, Tsou HK, Lin WC, Hung CH, Tsai CH, Hsu HC, Chen HT. A Minimally invasive endoscopic surgery for infectious spondylodiscitis of the thoracic and upper lumbar spine in immunocompromised patients. Biomed Res Int. 2015;2015:780451.
47. Yang S-C, Chiu Y-C, Chen H-S, Kao Y-H, Jou I-M, Yuan-Kun T. Percutaneous endoscopic debridement and drainage for the treatment of instrumented lumbar spine infection. J Orthop Surg. 2019;27(3):1–7.
48. Fu TS, Wang YC, Lin TY, Chang CW, Wong CB, Su JY. Comparison of percutaneous endoscopic surgery and traditional anterior open surgery for treating lumbar infectious spondylitis. J Clin Med. 2019;8(9):1356.
49. Mao Y, Yang L, Cui X. Percutaneous endoscopic debridement and drainage for spinal infection: systemic review and meta-analysis. Pain Physician. 2019;22:323–30.
50. Hsu L-C, Tseng T-M, Yang S-C, Chen H-S, Yen C-Y, Tu Y-K. Bilateral portal percutaneous endoscopic debridement and lavage for lumbar pyogenic spondylitis. Orthopedics. 2015;38(10):e856–63.
51. Yang SC, Fu TS, Chen HS, Kao YH, Yu SW, Tu YK. Minimally invasive endoscopic treatment for lumbar infectious spondylitis: a retrospective study in a tertiary referral center. BMC Musculoskelet Disord. 2014;15:105.
52. Leu HF, Hauser RK. Percutaneous endoscopic lumbar spine fusion. Neurosurg Clin N Am. 1996 Jan;7(1):107–17.
53. Osman SG. Endoscopic transforaminal decompression, interbody fusion, and percutaneous pedicle screw implantation of the lumbar spine: a case series report. Int J Spine Surg. 2012;6:157–66.
54. Liu J, Liu D, An G, et al. Clinical outcomes of percutaneous endoscopic debridement and drainage combined with percutaneous pedicle screw fixation for the treatment of infective spondylodiscitis. Res Square. 2020; https://doi.org/10.21203/rs.3.rs-23766/v1.
55. Choi E-J, Kim S-Y, Kim H-G, Shon H-S, Kim T-K, Kim K-H. Percutaneous endoscopic debridement and drainage with four different approach methods for the treatment of spinal infection. Pain Physician. 2017;20:E933–40.

Chapter 24
Surgical Treatment of TB Kyphosis

Rudra Narayan Mukherjee, Archit Goyal, and Bhavuk Garg

Abstract Post-tubercular kyphotic deformity poses a significant challenge to spine surgeons with a high rate of complications even in experienced hands. Identification of risk factors can help in prevention of post-tubercular kyphotic deformity by performing surgery during active stages in these patients. However, a spine surgeon is still likely to encounter these severe post-tubercular deformity during his practice and should be well versed with the different surgical approaches and osteotomies. This chapter focuses on the risk factors for post-tubercular kyphotic deformity, the classification of tubercular kyphosis, indications for surgery, different surgical approaches for treatment, and the type of osteotomies performed for post-tubercular kyphosis.

Keywords Tuberculosis · Kyphosis · Pott's spine · Deformity · Spinal osteotomy

24.1 Introduction

Kyphotic deformity is one of the most worrying complications of tuberculosis of spine. Almost 3–5% of patients with spinal tuberculosis develops severe kyphosis of spine [1, 2]. Progressive deformity may be prevented by treatment in early stages of disease. Failure to treat adequately may result in progression of deformity. It is believed that kyphotic deformity develops and progresses in spite of treatment with modern antitubercular drugs [3]. Patients with severe kyphotic deformity develops cardio-pulmonary dysfunction, painful costo-pelvic impingement, spinal canal stenosis, and spinal cord compression [4]. The risk of progression is believed to be low in adults. Despite the success of conservative management, a mean increase of 15° kyphosis is seen in 3–5% patients who progress to deformities >60° [2, 5].

R. N. Mukherjee · A. Goyal · B. Garg (✉)
All India Institute of Medical Sciences, New Delhi, India

S. S. Dhatt, V. Kumar (eds.), *Tuberculosis of the Spine*,
https://doi.org/10.1007/978-981-16-9495-0_24

The most dreaded complication of severe kyphotic deformity is the neurological deficit. Paraplegia in early stages of tubercular disease may need chemotherapy and surgery [2]. Clinically, patients who develop neurological deficit in active stage of disease fare better than those patients who develop neurological deficit in healed tuberculosis. Careful consideration is needed to identify patients in whom kyphosis increases on treatment leading to severe deformity. Late paraplegia is prevented by predicting the kyphotic deformity and restricting the progression by early surgical stabilization during active stage of disease [3, 6]. Correction of severe post-tubercular kyphotic deformity is a challenging surgery even for experienced surgeons with a high rate of complications.

24.2 Pathology

Anterior elements of the vertebral column are affected in majority of cases of spinal tuberculosis. The tuberculous lesion begins at the paradiscal area and gradually progresses to involve the vertebral endplates eventually weakening the structural integrity. The intervertebral disc balloons and herniates through these softened endplates. The line of weight transmission is situated anteriorly through the anterior half of vertebral bodies in thoracic vertebrae. This leads to local angular kyphosis and exaggeration of thoracic kyphosis. However, in the cervical and lumbar spine, the line of weight transmission passes through the posterior half of the vertebral bodies. In addition to it, the relatively large transverse process and pre-existing lordotic curve in cervical spine minimizes kyphosis. Large vertebral body and vertical orientation of the posterior articular facets of lumbar vertebrae predispose them to telescope early than to angulate. Thus, there is obliteration of natural lumbar and cervical lordosis first followed by gradual occurrence of kyphotic deformity. Hence, thoracic and thoracolumbar tuberculosis have higher risk of deformity with propensity to progress compared to lumbar and cervical disease. Severity of loss of vertebral body height, number of vertebral bodies involved, age of onset and the spinal segment affected are some of the factors that determine the severity of kyphotic deformity [1, 4, 7]. It is believed that 95% of patients present with clinically detectable kyphosis or loss of normal lordotic curve when they report to specialized centers for treatment in developing countries [1].

24.3 Behavior of Deformity in Adults

Normal stresses and strains in a diseased and weakened vertebral body due to daily activities result in pathological fracture and kyphotic collapse. Kyphotic deformity continues to grow even after administration of modern antitubercular drugs. This progression can be curtailed by utilization of appropriate spinal braces. Kyphosis is also believed to increase in surgically decompressed and bone grafted tubercular spine. Since the grafted bone is weak during the first few days of implantation, it is prone to complications such as graft slippage and graft breakage. This results in kyphotic deformity and its subsequent progression [8, 9]. The increase in deformity following surgical decompression is more in patients with long segment disease wherein longer bone grafts are used in thoracic and thoracolumbar spine. Once healed with bony ankylosis, the progression of deformity is not frightful in adult life. However, when healing with fibrous or fibro-osseous ankylosis occurs, the deformity may progress [4].

24.4 Behavior of Deformity in Children

When the disease occurs in early childhood, there is arrest of anterior growth plate of vertebral body in addition to intervertebral disc destruction and buckling collapse of the vertebrae. This results in retarded growth potential of the affected vertebrae. When the balance between the growth of the anterior and posterior growth plates is altered with continued growth of posterior vertebra, progressive kyphosis results even after the disease heals [1]. Pretreatment angle of kyphosis, level of lesion, number of vertebrae involved, pretreatment vertebral body loss and instability are strong predictors of progression of deformity [10]. Rajasekaran suggested a formula $Y = a + bx$ to predict the kyphotic deformity where Y is the value of predicted kyphotic angle, a and b are constants with values of 5.5 and 30.5, respectively, and x stands for the initial loss of vertebral body height [9]. As disease progresses and severity increases, posterior arch is disrupted in some children. This leads to spinal instability with radiological features such as separation of facet joints at multiple level, posterior retropulsion of diseased vertebral segment, lateral subluxation of the vertebral column and toppling of superior normal vertebral segment. These radiological signs were termed as "spine at risk" signs by Rajasekaran [10]. Approximation of anterior surface of several vertebral segments above and below the deformity occurs in an attempt to stabilize the vertebra. This leads to horizontal orientation of vertebral segments resulting in stress shielding of the growth plates which causes overgrowth of the vertebral segments. This overgrowth leads to stretching of the cord at the apex and may result in late onset paraplegia [7, 10, 11].

24.5 Surgical Management

Correction of deformity requires instrumentation of spine combined with or without radical debridement and chemotherapy [12]. Debridement is generally performed anteriorly as the disease foci are primarily anterior. Anterior debridement is quintessential when patient has neurological deficit, severe abscess formation or multilevel involvement [13]. Bone graft may be used to perform anterior reconstruction, either using an anterior or posterior approach. For larger deformities and stiffer curves with less than 25% flexibility, many types of corrective osteotomies has been recommended.

24.6 Classification

Rajasekaran et al. proposed a classification which was based on deficiency of anterior or posterior column, flexibility of disc-spaces, magnitude of the curve and requirement of osteotomy [14].

Type I: Intact anterior and posterior column

- I A: Mobile disc spaces
- I B: Ankylosed segments

Type II: Deficiency of any one column

- II A: Anterior column deficiency
- II B: Posterior column deficiency

Type III: Deficiency of both columns

- III A: Kyphosis ≤60°
- III B: Kyphosis ≥60°
- III C: Buckling collapse

The classification includes two modifiers—global sagittal balance (M) and coronal deformity (C). Global sagittal balance is assigned of the basis of sagittal vertical axis (SVA). Patients with SVA <5 cm are assigned M−, whereas patients with SVA >5 cm are assigned M+. Coronal Modifier of C− is assigned in cases of coronal Cobb angle <20° and C+ in cases of Cobb angle > 20°.

24.7 Indication for Surgery

The indications for surgery in spinal tuberculosis include:

1. Progressive neurological deficit
2. Persistent pain due to instability
3. Severe kyphotic deformity

Identifying the patients at risk for progression of deformity is important as early surgical intervention in such cases would prevent severe deformity. Following are the risk factors to predict progression of deformity [5, 10, 11]:

1. Age less than 10 years with loss of greater than one and a half vertebrae.
2. A pretreatment kyphosis angle of greater than 30°.
3. Cervicothoracic and thoracolumbar junctional kyphosis.
4. Presence of "spine at risk" signs [10].

24.8 Surgery in Active Disease

All patients who report for the first time with kyphotic deformity of 50° or more may be taken up for deformity correction surgery. In active tubercular spine, vertebral bodies are diseased, and anterior vertebral body height is decreased. Adjacent vertebral bodies may be inflamed. There may be compression of the spinal cord anteriorly with disc, granulation tissue, and debris. Meninges may show evidence of inflammation, which predisposes for deterioration of neurology. Intercostal blood vessels, epidural vessels, and anterior spinal arteries may be thrombosed [4].

Surgical considerations:

1. There is disc retropulsion, granulation tissue, and bony sequestrum in spinal tuberculosis lesion. Any deformity correction without addressing the diseased area or without decompressing anteriorly will produce devastating spinal cord indentation by posterior vertebral body (internal gibbus) and further neurological deterioration. Hence, internal gibbus should be addressed by thorough anterior debridement and corpectomy [15].
2. In long-standing kyphosis, vertebral column is shortened anteriorly with adjustment of spinal cord. Hence, any sudden correction of this deformity may lead to anterior column lengthening and consequent stretching of spinal cord. Thus, posterior column shortening is desired [15].
3. Instability is seen following anterior corpectomy and posterior column shortening. Hence, rigid instrumented stabilization followed by anterior grafting and posterior fusion is preferred [15].
4. Posterior instrumentation is recommended as anterior implant may not have a strong hold with limited span to withstand deforming forces [4].
5. It is preferable to perform anterior decompression (anterior corpectomy), posterior column shortening, posterior instrumentation and anterior and posterior bone grafting in the same sitting [16].
6. Throughout the procedure, spinal cord should be kept under vision, and deformity correction should be gentle to prevent any elongation of the spinal cord [4].

Techniques for kyphotic deformity correction in TB spine:

a. Single-stage transpedicular approach
b. Single- or two-stage anterior and posterior surgery
c. Single-stage kyphosis correction by extra-pleural anterolateral approach

24.8.1 Single-Stage Transpedicular Approach

This procedure is primarily performed to prevent progression of kyphotic deformity following surgery [13]. The reported loss of deformity correction till healing of the disease with this approach is 3.2°–3.4° [13, 16]. Posterolateral approach is used. A midline incision centering at kyphosis is made. A costotransversectomy and pedicle excision is performed at the apex of the kyphosis. Drainage of the abscess is performed along with debridement of the granulation tissue, and bony sequestrum and decompression of the spinal cord is achieved. Spinal instrumentation is done with pedicle screws or Hartshill loop with sublaminar wires, and kyphosis is gently corrected after removing bony and soft tissue structures preventing kyphosis correction. The anterior defect is subsequently grafted [4, 16].

24.8.2 Single- or Two-Stage Anterior and Posterior Surgery

Here kyphotic deformity correction is achieved by anterior decompression followed by posterior instrumentation. Transthoracic trans-pleural or retroperitoneal approach may be used for anterior decompression, and the anterior gap is filled with bone graft. This was followed by posterior instrumentation 2–3 weeks later or during the same procedure [4, 17, 18]. Shortening of the posterior column can be combined to achieve adequate deformity correction [17].

24.8.3 Single-Stage Kyphosis Correction by Extra-pleural Anterolateral Approach

Here, deformity correction is done by extra-pleural anterolateral approach. A mean kyphotic correction of 27.3° was obtained by Jain et al. [15]. T-shaped posterior incision is given. The straight arm of the incision is about 14–15 cm and is centered at the apex of the kyphosis. The transverse part of the incision is about 8 cm and perpendicular to the straight arm at the apex of kyphosis on left side. The posterior 6–8 cm of 2–3 ribs at the apex of the lesion is removed and anterolateral decompression performed. The diseased vertebral body is taken out as far as possible. The anterior wound is then packed. Three segments either side of the apex vertebrae are exposed through paraspinal exposure. Removal of the spinous process, laminae and pedicle at the apex of the deformity is performed. The posterior part of the right rib attached to the apex vertebra is also removed. Jain et al. reported the use of sublaminar wire with Hartshill rectangle to correct the kyphotic deformity. Anterior bone grafting is done after achieving correction using iliac crest bone graft and ribs are used as bone graft for posterior spinal fusion [4, 15].

24.9 Surgery in Healed Disease

Surgery to correct kyphotic deformities in healed tuberculosis is difficult and challenging. It is hazardous with high rate of complication [19]. Earlier staged surgical techniques were widely followed [19]. However, with development of newer approaches, advent of rigid instrumentation and refinement of surgical techniques, single-stage corrections were proposed to adequately correct deformity with good safety profile [15, 20].

24.10 Osteotomies and Vertebral Column Resection

Kyphotic segment is rigid and not amenable to correction in certain cases. Hence, osteotomies are performed to increase the spinal column flexibility. However, the complication rates of these procedures are higher which include greater bleeding and neurological injury. In severe thoracic kyphotic deformities, approaching the concavity of spine is challenging through the anterior transthoracic approach. Compromised lung function, adhesions and fibrosis multiply the morbidity. Anterior graft-related problems appear to be less with combined anterior and posterior surgery, and they result in a good correction of deformity [21–23]. However single-stage posterior approach for surgical procedures has been found to be viable and efficient as it eliminates the need for two surgical approaches, has lesser blood loss, lesser surgical time, and lower infection rates [23, 24].

24.10.1 Transpedicular Decancellation Osteotomy

This technique can be effectively used to achieve deformity correction of up to 20°–30° [20, 25, 26]. Correction obtained through single level transpedicular decancellation osteotomy is usually more than the correction achieved with single level Smith-Petersen osteotomy. However, the overall correction obtained is significantly more in Smith-Petersen osteotomy as it can be performed at multiple levels. Transpedicular decancellation osteotomy results in the contact of two broad cancellous surfaces resulting in increased fusion rates with less chances of pseudoarthrosis [20, 27]. The osteotomy is performed at the level of maximum deformity. Standard posterior incision is chosen, following adequate dissection and exposure of pedicles, decancellation is done through the pedicles using serial sized curettes. Lateral and medial wall of pedicle are removed, and vertebral body is curetted to complete decancellation. Contoured rods are placed, and reduction is carried out via sequential correction until the posterior elements are touching. Compression is performed across the fixation along with placement of bone graft over the lamina and spinous process.

24.10.2 Three Column Pedicle Subtraction Osteotomy

This procedure can be performed in both the lumbar and thoracic spine. When performed in thoracic spine, it is combined with resection of ribs to help approach the vertebral body more laterally. However, it is widely performed around L2 and L3 vertebra [28, 29]. Correction of up to 30°–40° can be obtained with the use of three column pedicle subtraction osteotomy [30, 31] (Figs. 24.1, 24.2, 24.3, and 24.4).

Standard posterior midline incision is used; two levels above and below the apex of the deformity are instrumented. Facetectomies are performed at each level to improve the mobility of spine and enhance intra-articular fusion. Bilateral wide laminectomy is carried out at the apex of the deformity which can be extended above and below as needed. In thoracic region, a 3–4 cm portion of the rib along with transverse process is removed. Following localization of the pedicle, a plane is developed on the lateral side of the pedicle and vertebral body using blunt dissection

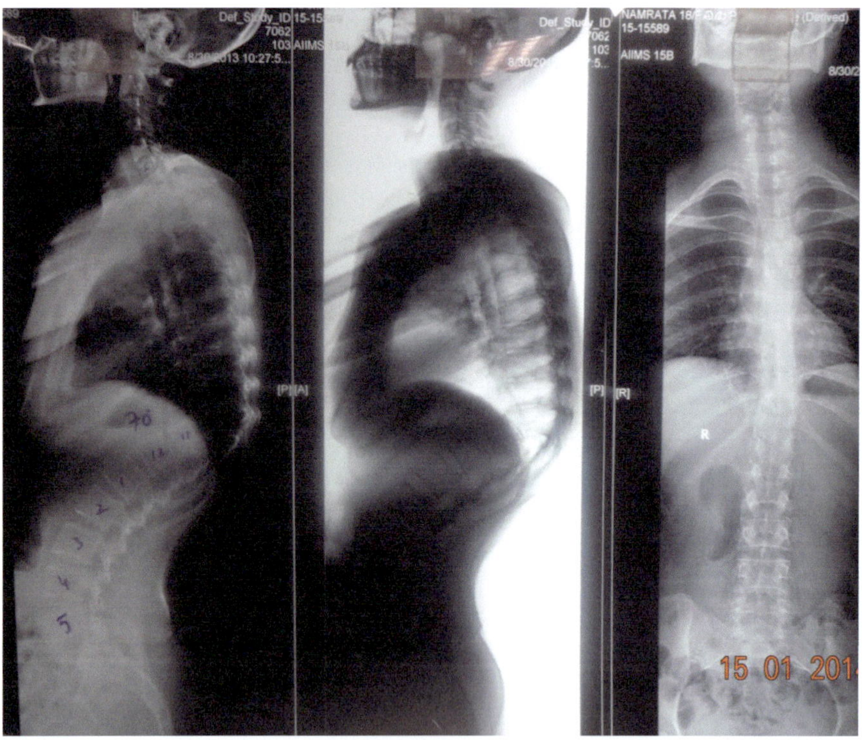

Fig. 24.1 Pre-operative radiograph, post-operative radiograph, and intra-operative images of a 20-year-old female with thoracic kyphotic deformity following healed tubercular disease involving D9 vertebrae who underwent Pedicle Subtraction Osteotomy for deformity correction with posterior instrumentation. Preoperative radiograph of a 20-year-old female with post-tubercular kyphotic deformity involving D9 vertebrae

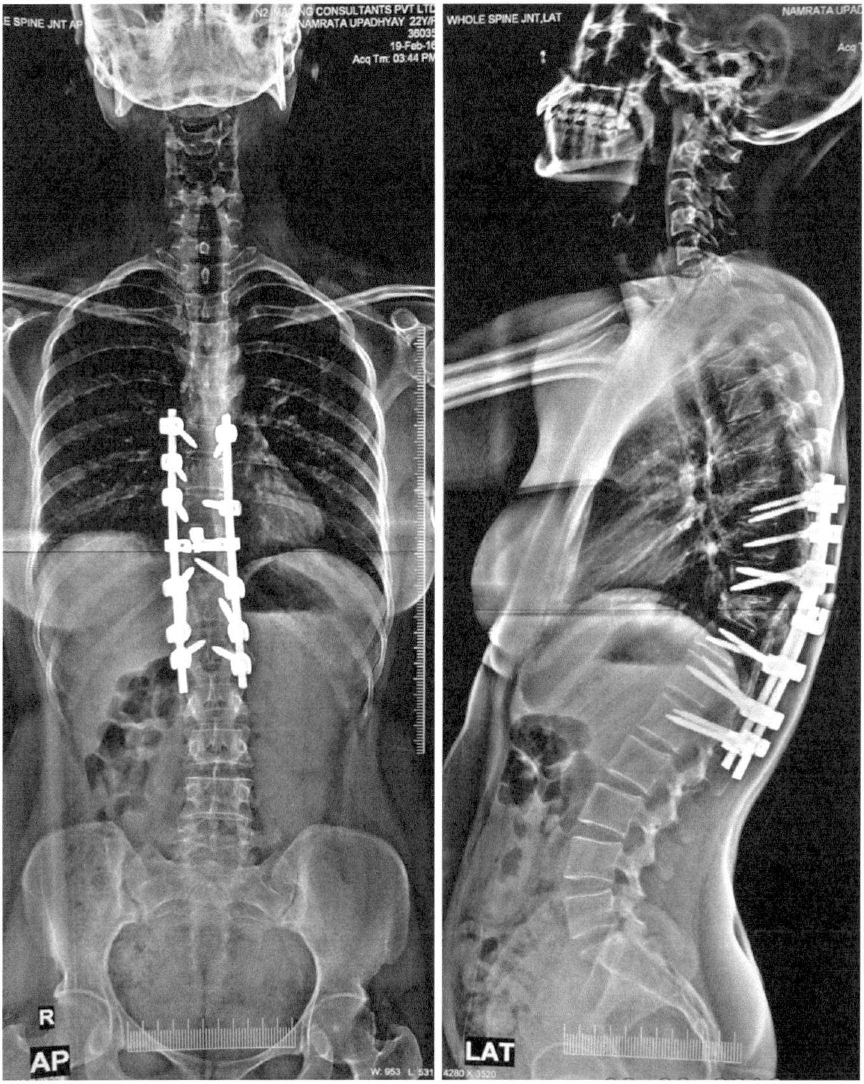

Fig. 24.2 Post-operative radiograph of the patient following pedicle subtraction osteotomy with posterior instrumentation

and packed with gauges. The pedicle is removed along with a wedge of vertebral body with its apex at the level of the anterior longitudinal ligament. The wedge is closed posteriorly with the help of a precontoured rod. Author also has experience in other three column osteotomies such as disc bone osteotomy (DBO), posterior vertebral column resection (PVCR), and anterior opening posterior closing osteotomy (AOPC) through posterior only approach with excellent results.

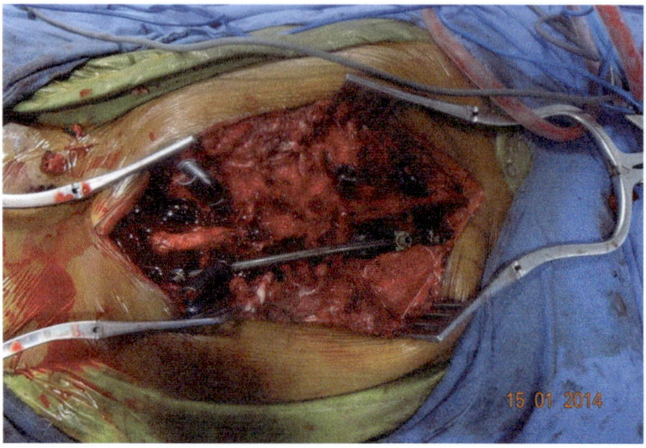

Fig. 24.3 Intraoperative radiograph of the above patient with temporary rod on one side and excised pedicle on the other side

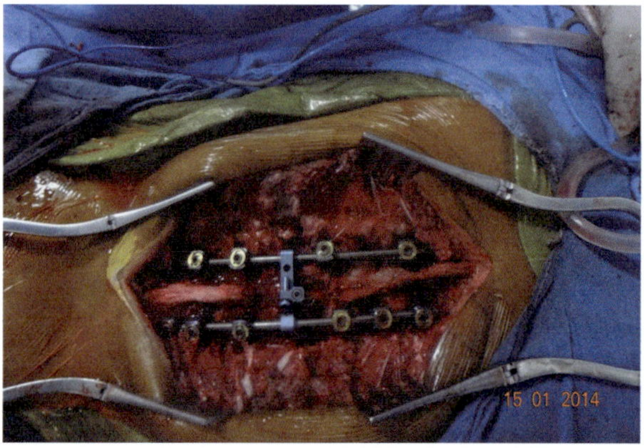

Fig. 24.4 Intraoperative picture showing final correction with contoured rods following pedicle subtraction osteotomy

24.10.3 Closing Opening Wedge Osteotomy

A deformity correction of 25°–52° has been reported using this technique [23, 32, 33]. Blunt dissection is used to obtain a plane between the vertebral body and pleura. Removal of a wedge from the vertebral body or fusion mass is carefully performed using a curette, rongeur, or a burr. Rajasekaran et al. recommend keeping the posterior vertebral cortex intact until the end to prevent excessive bleeding from epidural veins and injury to neural elements [23]. Shortening is carefully done using contoured rods to achieve a collapse of the wedge and correction of the deformity is achieved. Shortening is stopped at the first evidence of kinking or ballooning of the dura. The anterior column defect created during the posterior shortening is measured and a vertebral spacer such as a mesh cage with autograft inserted.

24.10.4 Posterior Vertebral Column Resection (PVCR)

Posterior vertebral column resection is reserved for more severe deformities and involves resection of all the columns. After instrumentation of the spine a temporary rod is placed on one side. This is followed by removal of the posterior elements. The rib heads and portion of the rib posteriorly are excised. The parietal pleura or psoas muscle (in lumbar spine) is detached from the anterior aspect of the vertebral body. This is followed by removal of the pedicles and lateral portion of the vertebral body. The rest of the body is then removed along with the intervening disc in a piecemeal fashion. A thin shell of posterior vertebral wall is kept intact at this stage. This protects the neural tube during removal of the vertebral body and disc. The procedure is then carried out from the contralateral side in a similar fashion. This is followed by removal of the posterior wall after breaking it using a posterior wall subsider leading to circumferential exposure of the neural tube. This is followed by deformity correction by changing the temporary rod with a rod with a less kyphotic contour. In situ bending of the rod to correct kyphosis has also been described. This is followed by compression across the osteotomy site further improving kyphosis. Residual anterior gap is filled with a bone graft or a vertebral spacer like a mesh cage filled with autograft (Figs. 24.5, 24.6, 24.7, and 24.8).

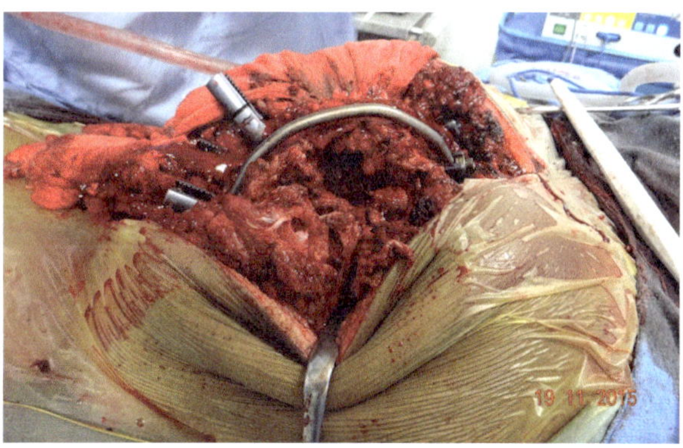

Fig. 24.5 Intra-operative images and post-operative radiograph of a 23-year-old male with thoracic kyphotic deformity involving D9-D10 vertebrae who underwent Vertebral Column Resection with deformity correction and posterior instrumentation. Intra-operative picture showing temporary rod contoured in preoperative kyphosis and vertebral body and disc resection being performed from the opposite side

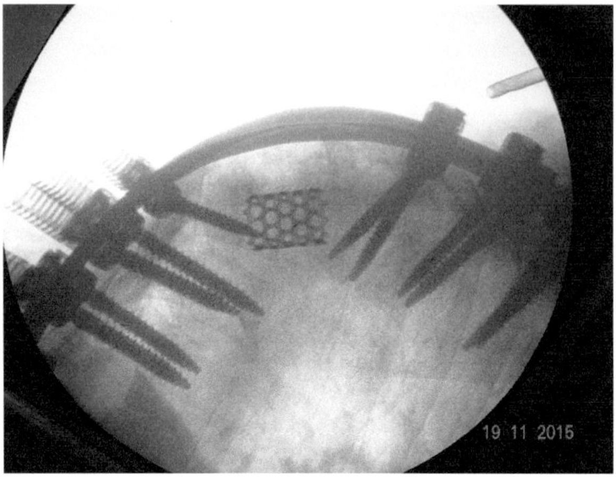

Fig. 24.6 Intra-operative lateral radiograph following vertebral column resection, correction using contoured rods, and placement of anterior mesh cage filled with autograft

Fig. 24.7 Post-operative radiograph of patient following vertebral column resection and deformity correction

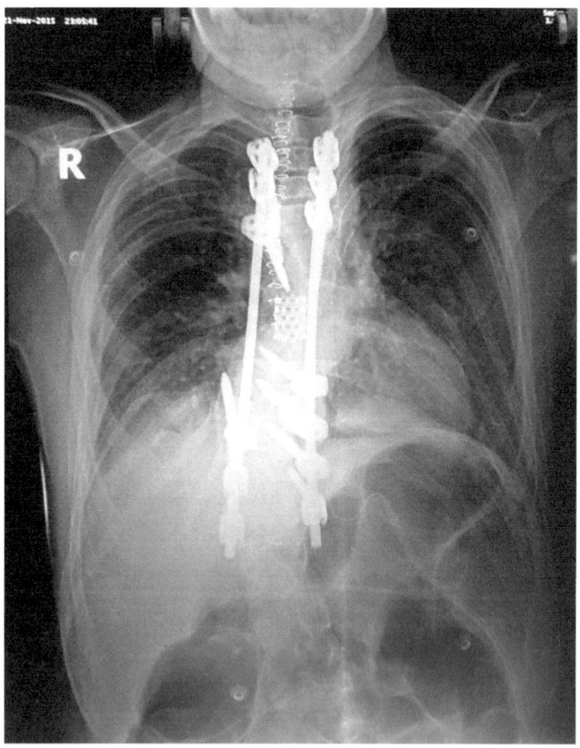

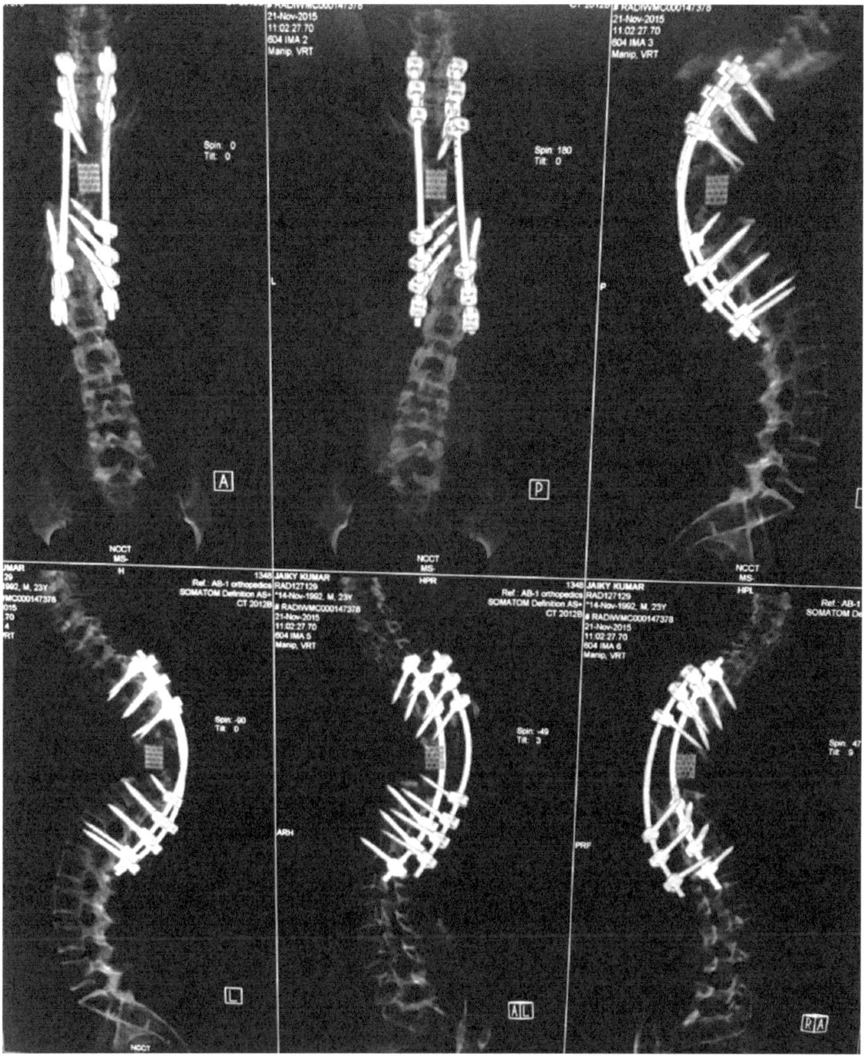

Fig. 24.8 Post-operative CT scan following vertebral column resection and deformity correction

24.10.5 *Modified Posterior Vertebral Column Resection (PVCR)*

A modification of the PVCR technique has been proposed by the senior author. Whereas a wide laminectomy is the first step in a conventional PVCR, the modified technique involves retaining the posterior elements till the other steps of the osteotomy are completed. The rationale behind this is that when a laminectomy is not performed, the cord remains gently suspended from the intact lamina due to epidural fat and veins. This prevents the ventral settling of the cord over the internal gibbus and prevents excessive handling of the cord during the osteotomy. The authors have noted lower complications with the modified PVCR compared to the conventional technique [34, 35].

24.11 Conclusion

Prevention of deformity and neurological deficit is the primary aim of the treatment of spinal tuberculosis. With the availability of potent anti-tuberculous drugs, uncomplicated tuberculosis has now become a medical disease. The most important factors influencing severity of deformity in spinal tuberculosis include the extent of vertebral destruction, number of vertebrae involved, level of the lesion and age of the patient with children and thoracolumbar spine lesion showing more severe deformities. The risk of disease progression is higher in children even with healed disease due to continued growth and thus may require surveillance till skeletal maturity. Children with pre-treatment kyphosis greater than 30° with two or more "spine at risk" signs are at a higher risk of developing severe deformity. Surgical procedures are simpler during active stage of the disease compared to a healed stage. Various surgical procedures are available for correction, and the choice depends on the severity of deformity and the preference and expertise of the surgeon.

References

1. Tuli SM. Severe kyphotic deformity in tuberculosis of the spine. Int Orthop. 1995;19(5):327–31.
2. Moon M-S, Moon Y-W, Moon J-L, Kim S-S, Sun D-H. Conservative treatment of tuberculosis of the lumbar and lumbosacral spine. Clin Orthop Relat Res. 2002 May;398:40–9.
3. Jain AK, Aggarwal PK, Arora A, Singh S. Behaviour of the kyphotic angle in spinal tuberculosis. Int Orthop. 2004 Apr;28(2):110–4.
4. Kyphosis in spinal tuberculosis – prevention and correction [Internet]. 2021 [cited 2021 Jan 7]. https://www.ncbi.nlm.nih.gov/pmc/articles/PMC2856387/.
5. Parthasarathy R, Sriram K, Santha T, Prabhakar R, Somasundaram PR, Sivasubramanian S. Short-course chemotherapy for tuberculosis of the spine. J Bone Joint Surg Br Vol. 1999;81-B(3):464–71.
6. Jain AK. Treatment of tuberculosis of the spine with neurologic complications. Clin Orthop Relat Res. 2002;398:75–84.
7. Rajasekaran S. Kyphotic deformity in spinal tuberculosis and its management. Int Orthop. 2012;36(2):359–65.
8. Rajasekaran S, Soundarapandian S. Progression of kyphosis in tuberculosis of the spine treated by anterior arthrodesis. J Bone Joint Surg Am. 1989;71(9):1314–23.
9. Rajasekaran S, Shanmugasundaram TK. Prediction of the angle of gibbus deformity in tuberculosis of the spine. J Bone Joint Surg Am. 1987;69(4):503–9.

10. Rajasekaran S. The natural history of post-tubercular kyphosis in children. Radiological signs which predict late increase in deformity. J Bone Joint Surg Br Vol. 2001;83:954–62.
11. Rajasekaran S. Buckling collapse of the spine in childhood spinal tuberculosis. Clin Orthop Relat Res. 2007;460:86–92.
12. Oga M, Arizono T, Takasita M, Sugioka Y. Evaluation of the risk of instrumentation as a foreign body in spinal tuberculosis. Clinical and biologic study. Spine (Phila Pa 1976). 1993;18(13):1890–4.
13. Güven O, Kumano K, Yalçin S, Karahan M, Tsuji S. A single stage posterior approach and rigid fixation for preventing kyphosis in the treatment of spinal tuberculosis. Spine (Phila Pa 1976). 1994;19(9):1039–43.
14. Rajasekaran S, Rajoli SR, Aiyer SN, Kanna R, Shetty AP. A classification for kyphosis based on column deficiency, curve magnitude, and osteotomy requirement. J Bone Joint Surg Am. 2018;100(13):1147–56.
15. Jain AK, Maheshwari AV, Jena S. Kyphus correction in spinal tuberculosis. Clin Orthop Relat Res. 2007;460:117–23.
16. Laheri VJ, Badhe NP, Dewnany GT. Single stage decompression, anterior interbody fusion and posterior instrumentation for tuberculous kyphosis of the dorso-lumbar spine. Spinal Cord. 2001;39(8):429–36.
17. Louw JA. Spinal tuberculosis with neurological deficit. Treatment with anterior vascularised rib grafts, posterior osteotomies and fusion. J Bone Joint Surg (Br). 1990;72(4):686–93.
18. Moon MS, Woo YK, Lee KS, Ha KY, Kim SS, Sun DH. Posterior instrumentation and anterior interbody fusion for tuberculous kyphosis of dorsal and lumbar spines. Spine (Phila Pa 1976). 1995;20(17):1910–6.
19. Yau AC, Hsu LC, O'Brien JP, Hodgson AR. Tuberculous kyphosis: correction with spinal osteotomy, halo-pelvic distraction, and anterior and posterior fusion. J Bone Joint Surg Am. 1974;56(7):1419–34.
20. Bezer M, Kucukdurmaz F, Guven O. Transpedicular decancellation osteotomy in the treatment of posttuberculous kyphosis. J Spinal Disord Tech. 2007;20(3):209–15.
21. Altman GT, Altman DT, Frankovitch KF. Anterior and posterior fusion for children with tuberculosis of the spine. Clin Orthop Relat Res. 1996;325:225–31.
22. Chen W-J, Wu C-C, Jung C-H, Chen L-H, Niu C-C, Lai P-L. Combined anterior and posterior surgeries in the treatment of spinal tuberculous spondylitis. Clin Orthop Relat Res. 2002;398:50–9.
23. Rajasekaran S, Vijay K, Shetty AP. Single-stage closing-opening wedge osteotomy of spine to correct severe post-tubercular kyphotic deformities of the spine: a 3-year follow-up of 17 patients. Eur Spine J. 2010;19(4):583–92.
24. Suk S-I, Kim J-H, Lee S-M, Chung E-R, Lee J-H. Anterior-posterior surgery versus posterior closing wedge osteotomy in posttraumatic kyphosis with neurologic compromised osteoporotic fracture. Spine (Phila Pa 1976). 2003;28(18):2170–5.
25. Murrey DB, Brigham CD, Kiebzak GM, Finger F, Chewning SJ. Transpedicular decompression and pedicle subtraction osteotomy (eggshell procedure): a retrospective review of 59 patients. Spine (Phila Pa 1976). 2002;27(21):2338–45.
26. Tian Sheng S. Modified decancellation posterior closing-wedge osteotomy for correction of traumatic thoracolumbar kyphotic deformity: a cadaveric and preliminary clinical study. Int J Phys Med Rehabil [Internet]. 2014. [cited 2021 Jan 14];02(05) https://www.omicsonline.org/open-access/modified-decancellation-posterior-closingwedge-osteotomy-for-correction-of-traumatic-2329-9096.1000227.php?aid=31794
27. Li F, Sagi HC, Liu B, Yuan HA. Comparative evaluation of single-level closing-wedge vertebral osteotomies for the correction of fixed kyphotic deformity of the lumbar spine: a cadaveric study. Spine (Phila Pa 1976). 2001;26(21):2385–91.
28. Gill JB, Levin A, Burd T, Longley M. Corrective osteotomies in spine surgery. J Bone Joint Surg Am. 2008;90(11):2509–20.

29. Bridwell KH. Decision making regarding Smith-Petersen vs. pedicle subtraction osteotomy vs. vertebral column resection for spinal deformity. Spine (Phila Pa 1976). 2006;31(19 Suppl):S171–8.
30. Kalra KP, Dhar SB, Shetty G, Dhariwal Q. Pedicle subtraction osteotomy for rigid post-tuberculous kyphosis. J Bone Joint Surg (Br). 2006;88(7):925–7.
31. Hong-Qi Z, Yong C, Jia H, Chaofeng G, Xiongke H. Modified pedicle subtraction osteotomies (mPSO) for thoracolumbar post-tubercular kyphosis in pediatric patients: retrospective clinical cases and review of the literature. Childs Nerv Syst. 2015 Aug;31(8):1347–54.
32. Kawahara N, Tomita K, Baba H, Kobayashi T, Fujita T, Murakami H. Closing-opening wedge osteotomy to correct angular kyphotic deformity by a single posterior approach. Spine (Phila Pa 1976). 2001;26(4):391–402.
33. Rajasekaran S, Kanna R, Shetty A. Closing-opening wedge osteotomy for severe, rigid, thoracolumbar post-tubercular kyphosis. Eur Spine J Off Publ Eur Spine Soc Eur Spinal Deform Soc Eur Section Cervical Spine Res Soc. 2011;20:343–8.
34. Papadopoulos EC, Boachie-Adjei O, Hess WF, Sanchez Perez-Grueso FJ, Pellisé F, Gupta M, et al. Early outcomes and complications of posterior vertebral column resection. Spine J. 2015;15(5):983–91.
35. Garg B, Mehta N. Modified posterior vertebral column resection for severe spinal deformity: a retrospective, comparative study. Spine J. 2020;20(9):1446–51.

Chapter 25
Head of Spine Surgery Post-tuberculosis Sagittal Balance of the Spine: Challenges and Approach

Martin Gehrchen

Abstract The chapter focuses mainly on the compensatory mechanisms of keeping an upright position and a horizontal gaze when the balance is affected in the sagittal plane post tuberculosis. The body's self-preservation and natural adaptation to any kyphosing event keeping the upright gait and horizontal gaze is the driver in these compensatory mechanisms. This chapter describes possible measures when dealing with post-tuberculosis affected sagittal balance.

The compensatory mechanisms are described with examples including illustrative figures.

Keywords Compensatory · Compensation · Sagittal balance

25.1 Introduction

The chapter will focus mainly on the compensatory mechanisms of keeping an upright position and a horizontal gaze when balance is affected in the sagittal plane post TB (PTB). The body's self-preservation and natural adaptation to any kyphosing event keeping the upright gait and horizontal gaze is the driver in these compensatory mechanisms.

The kyphosing event post TB can occur in any part of the spine affected, but this chapter focuses on the thoracolumbar (T/L) spine. The kyphosing events may occur over more segments or a few sometimes only one segment. To understand how to address the affection of sagittal balance post tuberculosis, it is necessary to understand the normal shapes of the spine as described by Roussouly [1]. According to the Roussouly classification of the normal spine shapes of asymptomatic individuals, five spinopelvic morphotypes were identified discriminating low pelvic

M. Gehrchen (✉)
Head of Spine Surgery Rigshospitalet, University of Copenhagen, Copenhagen, Denmark

S. S. Dhatt, V. Kumar (eds.), *Tuberculosis of the Spine*,
https://doi.org/10.1007/978-981-16-9495-0_25

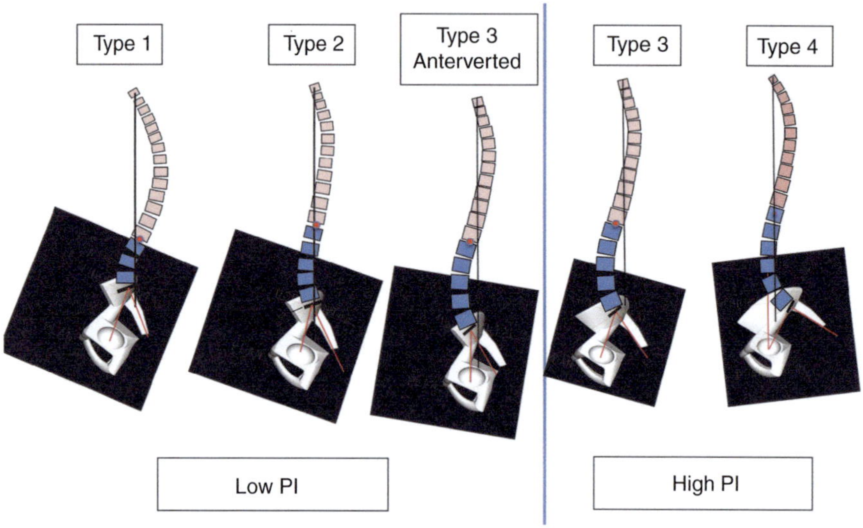

Fig. 25.1 The different types of the Roussouly classification. Note that types 1, 2, and the anteverted type are associated with low pelvic incidence (PI) values, and types 3 and 4 are associated with higher PI values. From Pierre Roussouly et al. [4]. Courtesy: these are from the personal collection of Dr. Bhavuk Garg, Additional Professor, Orthopaedics, AIIMS New Delhi

incidence (PI) (three types, one with anteversion of the pelvis) and high PI (two types) (Fig. 25.1). Furthermore, the anatomic demarcation of thoracic kyphosis and lumbar lordosis should be considered as spinal kyphosis (SK) and spinal lordosis (SL) not restricted to the anatomical location (i.e., L1-S1, etc.).

25.2 Understanding the Compensatory Mechanisms of a Post-tuberculosis Kyphosing Event

25.2.1 Pelvic Retroversion

The first well-known and described compensatory mechanism for a sagittal imbalance is **pelvic retroversion**. Duval Beaupere described the relation of the pelvic parameters—pelvic incidence (PI), pelvic tilt (PT) and sacral slope (SS)—and found a relation between PT and SS (PI = PT + SS) [2].

25.2.2 What Is the Mechanical Effect of Pelvic Retroversion?

The posterior pelvis rotation around the femoral heads induces a physical effect and a shape transformation. This includes reciprocal positioning of the hips (extension) and knees (flexion in pronounced retroversion). The kyphosing event in the spine will retrovert the pelvis counteracting this event and trying to move the body back to the gravity line position diminishing the gravity force anterior to the feet. At the same time, the SS and lumbar lordosis decrease.

25.2.3 How the Pelvic Shape Influences the Mechanism of Retroversion

Patients with a high PI may have more pelvic retroversion for compensation than a patient with low PI. Thus, in the standing position, there is a lesser ability of pelvic retroversion if PI is low, than with a high PI. In other words, to reach a high PT (strong retroversion), a patient must have a high PI. For example, if two patients are compared having the same amount of a kyphosing event, then the likelihood of a better global balance (C7 plumb line) is higher in the patient with a high PI compared to a patient with a low PI. A high level of retroversion is always linked to a pelvis with a high PI. Of course, if there is any pre-existing impairment of hip motion, knee extension will occur at a lower PI.

25.2.4 Gait

The retroversion of the pelvis can have an important effect on walking [3]. The hip extension must be free to maintain a balanced pelvis during gait. If the hips are locked in extension, the forward femoral tilt induces an anteverted pelvis positioning and a global forward tilt of the spine. Sometimes the compensatory mechanism of the pelvis (retroversion) is enough to keep the body in sagittal balance. However, in walking, this mechanism can lose its positive effect and strongly impair the sagittal balance since the hips cannot extend further (Fig. 25.2).

25.2.5 Spinal Extension Compensation

Another way of compensation is active extension of the spine above and below a kyphosing event. This mechanism exists only when the spine is flexible and when muscles are strong enough. This mechanism may be painful either by muscles overactivity and/or by posterior facets constraints. This mechanism may be located at any level of the spine. This can result in hyperlordosis where pre-existing lordosis is present (cervical or lumbar) in a flexible spine and is limited by the intervertebral extension ability. If the spine is rigid, sometimes an abnormal hyperextension can be seen with the development of a listhesis at its maximum. In the thoracic area, an inversion of the normal kyphosis can be seen and presents a lordosis as compensation (Fig. 25.3).

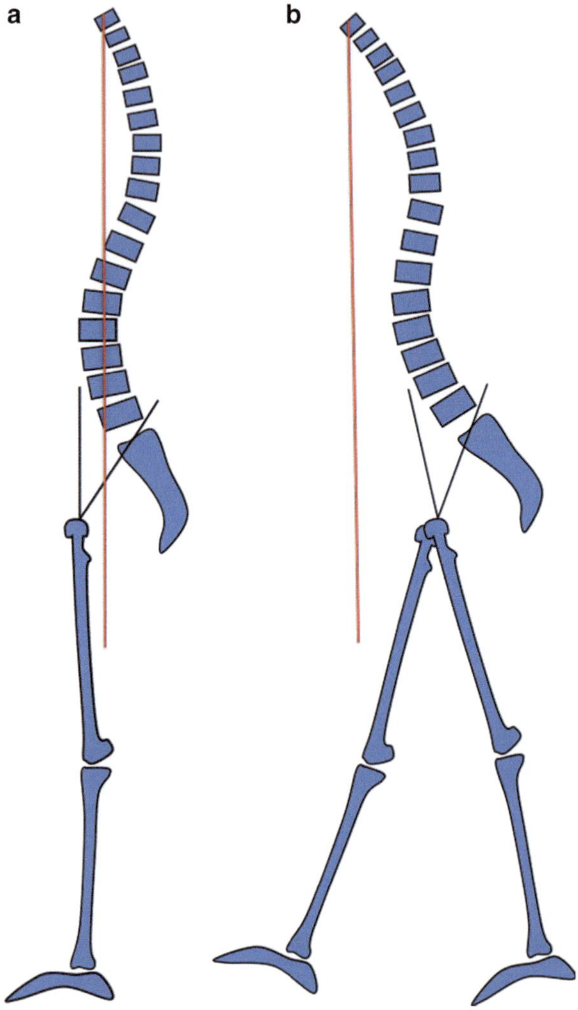

Fig. 25.2 (**a**) When the pelvis is retroverted in a standing position, the patient seems balanced. (**b**) When walking, the pelvis tilts forward driving by the femoral tilt during gait, impairing balance. From Pierre Roussouly et al. [4]. Courtesy: these are from the personal collection of Dr. Bhavuk Garg, Additional Professor, Orthopaedics, AIIMS New Delhi

There are different examples of compensatory mechanisms, as follows:

- Local kyphosation of segments such as after tuberculosis induces compensatory mechanisms and they are usually more pronounced due to the local process involving only a few segments compared to general kyphosation with multilevel involvement (like Scheuermann's disease (Fig. 25.4) or disc degeneration).
- Post-tuberculosis kyphosation in the thoracic region: induces extension (increased lordosis) below the kyphosation (and above in the cervical region). If

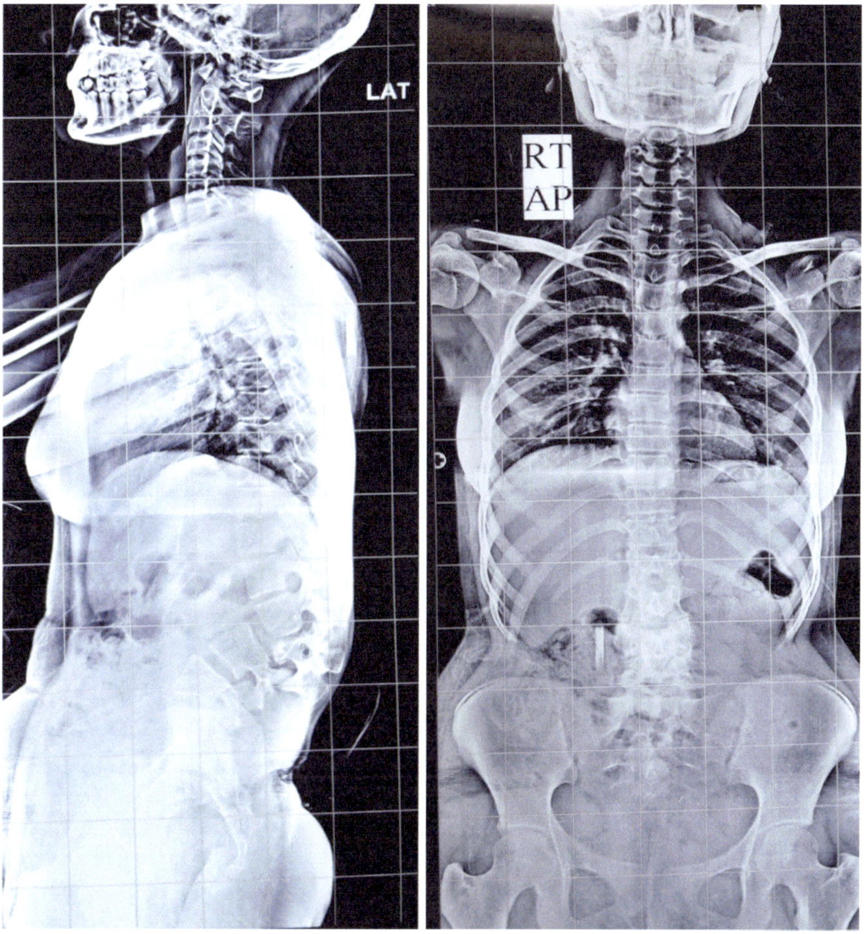

Fig. 25.3 Young patient with a localized post-tuberculosis kyphosis and flexible spine inducing a lordotic thoracic spine and hyperlordosis in the lumbar spine

the spine is flexible an increased lordosis will occur and this can further lead to severe muscle fatigue and increased load on the facet joints inducing further discomfort and pain. This applies also to the cervical region. The determinant of the compensatory mechanism is the magnitude of PI and, thereby, on the quantity of pelvic anteversion that can be reached. If the anteversion compensatory mechanism of the pelvis is exhausted and the kyphosation further increases, a retroversion of the pelvis can be seen trying to maintain the horizontal gaze. Any degeneration in the lumbar region at that point will result in retroversion of the pelvis. The same will happen in extended degeneration in the thoracic spine, and when the compensation is consumed, spinal lordosis will disappear producing a global kyphosis.

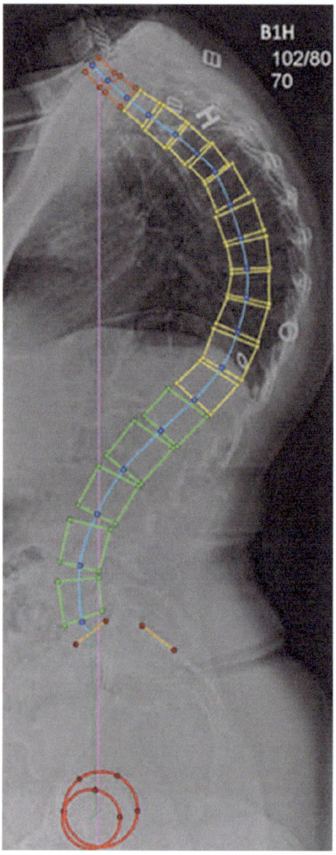

Fig. 25.4 Patient with a global Scheuermann's kyphosis.

- Post-tuberculosis in the thoracolumbar region: An increase of kyphosis induces extension (lordosis) below and above the kyphosation area and, thus, decrease of thoracic kyphosis and an increase of spinal lordosis in the flexible spine. In the rigid spine, a retroversion of the pelvis is seen.
- Post-tuberculosis in the lumbar region: When spinal lordosis is lost, extension of the segments above will occur if the spine is flexible. If the spine is rigid, the only compensatory possibility is retroversion of the pelvis.
- Post-tuberculosis in the lumbosacral region: This is highly complicated and the identification of PI can be quite difficult. The position of L5 relative to the sacrum may be an approximation in severe lumbosacral kyphosis. This situation will induce both pelvic retroversion and extension of the spine where the lordosis can reach the whole thoracic spine. After surgical correction of lumbosacral kyphosis, the compensatory mechanisms disappear spontaneously.

As illustrated above, the compensatory mechanisms are logical, however complex, and one must try different approaches to comprehend these mechanisms to understand fully the compensatory mechanisms.

25.3 Examples of Sagittal Balance After Post-tuberculosis Kyphosing Event of the Spine

Here presented are two cases of tuberculosis with a significant impact on the sagittal balance. One case with high PI and one case with low PI.

Case 1: High thoracic post-tuberculosis event with severe kyphosation in a 21-year-old female patient (Fig. 25.5). The shape of the spine according to the Roussouly classification is an anteverted type 4. The PI is high (64) with a negative PT and a SS of 65° (Fig. 25.6). The compensatory mechanisms are very clear on the X-ray as lined out:

(a) Extension of the thoracic spine (lordotic) above the post-tuberculosis kyphosing event and extension below inducing a prolonged and hyperlordotic spine.
(b) Immediate postoperatively there are still compensatory mechanisms in the work (i.e., extension of spine above and below), but usually this changes a bit after some months with reduction of lordosis and reduction of the extension above the lesion in young patients like this case (Fig. 25.7).

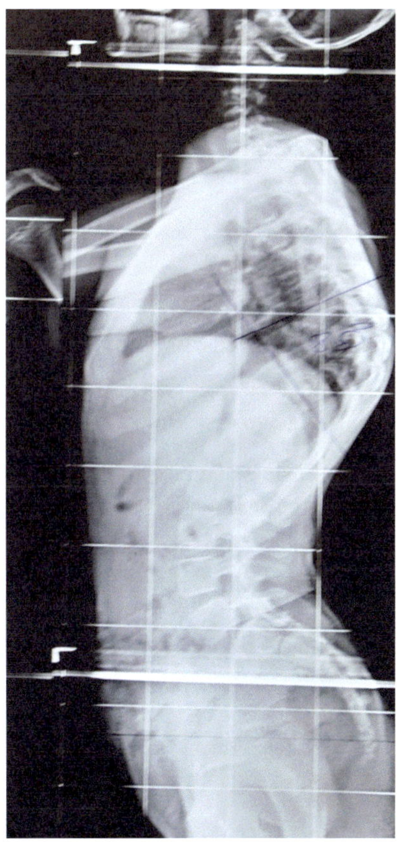

Fig. 25.5 Young patient with severe post-tuberculosis thoracic kyphosation

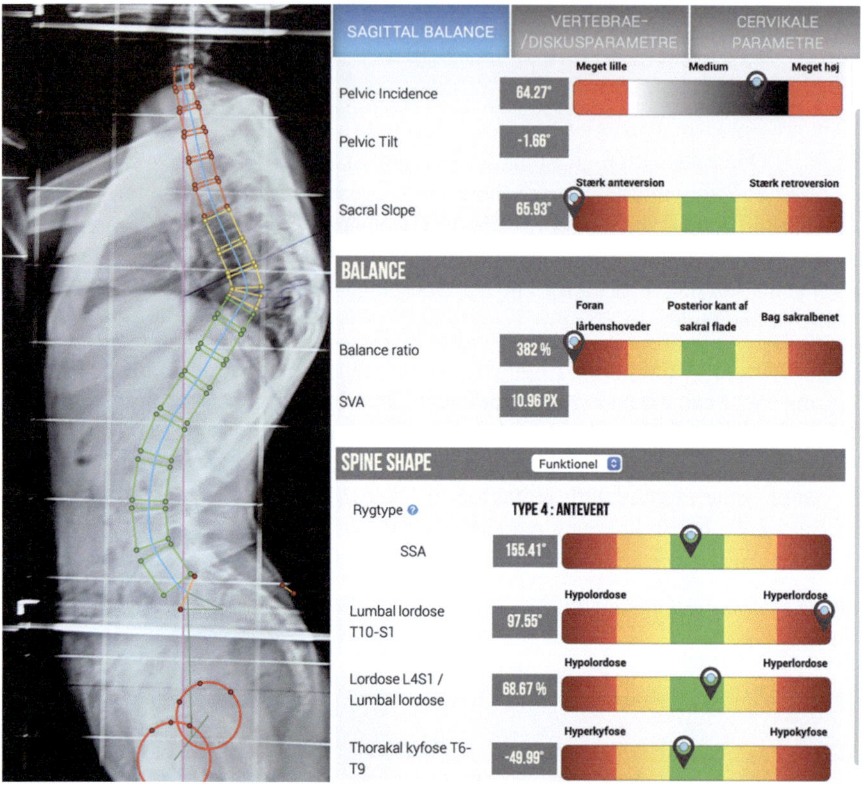

Fig. 25.6 Spinopelvic analysis of patient in Fig. 25.5 using KEOPs software

Case 2: Lumbar post-tuberculosis event producing a severe kyphosing event of around 90° in the lumbar spine (Fig. 25.3). The shape of spine according to the Roussouly classification is type 2. The PI is extremely low (29) with a PT of 28 and a SS of 1° indicating a very strong retroversion (Fig. 25.8). The compensatory mechanisms are very clear on the X-ray as lined out:

(a) Extension of the spine (lordotic in the thoracolumbar area) above the post-tuberculosis kyphosing event and below inducing a short hyperlordotic lumbar spine and a strongly retroverted pelvis below the event.
(b) Postoperatively there is still some compensatory mechanisms; however, there is a significant improvement of the preoperative compensatory mechanisms (Fig. 25.9). Thus, the PT is decreased significantly to 15 and SS increased to 15°. The lordosis at the thoracolumbar spine is gone and in the lumbar area there is now only a small hypolordosis. The type 2 spine according to Roussouly classification is a flat spine.

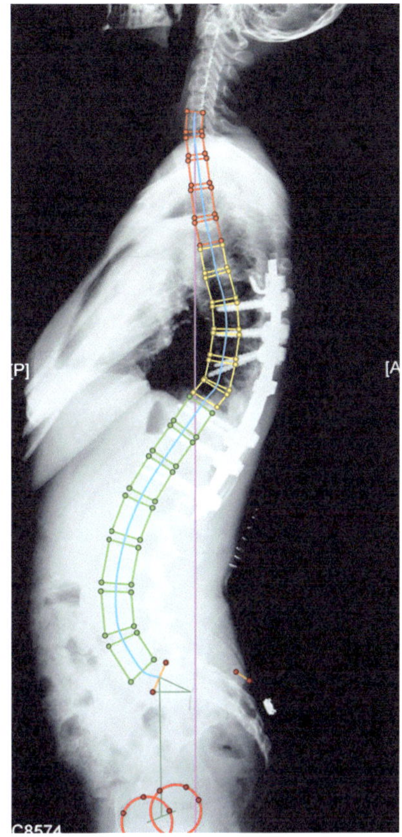

Fig. 25.7 Postoperative result after correction

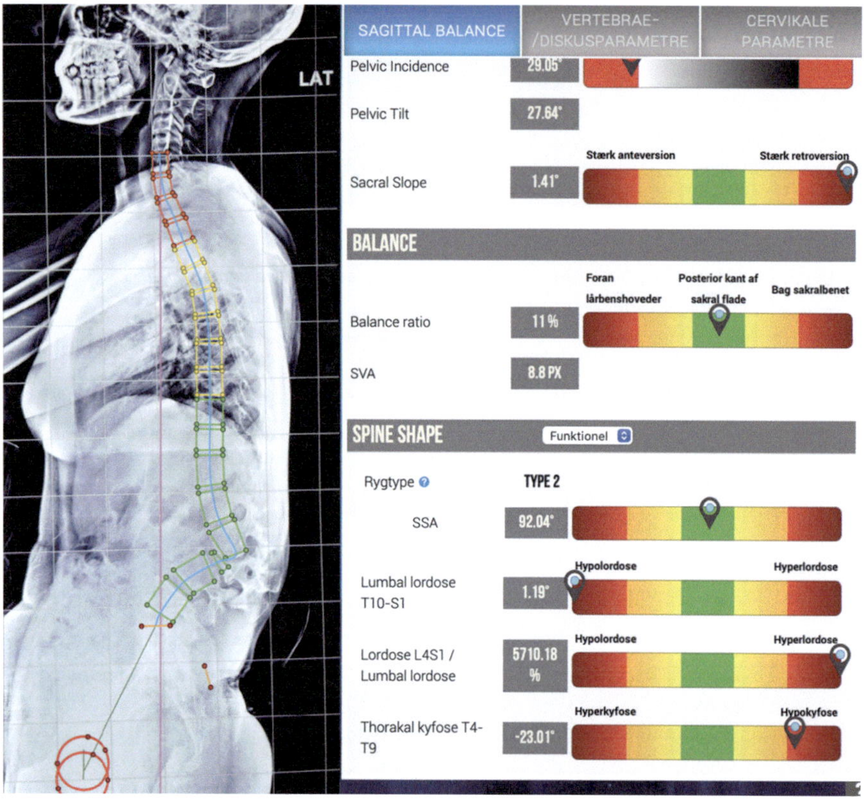

Fig. 25.8 Spinopelvic analysis of patient in Fig. 25.3 using KEOPs software

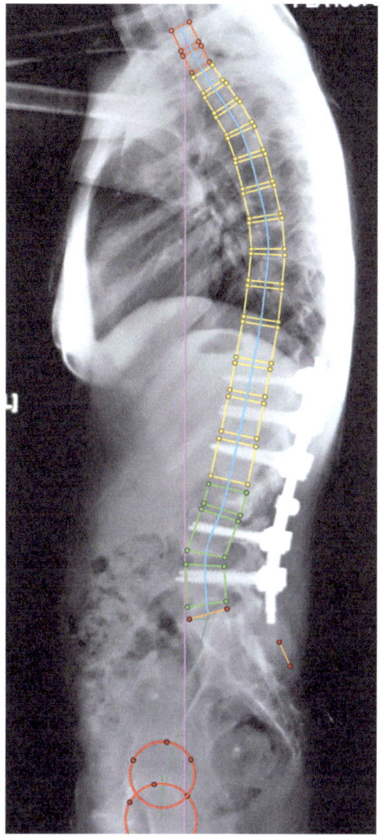

Fig. 25.9 Postoperative result after correction

References

1. Laouissat F, Sebaaly A, Gehrchen M, Roussouly P. Classification of normal sagittal spine alignment: refounding the Roussouly classification. Eur Spine J. 2018;27(8):2002–11. https://doi.org/10.1007/s00586-017-5111-x. Epub 2017 Apr 28
2. Legaye J, Duval-Beaupère G, Hecquet J, Marty C. Pelvic incidence: a fundamental pelvic parameter for three-dimensional regulation of spinal sagittal curves. Eur Spine J. 1998;7(2):99–103. https://doi.org/10.1007/s005860050038.
3. Lazennec JY, Brusson A, Rousseau MA. Hip-spine relations and sagittal balance clinical consequences. Eur Spine J. 2011;20(Suppl 5):686–98. https://doi.org/10.1007/s00586-011-1937-9. Epub 2011 Jul 28
4. Roussouly P, et al. Sagittal balance of the spine: from normal to pathology: a key for treatment strategy. New York, Stuttgart: Thieme Publishers; 2019. 256 pp, 259 illustrations, Hardcover, ISBN: 9781626237322

Chapter 26
TB Spine in Special Conditions

Ankit I. Mehta and Elsa Nico

Abstract Tuberculosis (TB) of the spine, or spinal TB, may present itself in the setting of various special conditions which include but are not limited to immunocompromised status, HIV, pregnancy, ankylosing spondylitis (AS) and other spondyloarthropathies, primary spinal tumors or spinal metastases, and polytrauma. These special conditions weaken the immune system and make it more susceptible to developing active TB or reactivating latent TB. HIV and immunosuppressive medications (i.e., TNF-alpha inhibitors) used to treat autoimmune disorders (i.e., ankylosing spondylitis, rheumatoid arthritis) deplete or inactivate crucial immune system modulators in containing TB, such as CD4+ T-cells and TNF-alpha, respectively. Spinal TB may mimic non-specific symptoms of inflammatory back pain in AS and fatigue or malaise in pregnancy. Spinal TB may also mimic primary spinal tumors or spinal metastases in radiographic imaging. For these reasons, spinal TB is often initially misdiagnosed, and treatment is delayed leading to progressive, more severe symptoms. There are, however, several signs specific to spinal TB that may aid clinicians in distinguishing it from AS and neoplasia in order to reach an accurate diagnosis and initiate proper treatment earlier.

Keywords HIV · Immunocompromised · Immunosuppressed · Pregnancy · Spondyloarthropathy · Ankylosing spondylitis · Spinal metastasis · Spinal tumor · Polytrauma · Multiple trauma

In most cases, tuberculosis (TB) presents primarily as a pulmonary disease; however, extra-pulmonary infection presents in 10–15% of patients as well. Of those extra-pulmonary infections, half are skeletal and 1–2% specifically involve the spine as "Pott's disease." As TB has become increasingly rare in the United States

A. I. Mehta (✉) · E. Nico
University of Illinois at Chicago, Chicago, IL, USA
e-mail: ankitm@uic.edu; enico2@uic.edu

S. S. Dhatt, V. Kumar (eds.), *Tuberculosis of the Spine*,
https://doi.org/10.1007/978-981-16-9495-0_26

and other non-endemic regions, the majority of cases seem to arise in the setting of special conditions that primarily involve an immunosuppressive state either through other diseases or medication side effects.

26.1 Immunocompromised Status

TB, and therefore TB of the spine, is associated with patients in an immunocompromised status from a weakened immune system. Various conditions may weaken the immune system including human immunodeficiency virus (HIV), cancer, malnutrition, and immunosuppressive medications for autoimmune disorders or organ transplantation.

26.1.1 HIV and M. tuberculosis *Co-infection*

HIV is a retrovirus transmitted from human-to-human through contact with infected blood, semen, or vaginal fluid. Epidemiological studies have demonstrated an increased risk of active TB infection during the course of HIV infection [1, 2]. When an individual is infected with HIV, during the early and chronic phases, the risk of acquiring active TB is 2–5 times greater than baseline. As HIV kills off more and more CD4+ T-cells and progresses into acquired immunodeficiency syndrome (AIDS), the risk of acquiring active TB jumps to at least 20-fold higher than baseline. Even after antiretroviral therapy (ART) has been administered to recover CD4+ T-cells, there is still an increased risk of acquiring active TB about fourfold above baseline. Figure 26.1 highlights the risk of acquiring active TB infection as HIV progresses [3]. HIV-positive patients have a 60% increased risk of developing skeletal TB [4, 5].

26.1.1.1 Pathogenesis of HIV and *M. tuberculosis* Co-infection

M. tuberculosis is a facultative intracellular organism of macrophages. Various *M. tuberculosis* virulence factors, including sulfatides and cord factor, are implicated in the pathogen's survival within macrophages and development of granulomas [6]. Granulomas are a collection of immune cells—epithelioid macrophages, multinucleated giant cells, and lymphocytes—that actively contain *M. tuberculosis* without completely eradicating or degrading it. Sulfatides are surface glycolipids on *M. tuberculosis* that inhibit phagolysosomal fusion, and therefore the degradation of *M. tuberculosis* contained within the phagosomes. Cord factor activates macrophages and promotes granuloma formation.

Mycobacterial antigens (i.e., lipids, lipoproteins, and nucleic acids) are sensed by pathogen recognition receptors (PRRs) within macrophages and presented to

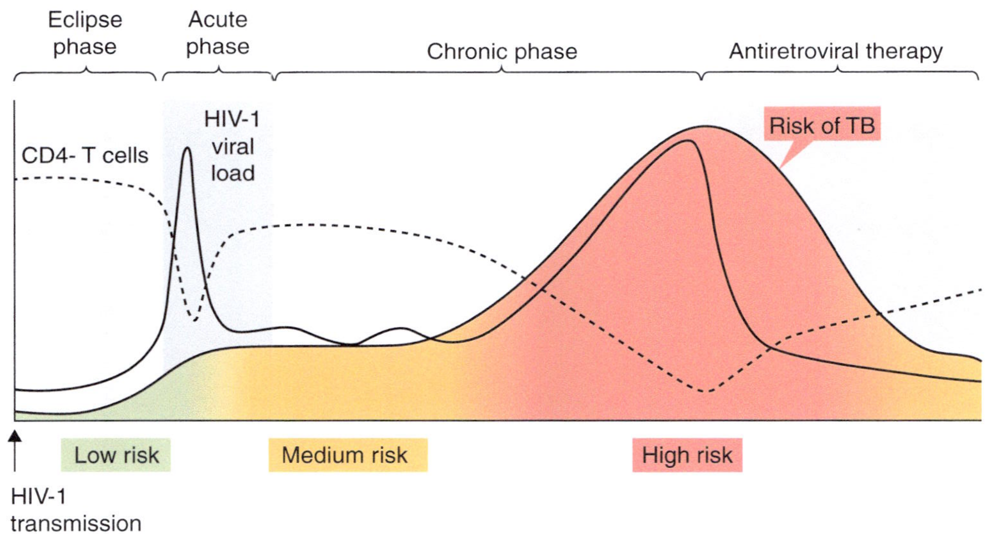

Fig. 26.1 HIV-1 and *M. tuberculosis* co-infection increases the risk of active tuberculosis: When an individual is infected with HIV, during the early and chronic phases, the risk of acquiring active TB is 2–5 times greater than baseline. As HIV kills off more and more CD4+ T-cells and progresses into acquired immunodeficiency syndrome (AIDS), the risk of acquiring active TB jumps to at least 20-fold higher than baseline. Even after antiretroviral therapy (ART) has been administered to recover CD4+ T-cells, there is still an increased risk of acquiring active TB about fourfold above baseline. (Reproduced from Bell et al. [3])

CD4+ T-cells which initiate an innate immune response and recruit even more immune cells [7, 8]. CD4+ T-cells, once presented with mycobacterial antigens, secrete IL-12. IL-12 is responsible for differentiating CD4+ T-cells into T_H1cells. T_H1cells secrete interferon-gamma (IFN-γ), which then activate macrophages into secreting various pro-inflammatory cytokines (i.e., TNF-alpha) and forming sequestering granulomas. These granulomas sequester, or restrict, *M. tuberculosis* within macrophages and confer immunological protection against *M. tuberculosis* dissemination. Genetic deficiencies in both IL-12 signaling and IFN-γ signaling present with an increased risk of TB infection [9].

HIV Disruption of *M. tuberculosis* Granuloma

HIV weakens the immune system, and therefore increases susceptibility to acquiring active TB or reactivating latent TB, by disrupting the immune response within granulomas [10–14]. These disruptions include (a) HIV preferential replication within CD4+ T-cells and macrophages co-infected with *M. tuberculosis* leading to (b) a depletion of CD4+ T-cells, (b) an impairment of macrophage function, and (c) an impairment of T-cell function [15]. With impairments in macrophage and T-cell functions and an overall decrease in CD4+ T-cell numbers, granulomas cannot effectively contain *M. tuberculosis*, which results in bacterial growth and spread.

HIV Replication in *M. Tuberculosis* Co-infected Immune Cells

In vitro studies have shown HIV replicates preferentially within *M. tuberculosis*-co-infected macrophages and CD4+ T-cells [16–25]. An increased viral load of both HIV and TB within activated CD4+ T-cells and macrophages may overwhelm these immune cells and the granulomas they are associated with, leading to disruption of the granuloma and its containment of TB.

Depletion of CD4+ T-Cells

HIV preferentially infects and depletes CD4+ T-cells [20–25]. By depleting one of the earliest players in granuloma formation, HIV directly disrupts granulomas and, therefore, increases the risk of active or reactivated TB infection [12, 26]. In individuals infected with both HIV and TB, CD4+ T-cells are depleted in peripheral blood, in the respiratory tract, and at the site of tuberculin skin test (TST) [27–29]. CD4+ T-cells which produce pro-inflammatory cytokines, like IFN-γ and TNF-alpha, involved in *M. tuberculosis* protection are also depleted [28]. Regardless of antiretroviral therapy, HIV+ individuals with lower CD4+ T-cell counts are more susceptible to TB than HIV+ individuals with higher CD4+ T-cell counts [30]. While CD4+ T-cell counts and cell-mediated immunity may be reduced, a compensatory humoral response with an increase in plasma cells, IgM, and IgG antibodies may be seen in co-infected tissue including co-infected spinal granulomas [31–33].

Changes in Macrophage Function

HIV impairs both apoptosis of TB-infected macrophages and acidification of TB-infected phagosomes [34–37]. *M. tuberculosis* itself, using sulfatides, inhibits phagolysosomal fusion and its ultimate degradation. Since phagolysosomal fusion is inhibited, apoptosis is used as a last resort by infected macrophages to kill the ingested pathogen. By reducing the ability of macrophages to form phagolysosomes and induce apoptosis, HIV virtually eliminates every possibility for macrophages to clear *M. tuberculosis*. Therefore, by impairing macrophage function HIV increases the likelihood of developing active or reactivated TB.

Changes in *M. tuberculosis*-Specific T-Cell Function

HIV decreases *M. tuberculosis*-specific T-cell responses. Individuals infected with both TB and HIV harbor T-cells that release less IFN-γ and TNF-alpha than individuals infected with TB alone [38, 39]. A reduction in pro-inflammatory cytokines, like IFN-γ and TNF-alpha, disrupts the integrity of granulomas and therefore increases the risk of developing active or reactivated TB.

Antiretroviral Therapy and Immune Reconstitution Inflammatory Syndrome

Antiretroviral therapy (ART) is administered to HIV patients to reduce the viral load, restore CD4+ T-cell counts and immune function, reduce complications, and improve overall survival. By restoring CD4+ T-cells and immunity, ART may induce immune reconstitution inflammatory syndrome (IRIS) in a subset of patients. IRIS represents an excessive immune response to and worsening of an existing infection or the appearance of a new infection [40]. Thus, IRIS may worsen active TB or reactivate latent TB [41].

26.1.1.2 Comparison of Radiological Findings Between HIV-Positive and HIV-Negative Patients

Radiological findings on magnetic resonance imaging (MRI) can help distinguish spinal TB presentation between HIV-positive and HIV-negative patients. HIV-negative patients show greater vertebral body destruction and subsequently a greater degree of kyphosis than HIV-positive patients [42–44]. HIV-positive patients, on the other hand, show greater abscess formation than HIV-negative patients [42, 44].

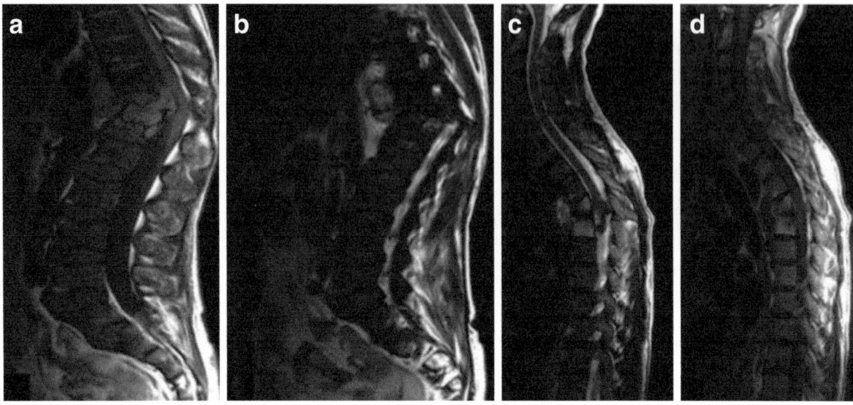

Fig. 26.2 MRI of an HIV-negative (**a**) and (**b**) and an HIV-positive (**c**) & (**d**) patient with spinal TB: The HIV-negative patient shows greater vertebral body destruction (T11/T12) and kyphosis. The HIV-positive patient shows significantly less vertebral body destruction and kyphosis. (Reproduced from Anley et al. [44])

Abscesses are larger in HIV-positive patients because HIV depletes CD4+ T-cells and their T-cell mediated immunity and therefore permits the underlying TB infection to induce a greater inflammatory response. Radiculomyelitis occurs more commonly in HIV-positive patients whereas spondylitis occurs more commonly in HIV-negative patients [43]. Figure 26.2 highlights some radiographic differences of spinal TB between HIV-positive and HIV-negative patients [44]. There is no difference between HIV-positive and HIV-negative patients in terms of number of vertebrae involved or skip lesions [42, 44]. Since HIV-positive patients have less vertebral body destruction and more abscess formation, a simple decompressive surgery may be preferred over decompression and fixation surgeries used to treat the larger vertebral destructions in HIV-negative patients.

26.1.2 Immunosuppressive Medications for Autoimmune Disorders

Inflammatory and autoimmune disorders, like rheumatoid arthritis and spondyloarthropathies, are often treated with non-specific immunosuppressive medications, such as methotrexate, cyclophosphamide, azathioprine, cyclosporine, and corticosteroids. These non-specific immunosuppressive agents, however, are associated with an increased risk and frequency of developing TB [45, 46]. Biological disease-modifying anti-rheumatic drugs (bDMARDs) like tumor necrosis factor alpha (TNF-alpha) inhibitors, for rheumatoid arthritis and spondyloarthropathies, are also linked to an increased risk of developing TB [47–58]. TNF-alpha inhibitors include anti-TNF-alpha monoclonal antibodies (i.e., infliximab, adalimumab) and

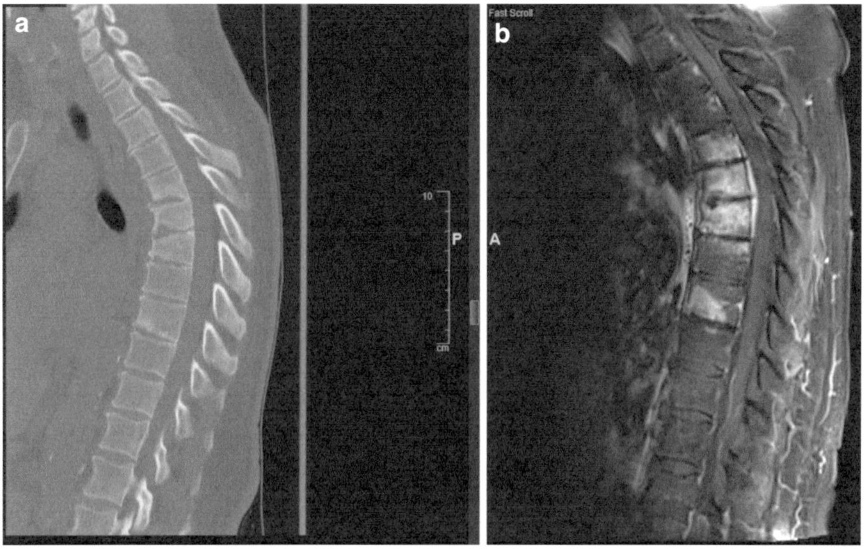

Fig. 26.3 (**a**) CT and (**b**) MRI T1-weighted of a rheumatoid arthritis patient on bDMARDs with spinal TB affecting thoracic spine T5-T9

etanercept – a fusion protein that serves as a decoy receptor for TNF-alpha. Interestingly, etanercept has a lower risk of developing TB than the anti-TNF-alpha monoclonal antibodies [51, 56, 59]. Figure 26.3 demonstrates the CT and MRI findings of a patient with rheumatoid arthritis on bDMARDs who developed spinal TB.

26.1.2.1 TNF-Alpha and Host Defenses

Once infected with TB, the host immune system initiates chronic inflammation through a granulomatous response whereby TB bacilli are "walled off" in granulomas comprised of a central core of activated macrophages—epithelioid cells—surrounded by multinucleated giant cells, caseating necrotic debris, and lymphocytes [60]. TNF-alpha, a cytokine, maintains this granulomatous inflammation by recruiting and stimulating macrophages to form epithelioid and giant cells [61–63]. In addition, TNF-alpha aids macrophages in containing and growing TB bacilli [64, 65].

Therefore, TNF-alpha inhibitors can cause sequestering granulomas to break down and reactivate latent TB, or secondary tuberculosis. Secondary tuberculosis represents most cases of TB associated with TNF-alpha inhibitors; however, there are a minority of cases in which TNF-alpha inhibitors cause progressive primary tuberculosis especially in severely ill patients, like those with AIDS or malnutrition. Both instances may lead to bacteremia and dissemination to multiple organ systems, including the spine. In fact, patients with TB in association with immunosuppression including TNF-alpha inhibitors have a higher likelihood of presenting with extrapulmonary involvement and hematogenous spread compared to patients with TB in the absence of immunosuppression [66–69].

26.1.2.2 Ankylosing Spondylitis and Other Spondyloarthropathies

Ankylosing spondylitis (AS) is a type of inflammatory, seronegative spondyloarthropathy characterized by arthritic pain commonly affecting the sacroiliac joints and spine, leading to kyphosis [70, 71]. Just like in rheumatoid arthritis, TNF-alpha inhibitors may be used for treatment of AS. Hence, AS patients treated with TNF-alpha inhibitors may present with reactivation of latent TB [58]. Screening for latent TB infection prior to starting TNF-alpha inhibitors using a tuberculin skin test or chest X-ray may result in a false negative if patients are immunosuppressed, such as on steroid therapy. Thus, it is recommended to screen for latent TB infection prior to starting TNF-alpha inhibitors using the QuantiFERON test, especially in immunosuppressed patients.

Diagnosing spinal TB in AS patients may be difficult because non-specific complaints such as inflammatory back pain are treated initially for AS due to sacroiliitis and spondylitis. Common symptoms of AS with spinal TB include dorsalgia, impaired spinal mobility, low-grade fever, worsening kyphosis, weight loss, and partial paraplegia [72]. Out of all of these symptoms, dorsalgia is the most common. Patients with AS alone have an increased risk of fracturing the spine from normal loads and osteoporosis compared to a healthy spine [73]. Patients with AS and spinal TB, both affecting the anterior column predominantly, have an even greater risk of fracturing the spine from normal loads and minor trauma due to the added risk of spinal cord compression from the spinal TB [74, 75]. Thus, it is crucial to diagnose spinal TB in AS patients as early as possible.

26.2 Pregnancy

TB significantly impacts pregnant women around the world. In 2011, around 200,000 cases of active TB affected pregnant women. The majority of these cases were in Africa and Southeast Asia; however, a substantial number of these cases occurred in the United States as well [76]. From 2003–2011, 26.6 out of every 100,000 births in the United States were associated with TB during pregnancy [77].

Pregnancy does not appear to influence TB pathogenesis, the risk of progression from latent to active disease, or response to anti-mycobacterial treatment [78–84]. Maternal active TB and postpartum active TB, however, in rare cases may spread to infants and is associated with significant perinatal mortality [85].

Early diagnosis of spinal TB in pregnant women proves challenging. Radiographic imaging is often delayed in order to protect the fetus [86, 87]. MRI should be used as diagnostic imaging for spinal TB in pregnant women during any stage of pregnancy since the lack of ionizing radiation poses no threat to the fetus. Non-specific symptoms of malaise and fatigue can present in both pregnancy and active TB, making it easier for pregnancy to mask underlying TB and increase the likelihood of extra-pulmonary expansion and more severe disease manifestations, including spinal TB [88–93]. The weight loss that is typically noted with TB may also be "hidden" due to the normal weight gain associated with pregnancy. Because of these non-specific or masking symptoms of early pregnancy, most pregnant women with spinal TB do not seek medical advice until late in pregnancy with more severe symptoms present like lower back pain, spinal deformity and injury, or neurological signs [4]. If left untreated, severe neurological symptoms, like paraplegia, may increase the risk of developing other life-threatening conditions such as urinary tract infection, decubitus ulcers, preterm labor, and autonomic hyperreflexia [87].

26.2.1 Treatment of Pregnant Women with TB

26.2.1.1 General Treatment of TB in Pregnant Women

Treating the underlying TB infection in pregnant women depends on whether the infection is latent or active and whether the woman is co-infected with HIV or not. For latent TB infection, both HIV-uninfected women and HIV-infected women in low-incidence settings should be treated with the preferred treatment of isoniazid (5 mg/kg [up to 300 mg] daily) for 9 months [94]. For latent TB infection in HIV-infected women in high-incidence settings, the preferred daily dose for isoniazid should be administered for at least 36 months. Pregnant women who are diagnosed with active TB should be treated immediately; untreated active TB is associated with a greater risk of adverse maternal and fetal outcomes than is treatment with anti-mycobacterial therapy [95]. Pregnant women with active TB may be treated with a regimen of isoniazid, rifampin, and ethambutol for the first 2 months followed by only isoniazid and rifampin for another 7 months, for a total of 9 months of treatment [80, 96, 97]. Isoniazid, rifampin, and ethambutol are not associated with adverse effects in the mother or fetus [98]. Pyrazinamide is not usually given to pregnant women, nor is it necessary, in the United States due to limited teratogenic data; however, the World Health Organization recommends the use of pyrazinamide even in pregnant women [82, 99, 100]. Pyrazinamide may be considered as part of the regimen especially when pregnant women are co-infected with HIV or show extra-pulmonary involvement, including the spine.

26.2.1.2 Treatment for Spinal TB in Pregnant Women

Treatment of spinal TB in pregnant women involves the same regimen of anti-mycobacterial therapy used in the general treatment of active TB in pregnant women; however, we must also consider surgical intervention if neurological deficits are present. Pregnant women with spinal TB but no neurological deficits may be treated with the conservative anti-mycobacterial regiment and stabilized with a brace [101]. Early surgical decompression of spinal TB, even during pregnancy, to prevent severe vertebral instability and paralysis may result in favorable prognosis and a stable outcome of pregnancy [102–104]. In pregnant women with spinal TB and progressive neurological deficits, there is no general consensus on the timing and nature of surgical intervention [103, 105]. Recommendations for spinal surgery, in general, for pregnant women with progressive neurological deficits include (a) induction of labor or C-section prior to spinal surgery at 34 weeks of gestation or later and (b) prepartum spinal surgery, in order to avoid morbidity in delivering a fetus prematurely, at gestation age earlier than 34 weeks [106].

There are various specific recommendations for performing surgery to treat pregnant women with spinal TB. In the first trimester, pregnant women can be placed in the ventral decubitus position [106]. In the second and third trimester, pregnant women should be placed on the left lateral decubitus position in order to avoid aortocaval compression syndrome by the gravid uterus when a pregnant woman lies on her back [106, 107]. Aortocaval compression syndrome may lead to severe hypotension and hemodynamic instability. A ventral debridement and posterior instrumented fusion is recommended [108]. If there is substantial vertebral body destruction and spinal instability, anterior reconstruction may be included [109, 110].

26.3 Spinal Metastasis or Spinal Primary Tumors

In higher income countries, where TB is not endemic, medical recognition of Pott's disease has decreased more than the incidence of spinal TB itself and is often overlooked in the differential diagnosis of spinal lesions leading to diagnostic delays, errors, morbidity, and even death [111–114]. Spinal TB is often overlooked in favor of spinal primary tumors or spinal metastasis even though spinal TB continues to be more common than primary spinal tumors, even in North America [114]. Spinal TB can mimic spinal metastasis from the prostate, thyroid, and lung [115–118]. If spinal TB is mistakenly diagnosed as neoplastic and chemotherapy is initiated, the chemotherapy-induced immunosuppression may further complicate the underlying TB. If spinal TB is caught too late, the disease may have progressed to severe neurologic complications like paresis or paraplegia.

26.3.1 Typical Features of Spinal TB

Classically, spinal TB presents as continuous involvement of two or more adjacent vertebral bodies and intervening vertebral discs. Vertebral lesions are typically paradiskal, and for that reason, tend to also involve the intervertebral discs and cause disc space narrowing. Paradiskal lesions involve the intervertebral disc directly or indirectly. Indirect involvement of the disc results from damage to the subchondral bone and disc herniation [116]. Spinal TB is typically located in the thoracolumbar region and rarely in the sacral region [119]. So, if a spinal lesion involves the sacral region, a diagnosis of chordoma or chondrosarcoma is made more often than one of spinal TB. Skip lesions, or noncontiguous involvement, is more common in neoplastic spinal disease. Grossly, spinal TB lesions usually present with paravertebral abscess or pus formation which helps distinguish from a solid spinal tumor. On imaging, spinal TB demonstrates predominantly anterior vertebral body destruction, reduced disc height, end plate erosion, sclerosis, paravertebral masses, and calcification of paraspinal masses [120]. Involvement from the vertebral bodies may extend to the pedicles and neural arch [113, 120]. Several case reports and case series, though, have demonstrated up to 25% of cases of spinal TB with atypical features rather than the classic presentation [111–114, 121–131].

26.3.2 Atypical Features of Spinal TB

Atypical features of spinal TB are rare and include (1) involvement of the posterior components (neural arch) of the vertebral column with or without involvement of the typical anterior components (vertebral bodies and discs) [111–113, 121–133], (2) skip lesions, where two or more sections of spinal TB are separated by uninvolved vertebrae [121, 122, 129, 132–134], (3) extradural compression of the spinal cord with no radiographic proof of bony involvement [112, 122], (4) single body disease [112, 114], and (5) a palpable pelvic mass and consequent destruction of the sacrum [123]. Involvement of only the neural arch and noncontiguous vertebral involvement with a large enough separation to involve only the two extremities of the spine, cervical and sacral, are even rarer [123]. If only the neural arch is involved, hence no involvement of the vertebral bodies or intervertebral discs, these patients may not present with the classic presentation of vertebral collapse, compression fracture, vertebral wedging, or kyphosis or the classic symptoms of nerve root compression or intercostal pain [111–113, 123]. One case report demonstrated a single patient presenting with spinal TB with four of these five atypical features – involvement of the neural arch only, skip lesions including both the sacrum and cervical spine, extradural compression of the spinal cord with no bony involvement on radiography, and a destructive, palpable mass in the sacrum [123]. Atypical spinal TB lesions may further confuse clinicians and point to a tumor rather than TB if the lesions do not present with abscess or pus formation [123, 134]. Other atypical findings may include anterior subperiosteal lesions, central vertebral lesions, reactive sclerosis, intra-spinal lesions, and syrinx formation [135–137]. Anterior vertebral lesions degrade the periosteum across several vertebral segments resulting in avascularity and anterior scalloping. Central lesions may collapse the vertebrae while preserving the disc, mimicking lymphoma or metastasis [116]. Figure 26.4 highlights several atypical features of spinal TB including sacral involvement, isolated involvement of the neural arch, and skip lesions [123, 138, 139].

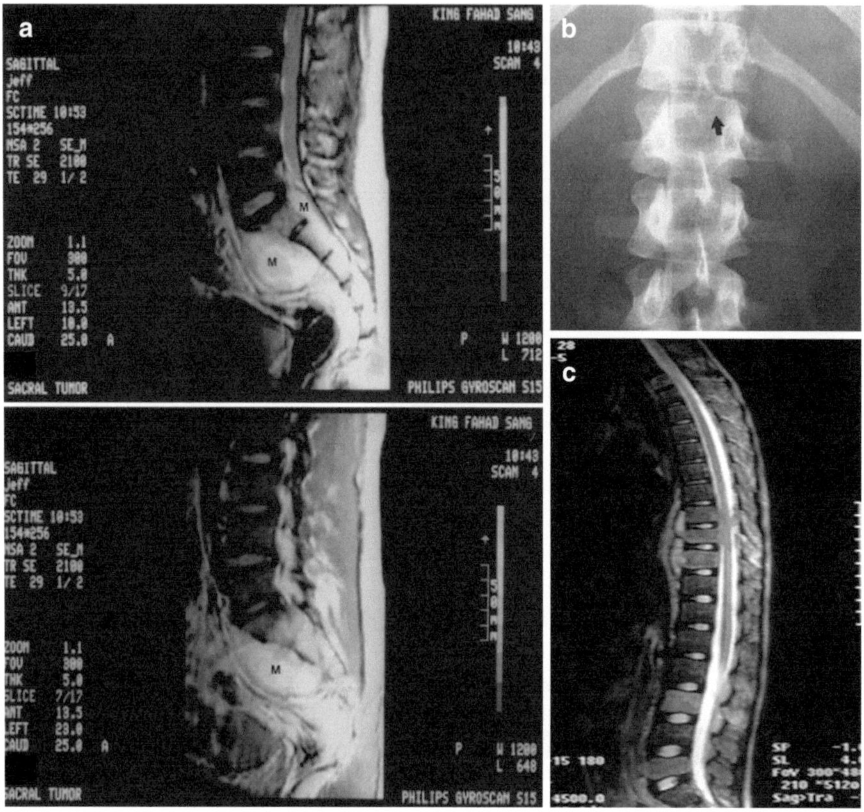

Fig. 26.4 Atypical features of spinal TB: (**a**) shows involvement and erosion of the sacrum, (**b**) shows isolated involvement of the neural arch including the spinous process and left lamina, and (**c**) shows multiple skip lesions. (Reproduced from Naim-Ur-Rahman et al. [123], Ragland et al. [138], and Sharma et al. [139])

As a result of increasing rates of immigration from TB-endemic countries and increasing prevalence of immunocompromised patients, clinicians should have TB on their differential diagnosis of spinal lesions. Spinal surgeons across the world, even where TB is less endemic, must recognize both typical and atypical spinal presentations of TB in order to include spinal TB in their differential diagnosis of primary and metastatic spinal tumors. If there is any suspicion of spinal TB, clinicians should biopsy the lesion(s) and assess the histopathology and culture. By expanding the differential diagnosis to include atypical spinal TB presentations, patients with atypical spinal TB may receive a diagnosis at an earlier stage of the disease rather than at a later stage of irreversible neurological impairments and spinal deformities.

26.4 Polytrauma

Polytrauma is a term used to describe multiple severe injuries in multiple parts of the body leading to shock and/or hemorrhagic hypotension [140]. In rare cases, polytrauma involving the spine has been associated with the development of spinal TB [141]. Polytrauma may increase the likelihood of developing spinal TB, or TB in general, since trauma suppresses CD4+ T-cell responses which are crucial in the containment of TB [142–145].

References

1. Sonnenberg P, Glynn JR, Fielding K, Murray J, Godfrey-Faussett P, Shearer S. How soon after infection with HIV does the risk of tuberculosis start to increase? a retrospective cohort study in South African gold miners. J Infect Dis. 2005;191(2):150–8. https://doi.org/10.1086/426827. Epub 2004 Dec 13
2. Getahun H, Gunneberg C, Granich R, Nunn P. HIV infection-associated tuberculosis: the epidemiology and the response. Clin Infect Dis. 2010;50(Suppl 3):S201–7. https://doi.org/10.1086/651492.
3. Bell LCK, Noursadeghi M. Pathogenesis of HIV-1 and Mycobacterium tuberculosis co-infection. Nat Rev Microbiol. 2018;16(2):80–90. https://doi.org/10.1038/nrmicro.2017.128. Epub 2017 Nov 7
4. Garg RK, Somvanshi DS. Spinal tuberculosis: a review. J Spinal Cord Med. 2011;34(5):440–54. https://doi.org/10.1179/2045772311Y.0000000023.
5. Agrawal V, Patgaonkar PR, Nagariya SP. Tuberculosis of spine. J Craniovertebr Junction Spine. 2010;1(2):74–85. https://doi.org/10.4103/0974-8237.77671.
6. Peddireddy V, Doddam SN, Ahmed N. Mycobacterial dormancy systems and host responses in tuberculosis. Front Immunol. 2017;8:84. https://doi.org/10.3389/fimmu.2017.00084.
7. Kleinnijenhuis J, Oosting M, Joosten LA, Netea MG, Van Crevel R. Innate immune recognition of Mycobacterium tuberculosis. Clin Dev Immunol. 2011;2011:405310. https://doi.org/10.1155/2011/405310. Epub 2011 Apr 7
8. Watson RO, Bell SL, MacDuff DA, Kimmey JM, Diner EJ, Olivas J, Vance RE, Stallings CL, Virgin HW, Cox JS. The cytosolic sensor cGAS detects Mycobacterium tuberculosis DNA to induce type I interferons and activate autophagy. Cell Host Microbe. 2015;17(6):811–9. https://doi.org/10.1016/j.chom.2015.05.004. Epub 2015 Jun 2
9. Al-Muhsen S, Casanova JL. The genetic heterogeneity of mendelian susceptibility to mycobacterial diseases. J Allergy Clin Immunol. 2008;122(6):1043–51; quiz 1052-3. https://doi.org/10.1016/j.jaci.2008.10.037.
10. Bezuidenhout J, Roberts T, Muller L, van Helden P, Walzl G. Pleural tuberculosis in patients with early HIV infection is associated with increased TNF-alpha expression and necrosis in granulomas. PLoS One. 2009;4(1):e4228. https://doi.org/10.1371/journal.pone.0004228. Epub 2009 Jan 19
11. de Noronha AL, Báfica A, Nogueira L, Barral A, Barral-Netto M. Lung granulomas from Mycobacterium tuberculosis/HIV-1 co-infected patients display decreased in situ TNF production. Pathol Res Pract. 2008;204(3):155–61. https://doi.org/10.1016/j.prp.2007.10.008. Epub 2007 Dec 21
12. Lawn SD, Butera ST, Shinnick TM. Tuberculosis unleashed: the impact of human immunodeficiency virus infection on the host granulomatous response to Mycobacterium tuberculosis. Microbes Infect. 2002;4(6):635–46. https://doi.org/10.1016/s1286-4579(02)01582-4.

13. Safi H, Gormus BJ, Didier PJ, Blanchard JL, Lakey DL, Martin LN, Murphey-Corb M, Vankayalapati R, Barnes PF. Spectrum of manifestations of Mycobacterium tuberculosis infection in primates infected with SIV. AIDS Res Hum Retrovir. 2003;19(7):585–95. https://doi.org/10.1089/088922203322230950.
14. Shen JY, Barnes PF, Rea TH, Meyer PR. Immunohistology of tuberculous adenitis in symptomatic HIV infection. Clin Exp Immunol. 1988;72(2):186–9.
15. Diedrich CR, Flynn JL. HIV-1/mycobacterium tuberculosis coinfection immunology: how does HIV-1 exacerbate tuberculosis? Infect Immun. 2011;79(4):1407–17. https://doi.org/10.1128/IAI.01126-10. Epub 2011 Jan 18
16. Goletti D, Weissman D, Jackson RW, Collins F, Kinter A, Fauci AS. The in vitro induction of human immunodeficiency virus (HIV) replication in purified protein derivative-positive HIV-infected persons by recall antigen response to Mycobacterium tuberculosis is the result of a balance of the effects of endogenous interleukin-2 and proinflammatory and antiinflammatory cytokines. J Infect Dis. 1998;177(5):1332–8. https://doi.org/10.1086/515276.
17. Hoshino Y, Hoshino S, Gold JA, Raju B, Prabhakar S, Pine R, Rom WN, Nakata K, Weiden M. Mechanisms of polymorphonuclear neutrophil-mediated induction of HIV-1 replication in macrophages during pulmonary tuberculosis. J Infect Dis. 2007;195(9):1303–10. https://doi.org/10.1086/513438. Epub 2007 Mar 19
18. Hoshino Y, Nakata K, Hoshino S, Honda Y, Tse DB, Shioda T, Rom WN, Weiden M. Maximal HIV-1 replication in alveolar macrophages during tuberculosis requires both lymphocyte contact and cytokines. J Exp Med. 2002;195(4):495–505. https://doi.org/10.1084/jem.20011614.
19. Ranjbar S, Boshoff HI, Mulder A, Siddiqi N, Rubin EJ, Goldfeld AE. HIV-1 replication is differentially regulated by distinct clinical strains of Mycobacterium tuberculosis. PLoS One. 2009;4(7):e6116. https://doi.org/10.1371/journal.pone.0006116.
20. Brenchley JM, Schacker TW, Ruff LE, Price DA, Taylor JH, Beilman GJ, Nguyen PL, Khoruts A, Larson M, Haase AT, Douek DC. CD4+ T cell depletion during all stages of HIV disease occurs predominantly in the gastrointestinal tract. J Exp Med. 2004;200(6):749–59. https://doi.org/10.1084/jem.20040874. Epub 2004 Sep 13
21. Centlivre M, Sala M, Wain-Hobson S, Berkhout B. In HIV-1 pathogenesis the die is cast during primary infection. AIDS. 2007;21(1):1–11. https://doi.org/10.1097/QAD.0b013e3280117f7f.
22. Li Q, Duan L, Estes JD, Ma ZM, Rourke T, Wang Y, Reilly C, Carlis J, Miller CJ, Haase AT. Peak SIV replication in resting memory CD4+ T cells depletes gut lamina propria CD4+ T cells. Nature. 2005;434(7037):1148–52. https://doi.org/10.1038/nature03513.
23. Mattapallil JJ, Douek DC, Hill B, Nishimura Y, Martin M, Roederer M. Massive infection and loss of memory CD4+ T cells in multiple tissues during acute SIV infection. Nature. 2005;434(7037):1093–7. https://doi.org/10.1038/nature03501.
24. Schneider T, Jahn HU, Schmidt W, Riecken EO, Zeitz M, Ullrich R. Loss of CD4 T lymphocytes in patients infected with human immunodeficiency virus type 1 is more pronounced in the duodenal mucosa than in the peripheral blood. Berlin Diarrhea/Wasting Syndrome Study Group Gut. 1995;37(4):524–9. https://doi.org/10.1136/gut.37.4.524.
25. Veazey RS, Tham IC, Mansfield KG, DeMaria M, Forand AE, Shvetz DE, Chalifoux LV, Sehgal PK, Lackner AA. Identifying the target cell in primary simian immunodeficiency virus (SIV) infection: highly activated memory CD4(+) T cells are rapidly eliminated in early SIV infection in vivo. J Virol. 2000;74(1):57–64. https://doi.org/10.1128/jvi.74.1.57-64.2000.
26. Law KF, Jagirdar J, Weiden MD, Bodkin M, Rom WN. Tuberculosis in HIV-positive patients: cellular response and immune activation in the lung. Am J Respir Crit Care Med. 1996;153(4 Pt 1):1377–84. https://doi.org/10.1164/ajrccm.153.4.8616569.
27. Bell LC, Pollara G, Pascoe M, Tomlinson GS, Lehloenya RJ, Roe J, Meldau R, Miller RF, Ramsay A, Chain BM, Dheda K, Noursadeghi M. In vivo molecular dissection of the effects of HIV-1 in active tuberculosis. PLoS Pathog. 2016;12(3):e1005469. https://doi.org/10.1371/journal.ppat.1005469.

28. Kalsdorf B, Scriba TJ, Wood K, Day CL, Dheda K, Dawson R, Hanekom WA, Lange C, Wilkinson RJ. HIV-1 infection impairs the bronchoalveolar T-cell response to mycobacteria. Am J Respir Crit Care Med. 2009;180(12):1262–70. https://doi.org/10.1164/rccm.200907-1011OC. Epub 2009 Sep 24
29. Geldmacher C, Ngwenyama N, Schuetz A, Petrovas C, Reither K, Heeregrave EJ, Casazza JP, Ambrozak DR, Louder M, Ampofo W, Pollakis G, Hill B, Sanga E, Saathoff E, Maboko L, Roederer M, Paxton WA, Hoelscher M, Koup RA. Preferential infection and depletion of Mycobacterium tuberculosis-specific CD4 T cells after HIV-1 infection. J Exp Med. 2010;207(13):2869–81. https://doi.org/10.1084/jem.20100090. Epub 2010 Nov 29
30. Lawn SD, Myer L, Edwards D, Bekker LG, Wood R. Short-term and long-term risk of tuberculosis associated with CD4 cell recovery during antiretroviral therapy in South Africa. AIDS. 2009;23(13):1717–25. https://doi.org/10.1097/QAD.0b013e32832d3b6d.
31. Montezuma-Rusca JM, Moir S, Kardava L, Buckner CM, Louie A, Kim LJ, Santich BH, Wang W, Fankuchen OR, Diaz G, Daub JR, Rosenzweig SD, Chun TW, Li Y, Braylan RC, Calvo KR, Fauci AS. Bone marrow plasma cells are a primary source of serum HIV-1-specific antibodies in chronically infected individuals. J Immunol. 2015;194(6):2561–8. https://doi.org/10.4049/jimmunol.1402424. Epub 2015 Feb 13
32. Tomaras GD, Haynes BF. HIV-1-specific antibody responses during acute and chronic HIV-1 infection. Curr Opin HIV AIDS. 2009;4(5):373–9. https://doi.org/10.1097/COH.0b013e32832f00c0.
33. Bhattacharya D, Danaviah S, Muema DM, Akilimali NA, Moodley P, Ndung'u T, Das G. Cellular architecture of spinal granulomas and the immunological response in tuberculosis patients coinfected with HIV. Front Immunol. 2017;8:1120. https://doi.org/10.3389/fimmu.2017.01120.
34. Patel NR, Swan K, Li X, Tachado SD, Koziel HM. Impaired tuberculosis-mediated apoptosis in alveolar macrophages from HIV+ persons: potential role of IL-10 and BCL-3. J Leukoc Biol. 2009;86(1):53–60. https://doi.org/10.1189/jlb.0908574. Epub 2009 Apr 21
35. Patel NR, Zhu J, Tachado SD, Zhang J, Wan Z, Saukkonen J, Koziel H. HIV impairs TNF-alpha mediated macrophage apoptotic response to Mycobacterium tuberculosis. J Immunol. 2007;179(10):6973–80. https://doi.org/10.4049/jimmunol.179.10.6973.
36. Deretic V, Vergne I, Chua J, Master S, Singh SB, Fazio JA, Kyei G. Endosomal membrane traffic: convergence point targeted by Mycobacterium tuberculosis and HIV. Cell Microbiol. 2004;6(11):999–1009. https://doi.org/10.1111/j.1462-5822.2004.00449.x.
37. Mwandumba HC, Russell DG, Nyirenda MH, Anderson J, White SA, Molyneux ME, Squire SB. Mycobacterium tuberculosis resides in nonacidified vacuoles in endocytically competent alveolar macrophages from patients with tuberculosis and HIV infection. J Immunol. 2004;172(7):4592–8. https://doi.org/10.4049/jimmunol.172.7.4592.
38. Zhang M, Gong J, Iyer DV, Jones BE, Modlin RL, Barnes PF. T cell cytokine responses in persons with tuberculosis and human immunodeficiency virus infection. J Clin Invest. 1994;94(6):2435–42. https://doi.org/10.1172/JCI117611.
39. Hertoghe T, Wajja A, Ntambi L, Okwera A, Aziz MA, Hirsch C, Johnson J, Toossi Z, Mugerwa R, Mugyenyi P, Colebunders R, Ellner J, Vanham G. T cell activation, apoptosis and cytokine dysregulation in the (co)pathogenesis of HIV and pulmonary tuberculosis (TB). Clin Exp Immunol. 2000;122(3):350–7. https://doi.org/10.1046/j.1365-2249.2000.01385.x.
40. Shelburne SA 3rd, Hamill RJ, Rodriguez-Barradas MC, Greenberg SB, Atmar RL, Musher DW, Gathe JC Jr, Visnegarwala F, Trautner BW. Immune reconstitution inflammatory syndrome: emergence of a unique syndrome during highly active antiretroviral therapy. Medicine (Baltimore). 2002;81(3):213–27. https://doi.org/10.1097/00005792-200205000-00005.
41. Leonard JM. Central nervous system tuberculosis. Microbiol Spectr. 2017;5(2) https://doi.org/10.1128/microbiolspec.TNMI7-0044-2017.
42. Sagane SS, Patil VS, Bartakke GD, Kale KY. Assessment of clinical and radiological parameters in spinal tuberculosis: comparison between human immunodeficiency virus-positive

and human immunodeficiency virus-negative patients. Asian Spine J. 2020;14(6):857–63. https://doi.org/10.31616/asj.2019.0251. Epub 2020 Mar 13

43. Marais S, Roos I, Mitha A, Mabusha SJ, Patel V, Bhigjee AI. Spinal tuberculosis: clinicoradiological findings in 274 patients. Clin Infect Dis. 2018;67(1):89–98. https://doi.org/10.1093/cid/ciy020.
44. Anley CM, Brandt AD, Dunn R. Magnetic resonance imaging findings in spinal tuberculosis: comparison of HIV positive and negative patients. Indian J Orthop. 2012;46(2):186–90. https://doi.org/10.4103/0019-5413.93688.
45. Chung TT, Ko HJ, Lau CS, Chung HY. A retrospective study on the risk of tuberculosis in patients with rheumatoid arthritis. Rheumatol Int. 2020;40(6):983–90. https://doi.org/10.1007/s00296-020-04583-8.
46. Carmona L, Hernández-García C, Vadillo C, Pato E, Balsa A, González-Alvaro I, Belmonte MA, Tena X, Sanmartí R, EMECAR Study Group. Increased risk of tuberculosis in patients with rheumatoid arthritis. J Rheumatol. 2003;30(7):1436–9.
47. Bongartz T, Sutton AJ, Sweeting MJ, Buchan I, Matteson EL, Montori V. Anti-TNF antibody therapy in rheumatoid arthritis and the risk of serious infections and malignancies: systematic review and meta-analysis of rare harmful effects in randomized controlled trials. JAMA. 2006;295(19):2275–85. https://doi.org/10.1001/jama.295.19.2275. Erratum in: JAMA. 2006 Jun 7;295(21):2482
48. Keane J, Gershon S, Wise RP, Mirabile-Levens E, Kasznica J, Schwieterman WD, Siegel JN, Braun MM. Tuberculosis associated with infliximab, a tumor necrosis factor alpha-neutralizing agent. N Engl J Med. 2001;345(15):1098–104. https://doi.org/10.1056/NEJMoa011110.
49. Gómez-Reino JJ, Carmona L, Valverde VR, Mola EM. Montero MD; BIOBADASER Group. Treatment of rheumatoid arthritis with tumor necrosis factor inhibitors may predispose to significant increase in tuberculosis risk: a multicenter active-surveillance report. Arthritis Rheum. 2003;48(8):2122–7. https://doi.org/10.1002/art.11137.
50. Fonseca JE, Canhão H, Silva C, Miguel C, Mediavilla MJ, Teixeira A, Castelão W, Nero P, Bernardes M, Bernardo A, Mariz E, Godinho F, Santos MJ, Bogas M, Oliveira M, Saavedra MJ, Barcelos A, Cruz M, Santos RA, Maurício L, Rodrigues M, Figueiredo G, Quintal A, Patto JV, Malcata A, da Silva JC, Araújo D, Ventura F, Branco J, Queiroz MV. Grupo de Estudos de Artrite Reumatóide da Sociedade Portuguesa de Reumatologia. Tubereulose em doentes reumáticos tratados com antagonistas do factor de necrose tumoral alfa: a experiência Portuguesa [Tuberculosis in rheumatic patients treated with tumour necrosis factor alpha antagonists: the Portuguese experience]. Acta Reumatol Port. 2006;31(3):247–53. Portuguese
51. Brassard P, Kezouh A, Suissa S. Antirheumatic drugs and the risk of tuberculosis. Clin Infect Dis. 2006;43(6):717–22. https://doi.org/10.1086/506935. Epub 2006 Aug 10
52. Wallis RS, Broder MS, Wong JY, Hanson ME, Beenhouwer DO. Granulomatous infectious diseases associated with tumor necrosis factor antagonists. Clin Infect Dis. 2004;38(9):1261–5. https://doi.org/10.1086/383317. Epub 2004 Apr 15
53. Wallis RS, Broder M, Wong J, Beenhouwer D. Granulomatous infections due to tumor necrosis factor blockade: correction. Clin Infect Dis. 2004;39(8):1254–5. https://doi.org/10.1086/424455.
54. Askling J, Fored CM, Brandt L, Baecklund E, Bertilsson L, Cöster L, Geborek P, Jacobsson LT, Lindblad S, Lysholm J, Rantapää-Dahlqvist S, Saxne T, Romanus V, Klareskog L, Feltelius N. Risk and case characteristics of tuberculosis in rheumatoid arthritis associated with tumor necrosis factor antagonists in Sweden. Arthritis Rheum. 2005;52(7):1986–92. https://doi.org/10.1002/art.21137.
55. Dixon WG, Watson K, Lunt M, Hyrich KL, Silman AJ, Symmons DP, British Society for Rheumatology Biologics Register. Rates of serious infection, including site-specific and bacterial intracellular infection, in rheumatoid arthritis patients receiving anti-tumor necrosis factor therapy: results from the British Society for Rheumatology Biologics Register. Arthritis Rheum. 2006;54(8):2368–76. https://doi.org/10.1002/art.21978.

56. Tubach F, Salmon D, Ravaud P, Allanore Y, Goupille P, Bréban M, Pallot-Prades B, Pouplin S, Sacchi A, Chichemanian RM, Bretagne S, Emilie D, Lemann M, Lortholary O, Mariette X, Research Axed on Tolerance of Biotherapies Group. Risk of tuberculosis is higher with anti-tumor necrosis factor monoclonal antibody therapy than with soluble tumor necrosis factor receptor therapy: The three-year prospective French Research Axed on Tolerance of Biotherapies registry. Arthritis Rheum. 2009;60(7):1884–94. https://doi.org/10.1002/art.24632. Erratum in: Arthritis Rheum. 2009 Aug;60(8):2540. Lorthololary, O [corrected to Lortholary, O]
57. Winthrop KL, Baxter R, Liu L, Varley CD, Curtis JR, Baddley JW, McFarland B, Austin D, Radcliffe L, Suhler E, Choi D, Rosenbaum JT, Herrinton LJ. Mycobacterial diseases and antitumour necrosis factor therapy in USA. Ann Rheum Dis. 2013;72(1):37–42. https://doi.org/10.1136/annrheumdis-2011-200690. Epub 2012 Apr 20
58. Yoo WH. Multiple organ tuberculosis of lung, pleura, and peritoneum in ankylosing spondylitis during adalimumab therapy. Rheumatol Int. 2012;32(3):787–90. https://doi.org/10.1007/s00296-009-1357-x. Epub 2010 Jan 5
59. Dixon WG, Hyrich KL, Watson KD, Lunt M, Galloway J, Ustianowski A, B S R B R Control Centre Consortium, Symmons DP, BSR Biologics Register. Drug-specific risk of tuberculosis in patients with rheumatoid arthritis treated with anti-TNF therapy: results from the British Society for Rheumatology Biologics Register (BSRBR). Ann Rheum Dis. 2010;69(3):522–8. https://doi.org/10.1136/ard.2009.118935. Epub 2009 Oct 22
60. Randhawa PS. Lymphocyte subsets in granulomas of human tuberculosis: an in situ immunofluorescence study using monoclonal antibodies. Pathology. 1990;22(3):153–5. https://doi.org/10.3109/00313029009063555.
61. Algood HM, Lin PL, Flynn JL. Tumor necrosis factor and chemokine interactions in the formation and maintenance of granulomas in tuberculosis. Clin Infect Dis. 2005;41(Suppl 3):S189–93. https://doi.org/10.1086/429994.
62. Gardam MA, Keystone EC, Menzies R, Manners S, Skamene E, Long R, Vinh DC. Anti-tumour necrosis factor agents and tuberculosis risk: mechanisms of action and clinical management. Lancet Infect Dis. 2003;3(3):148–55. https://doi.org/10.1016/s1473-3099(03)00545-0.
63. Lin PL, Myers A, Smith L, Bigbee C, Bigbee M, Fuhrman C, Grieser H, Chiosea I, Voitenek NN, Capuano SV, Klein E, Flynn JL. Tumor necrosis factor neutralization results in disseminated disease in acute and latent Mycobacterium tuberculosis infection with normal granuloma structure in a cynomolgus macaque model. Arthritis Rheum. 2010;62(2):340–50. https://doi.org/10.1002/art.27271.
64. Bekker LG, Freeman S, Murray PJ, Ryffel B, Kaplan G. TNF-alpha controls intracellular mycobacterial growth by both inducible nitric oxide synthase-dependent and inducible nitric oxide synthase-independent pathways. J Immunol. 2001;166(11):6728–34. https://doi.org/10.4049/jimmunol.166.11.6728.
65. Clay H, Volkman HE, Ramakrishnan L. Tumor necrosis factor signaling mediates resistance to mycobacteria by inhibiting bacterial growth and macrophage death. Immunity. 2008;29(2):283–94. https://doi.org/10.1016/j.immuni.2008.06.011.
66. Saliu OY, Sofer C, Stein DS, Schwander SK, Wallis RS. Tumor-necrosis-factor blockers: differential effects on mycobacterial immunity. J Infect Dis. 2006;194(4):486–92. https://doi.org/10.1086/505430. Epub 2006 Jul 10
67. Mohan AK, Coté TR, Block JA, Manadan AM, Siegel JN, Braun MM. Tuberculosis following the use of etanercept, a tumor necrosis factor inhibitor. Clin Infect Dis. 2004;39(3):295–9. https://doi.org/10.1086/421494. Epub 2004 Jul 16
68. Centers for Disease Control and Prevention (CDC). Tuberculosis associated with blocking agents against tumor necrosis factor-alpha—California, 2002–2003. MMWR Morb Mortal Wkly Rep. 2004;53(30):683–6.
69. Hill PC, Brookes RH, Fox A, Fielding K, Jeffries DJ, Jackson-Sillah D, Lugos MD, Owiafe PK, Donkor SA, Hammond AS, Otu JK, Corrah T, Adegbola RA, McAdam KP. Large-scale evaluation of enzyme-linked immunospot assay and skin test for diagnosis of Mycobacterium

tuberculosis infection against a gradient of exposure in The Gambia. Clin Infect Dis. 2004;38(7):966–73. https://doi.org/10.1086/382362. Epub 2004 Mar 16
70. Taurog JD, Chhabra A, Colbert RA. Ankylosing spondylitis and axial spondyloarthritis. N Engl J Med. 2016;375(13):1303. https://doi.org/10.1056/NEJMc1609622.
71. Xia Q, Fan D, Yang X, Li X, Zhang X, Wang M, Xu S, Pan F. Progression rate of ankylosing spondylitis in patients with undifferentiated spondyloarthritis: a systematic review and meta-analysis. Medicine (Baltimore). 2017;96(4):e5960. https://doi.org/10.1097/MD.0000000000005960.
72. Yin XH, Liu SC, Yang M, He BR, Liu ZK, Hao DJ. Posterior surgical treatment of ankylosing spondylitis with spinal tuberculosis: a case series and long-term follow-up. Medicine (Baltimore). 2018;97(34):e11925. https://doi.org/10.1097/MD.0000000000011925.
73. Cooper C, Carbone L, Michet CJ, Atkinson EJ, O'Fallon WM, Melton LJ 3rd. Fracture risk in patients with ankylosing spondylitis: a population based study. J Rheumatol. 1994;21(10):1877–82.
74. Hunter T, Dubo H. Spinal fractures complicating ankylosing spondylitis. Ann Intern Med. 1978;88(4):546–9. https://doi.org/10.7326/0003-4819-88-4-546.
75. Hunter T, Dubo HI. Spinal fractures complicating ankylosing spondylitis. A long-term followup study. Arthritis Rheum. 1983;26(6):751–9. https://doi.org/10.1002/art.1780260608.
76. Sugarman J, Colvin C, Moran AC, Oxlade O. Tuberculosis in pregnancy: an estimate of the global burden of disease. Lancet Glob Health. 2014;2(12):e710–6. https://doi.org/10.1016/S2214-109X(14)70330-4.
77. El-Messidi A, Czuzoj-Shulman N, Spence AR, Abenhaim HA. Medical and obstetric outcomes among pregnant women with tuberculosis: a population-based study of 7.8 million births. Am J Obstet Gynecol. 2016;215(6):797.e1–6. https://doi.org/10.1016/j.ajog.2016.08.009. Epub 2016 Aug 13
78. Snider D. Pregnancy and tuberculosis. Chest. 1984;86(3 Suppl):10S–3S. https://doi.org/10.1378/chest.86.3.10s.
79. Hamadeh MA, Glassroth J. Tuberculosis and pregnancy. Chest. 1992;101(4):1114–20. https://doi.org/10.1378/chest.101.4.1114.
80. Schaefer G, Zervoudakis IA, Fuchs FF, David S. Pregnancy and pulmonary tuberculosis. Obstet Gynecol. 1975;46(6):706–15.
81. Centers for Disease Control and Prevention (CDC). Tuberculosis among pregnant women—New York City, 1985–1992. MMWR Morb Mortal Wkly Rep. 1993;42(31):605, 611–2.
82. Davidson PT. Managing tuberculosis during pregnancy. Lancet. 1995;346(8969):199–200. https://doi.org/10.1016/s0140-6736(95)91263-0.
83. Espinal MA, Reingold AL, Lavandera M. Effect of pregnancy on the risk of developing active tuberculosis. J Infect Dis. 1996;173(2):488–91. https://doi.org/10.1093/infdis/173.2.488.
84. Miele K, Bamrah Morris S, Tepper NK. Tuberculosis in Pregnancy. Obstet Gynecol. 2020;135(6):1444–53. https://doi.org/10.1097/AOG.0000000000003890.
85. Loto OM, Awowole I. Tuberculosis in pregnancy: a review. J Pregnancy. 2012;2012:379271. https://doi.org/10.1155/2012/379271. Epub 2011 Nov 1
86. Jana N, Vasishta K, Saha SC, Ghosh K. Obstetrical outcomes among women with extrapulmonary tuberculosis. N Engl J Med. 1999;341(9):645–9. https://doi.org/10.1056/NEJM199908263410903.
87. Lowenstein L, Solt I, Fischer D, Drugan A. Spinal tuberculosis with paraplegia in pregnancy. Isr Med Assoc J. 2004;6(7):436–7.
88. Carter EJ, Mates S. Tuberculosis during pregnancy. The Rhode Island experience, 1987 to 1991. Chest. 1994;106(5):1466–70. https://doi.org/10.1378/chest.106.5.1466.
89. Ormerod P. Tuberculosis in pregnancy and the puerperium. Thorax. 2001;56(6):494–9. https://doi.org/10.1136/thorax.56.6.494.
90. Knight M, Kurinczuk JJ, Nelson-Piercy C, Spark P, Brocklehurst P, UKOSS. Tuberculosis in pregnancy in the UK. BJOG. 2009;116(4):584–8. https://doi.org/10.1111/j.1471-0528.2008.02097.x.

91. Kothari A, Mahadevan N, Girling J. Tuberculosis and pregnancy--Results of a study in a high prevalence area in London. Eur J Obstet Gynecol Reprod Biol. 2006;126(1):48–55. https://doi.org/10.1016/j.ejogrb.2005.07.025. Epub 2005 Sep 9
92. Wilson EA, Thelin TJ, Dilts PV Jr. Tuberculosis complicated by pregnancy. Am J Obstet Gynecol. 1973;115(4):526–9. https://doi.org/10.1016/0002-9378(73)90401-8.
93. Llewelyn M, Cropley I, Wilkinson RJ, Davidson RN. Tuberculosis diagnosed during pregnancy: a prospective study from London. Thorax. 2000;55(2):129–32. https://doi.org/10.1136/thorax.55.2.129.
94. American Thoracic Society. Targeted tuberculin testing and treatment of latent tuberculosis infection. MMWR Recomm Rep. 2000;49(RR-6):1–51.
95. Sobhy S, Babiker Z, Zamora J, Khan KS, Kunst H. Maternal and perinatal mortality and morbidity associated with tuberculosis during pregnancy and the postpartum period: a systematic review and meta-analysis. BJOG. 2017;124(5):727–33. https://doi.org/10.1111/1471-0528.14408. Epub 2016 Nov 11
96. Nahid P, Dorman SE, Alipanah N, Barry PM, Brozek JL, Cattamanchi A, Chaisson LH, Chaisson RE, Daley CL, Grzemska M, Higashi JM, Ho CS, Hopewell PC, Keshavjee SA, Lienhardt C, Menzies R, Merrifield C, Narita M, O'Brien R, Peloquin CA, Raftery A, Saukkonen J, Schaaf HS, Sotgiu G, Starke JR, Migliori GB, Vernon A. Official American Thoracic Society/Centers for Disease Control and Prevention/Infectious Diseases Society of America Clinical Practice Guidelines: Treatment of Drug-Susceptible Tuberculosis. Clin Infect Dis. 2016;63(7):e147–95. https://doi.org/10.1093/cid/ciw376. Epub 2016 Aug 10
97. Snider DE Jr, Layde PM, Johnson MW, Lyle MA. Treatment of tuberculosis during pregnancy. Am Rev Respir Dis. 1980;122(1):65–79. https://doi.org/10.1164/arrd.1980.122.1.65.
98. Mathad JS, Gupta A. Tuberculosis in pregnant and postpartum women: epidemiology, management, and research gaps. Clin Infect Dis. 2012;55(11):1532–49. https://doi.org/10.1093/cid/cis732. Epub 2012 Aug 31
99. Enarson DA, Rieder HL, Arnodottir T, Trebucq A. Management of tuberculosis: a guide for low income countries. 5th ed. Paris: International Union Against Tuberculosis and Lung Disease; 2000.
100. World Health Organization. Guidelines for treatment of tuberculosis, 4th edition. WHO, Geneva 2010. http://apps.who.int.proxy.cc.uic.edu/iris/bitstream/10665/44165/1/9789241547833_eng.pdf?ua=1&ua=1. Accessed 05 Oct 2016.
101. Rathod AK, Singh V, Patil P, Singh H. Is decompressive surgery the only treatment option? a case series of patients with spinal tuberculosis in advanced pregnancy. Eur Spine J. 2017;26(12):3170–7. https://doi.org/10.1007/s00586-017-5143-2. Epub 2017 May 22
102. Singh H, Singh J, Abdullah BT, Matthews A. Tuberculous paraplegia in pregnancy treated by surgery. Singap Med J. 2002;43(5):251–3.
103. Badve SA, Ghate SD, Badve MS, Rustagi T, Macchiwala T, Parekh AN, Shah SV. Tuberculosis of spine with neurological deficit in advanced pregnancy: a report of three cases. Spine J. 2011;11(1):e9–16. https://doi.org/10.1016/j.spinee.2010.11.003.
104. Kaul R, Chhabra HS, Kanagaraju V, Mahajan R, Tandon V, Nanda A, Sangondimath G, Patel N. Antepartum surgical management of Pott's paraplegia along with maintenance of pregnancy during second trimester. Eur Spine J. 2016;25(4):1064–9. https://doi.org/10.1007/s00586-015-4045-4. Epub 2015 Jun 25
105. Mak KC, Cheung KM. Surgical treatment of acute TB spondylitis: indications and outcomes. Eur Spine J. 2013;22(Suppl 4):603–11. https://doi.org/10.1007/s00586-012-2455-0. Epub 2012 Aug 16
106. Han IH, Kuh SU, Kim JH, Chin DK, Kim KS, Yoon YS, Jin BH, Cho YE. Clinical approach and surgical strategy for spinal diseases in pregnant women: a report of ten cases. Spine (Phila Pa 1976). 2008;33(17):E614–9. https://doi.org/10.1097/BRS.0b013e31817c6c7d.
107. Kanas M, Kunzle H, Martins DE, Kirsch LA, Puertas EB, Wajchenberg M. Diskectomy during pregnancy: case report and review of the literature. Global Spine J. 2015;5(2):130–4. https://doi.org/10.1055/s-0034-1387178. Epub 2014 Aug 6

108. Khoo LT, Mikawa K, Fessler RG. A surgical revisitation of Pott distemper of the spine. Spine J. 2003;3(2):130–45. https://doi.org/10.1016/s1529-9430(02)00410-2.
109. Khatri GR, Frieden TR. The status and prospects of tuberculosis control in India. Int J Tuberc Lung Dis. 2000;4(3):193–200.
110. Jain AK, Dhammi IK, Prashad B, Sinha S, Mishra P. Simultaneous anterior decompression and posterior instrumentation of the tuberculous spine using an anterolateral extrapleural approach. J Bone Joint Surg (Br). 2008;90(11):1477–81. https://doi.org/10.1302/0301-620X.90B11.20972.
111. Naim-ur-Rahman. Atypical forms of spinal tuberculosis. J Bone Joint Surg (Br). 1980;62-B(2):162–5. https://doi.org/10.1302/0301-620X.62B2.7364827.
112. Naim-Ur-Rahman A-AKM, Khan FA. Atypical forms of spinal tuberculosis. Acta Neurochir. 1987;88(1-2):26–33. https://doi.org/10.1007/BF01400511.
113. Naim-Ur-Rahman, Jamjoom A, Jamjoom ZA, Al-Tahan AM. Neural arch tuberculosis: radiological features and their correlation with surgical findings. Br J Neurosurg. 1997;11(1):32–8. https://doi.org/10.1080/02688699746663.
114. Weaver P, Lifeso RM. The radiological diagnosis of tuberculosis of the adult spine. Skelet Radiol. 1984;12(3):178–86. https://doi.org/10.1007/BF00361084.
115. Gupta N, Elumalai RK, Verma R, Belho ES, Dhawan S. Spinal tuberculosis mimicking as prostate cancer metastases in Ga-68 prostate-specific membrane antigen positron-emission tomography/computed tomography. Indian J Nucl Med. 2020;35(3):271–3. https://doi.org/10.4103/ijnm.IJNM_56_20. Epub 2020 Jul 1
116. Young A, Maitra S, Ho S, Wang RC. Pott's disease mimicking thyroid carcinoma with spinal metastasis. OTO Open. 2020;4(3) https://doi.org/10.1177/2473974X20948837.
117. Sakamoto T, Takahashi H, Saito J, Matsuzawa Y, Aoki Y, Nakajima A, Sonobe M, Akatsu Y, Yamada M, Akiyama Y, Iwai T, Yanagisawa K, Shiga Y, Inage K, Orita S, Eguchi Y, Maki S, Furuya T, Akazawa T, Koda M, Yamazaki M, Ohtori S, Nakagawa K. Surgical treatment for spinal tuberculosis without elevation of inflammatory biomarkers at the initial visit mimicking spinal metastasis. Case Rep Orthop. 2020;2020:8873170. https://doi.org/10.1155/2020/8873170.
118. Ringshausen FC, Tannapfel A, Nicolas V, Weber A, Duchna HW, Schultze-Werninghaus G, Rohde G. A fatal case of spinal tuberculosis mistaken for metastatic lung cancer: recalling ancient Pott's disease. Ann Clin Microbiol Antimicrob. 2009;8:32. https://doi.org/10.1186/1476-0711-8-32.
119. Ansari S, Amanullah MF, Ahmad K, Rauniyar RK. Pott's spine: diagnostic imaging modalities and technology advancements. N Am J Med Sci. 2013;5(7):404–11. https://doi.org/10.4103/1947-2714.115775.
120. Jevtic V. Vertebral infection. Eur Radiol. 2004;14(Suppl 3):E43–52. https://doi.org/10.1007/s00330-003-2046-x.
121. Obisesan AA, Lagundoye SB, Lawson EA. Radiological features of tuberculosis of the spine in Ibadan. Nigeria Afr J Med Med Sci. 1977;6(2):55–67.
122. Jain AK. Tuberculosis of the spine: a fresh look at an old disease. J Bone Joint Surg (Br). 2010;92(7):905–13. https://doi.org/10.1302/0301-620X.92B7.24668.
123. Naim-Ur-Rahman, El-Bakry A, Jamjoom A, Jamjoom ZA, Kolawole TM. Atypical forms of spinal tuberculosis: case report and review of the literature. Surg Neurol. 1999;51(6):602–7. https://doi.org/10.1016/s0090-3019(98)00101-3.
124. Bell D, Cockshott WP. Tuberculosis of the vertebral pedicles. Radiology. 1971;99(1):43–8. https://doi.org/10.1148/99.1.43.
125. Haacke EM, Brown RW, Thompson MR, Venkatesan R. Magnetic resonance imaging: physical principles and sequence design. New York: Wiley-Liss; 1999.
126. Dolin PJ, Raviglione MC, Kochi A. Global tuberculosis incidence and mortality during 1990-2000. Bull World Health Organ. 1994;72(2):213–20.
127. Elghazawi AK. Clinical syndromes and differential diagnosis of spinal disorders. Radiol Clin N Am. 1991;29(4):651–63.

128. Esses SI. Infections of the spine. Textbook of Spinal Disorders. Philadelphia: JB Lippincott; 1995. p. 229–41.
129. Jacobs P. Some lesions of the spine in immigrants. Proc R Soc Med. 1974;67(9):862–6.
130. Maher D, Harries A. Organisation of an effective national tuberculosis control programme. Postgraduate Doctor Middle Eastern Ed. 1996;19:292–7.
131. McKee DF, Barr WM, Bryan CS, Lunceford EM Jr. Primary aspergillosis of the spine mimicking Pott's paraplegia. J Bone Joint Surg Am. 1984;66(9):1481–3.
132. Thammaroj J, Kitkhuandee A, Sawanyawisuth K, Chowchuan P, Promon K. MR findings in spinal tuberculosis in an endemic country. J Med Imaging Radiat Oncol. 2014;58(3):267–76. https://doi.org/10.1111/1754-9485.12157. Epub 2014 Feb 14
133. Wang LN, Wang L, Liu LM, Song YM, Li Y, Liu H. Atypical spinal tuberculosis involved noncontiguous multiple segments: case series report with literature review. Medicine (Baltimore). 2017;96(14):e6559. https://doi.org/10.1097/MD.0000000000006559.
134. Sharif HS, Aideyan OA, Clark DC, Madkour MM, Aabed MY, Mattsson TA. al-Deeb SM, Moutaery KR. Brucellar and tuberculous spondylitis: comparative imaging features. Radiology. 1989;171(2):419–25. https://doi.org/10.1148/radiology.171.2.2704806.
135. Khattry N, Thulkar S, Das A, Khan SA, Bakhshi S. Spinal tuberculosis mimicking malignancy: atypical imaging features. Indian J Pediatr. 2007;74(3):297–8. https://doi.org/10.1007/s12098-007-0049-3.
136. Moore SL, Rafii M. Imaging of musculoskeletal and spinal tuberculosis. Radiol Clin N Am. 2001;39(2):329–42. https://doi.org/10.1016/s0033-8389(05)70280-3.
137. Mittal S, Khalid M, Sabir AB, Khalid S. Comparison of magnetic resonance imaging findings between pathologically proven cases of atypical tubercular spine and tumour metastasis: a retrospective study in 40 patients. Asian Spine J. 2016;10(4):734–43. https://doi.org/10.4184/asj.2016.10.4.734. Epub 2016 Aug 16
138. Ragland RL, Abdelwahab IF, Braffman B, Moss DS. Posterior spinal tuberculosis: a case report. AJNR Am J Neuroradiol. 1990;11(3):612–3.
139. Sharma D, Swaminathan A, Suri D, Saxena AK, Kumar A, Nijhawan R, Singh S. Tuberculosis spine presenting as multiple skip lesions and non-contiguous paraspinal abscesses: an atypical presentation. Indian J Pediatr. 2014;81(9):961–2. https://doi.org/10.1007/s12098-013-1210-9. Epub 2013 Sep 21
140. Kroupa JK. definici polytraumatu a polytraumatismu [Definition of "polytrauma" and "polytraumatism"]. Acta Chir Orthop Traumatol Cechoslov. 1990;57(4):347–60. Czech
141. Kedous MA, Msakni A, Chebbi W, Zaraa M, Trabelsi M. Unusual circumstances to diagnose cervical Pott's disease. Skelet Radiol. 2018;47(5):723–7. https://doi.org/10.1007/s00256-017-2841-0. Epub 2017 Dec 7
142. Lederer JA, Rodrick ML, Mannick JA. The effects of injury on the adaptive immune response. Shock. 1999;11(3):153–9. https://doi.org/10.1097/00024382-199903000-00001.
143. Zedler S, Bone RC, Baue AE, von Donnersmarck GH, Faist E. T-cell reactivity and its predictive role in immunosuppression after burns. Crit Care Med. 1999;27(1):66–72. https://doi.org/10.1097/00003246-199901000-00028.
144. Faunce DE, Gamelli RL, Choudhry MA, Kovacs EJ. A role for CD1d-restricted NKT cells in injury-associated T cell suppression. J Leukoc Biol. 2003;73(6):747–55. https://doi.org/10.1189/jlb.1102540.
145. Pinheiro HS, Camara NO, Noronha IL, Maugeri IL, Franco MF, Medina JO, Pacheco-Silva A. Contribution of CD4+ T cells to the early mechanisms of ischemia-reperfusion injury in a mouse model of acute renal failure. Braz J Med Biol Res. 2007;40(4):557–68. https://doi.org/10.1590/s0100-879x2007000400015.

Chapter 27
Advancements in the Surgical Management of Spinal Tuberculosis

Vamsi Reddy and Viren Vasudeva

Abstract Spinal tuberculosis or Pott's disease is the most common musculoskeletal pathology in tuberculosis (TB) patients. Presently, spine intervention for TB is largely reserved for adequately managing the complications (e.g., neurovascular compression). Antitubercular therapy (ATT) remains the mainstay of an efficient management of spinal TB. Regardless, surgical intervention is still often required when a combination of these two treatment modalities offers the best outcome. In this chapter, the authors discuss advances in imaging modalities, interventional therapies, surgical techniques, and medical management for spinal TB.

Keywords Spinal tuberculosis · Pott's disease · Radiography · Spinal fusion surgery · Disease eradication

27.1 Introduction

Tuberculosis (TB) is a multisystem disorder that remains endemic in less developed countries of the world. Musculoskeletal manifestations constitute a characteristic feature of extrapulmonary TB in up to 10% of the infected cases [1, 2]. Spinal tuberculosis, being the most common musculoskeletal pathology, affects nearly 1–2% of all the TB patients [1]. TB spine, usually referred to as Pott's disease, is a seriously debilitating condition, and needs a multidisciplinary approach for efficient case management. In the recent years, immense progress has been made in terms of its surgical management, thereby rendering the overall prognosis of spinal disease excellent.

V. Reddy
Medical College of Georgia, Augusta University, Augusta, GA, USA

V. Vasudeva (✉)
Georgia Neurological Surgery and Comprehensive Spine, Athens, GA, USA
e-mail: vvasudeva@georgianeuro.com

S. S. Dhatt, V. Kumar (eds.), *Tuberculosis of the Spine*,
https://doi.org/10.1007/978-981-16-9495-0_27

27.2 TB Spine: A Historical Perspective

Spinal TB has been described as a historical disease where Egyptian mummies, as ancient as 3000 BC, have been diagnosed with vertebral deformities characteristic of TB. In the eighteenth century, Percival Pott coined the term Pott's disease to describe the classical findings of a tuberculous spine. In the earlier times, spinal tuberculosis was conservatively managed with the help of spinal immobilization by the means of body casts or braces. However, surgeons soon commenced operative intervention which was aimed at stabilizing the damaged vertebral segments through spine fusion techniques. Thus, posterior spinal fusion was first introduced by Hibbs et al. In addition, some schools of thought also encouraged a total excision of the diseased spinal segments which resulted in a markedly better patient outcome. In the mid-twentieth century, anti-tubercular therapy (ATT) became widely available, and owing to its brilliant success in treating the diseased spine, the use of spine surgery declined gradually. Moreover, the nature of surgical treatment has also become far less invasive over time [3, 4].

Presently, spine intervention for TB is largely reserved for adequately managing the complications (e.g., neurovascular compression) that are directly associated with Pott's disease.

27.3 Natural History and Clinical Correlations

Spinal TB follows an insidious, chronic course. Less than one-third of the patients develop non-specific manifestations while the remaining are prone to pathogenesis of the following debilitating clinical features [5]:

1. Cold abscess formation
2. Spine deformities
3. Neurological deficit

27.3.1 Cold Abscesses

The vertebral bodies can acquire tuberculous bacteria via hematogenous dissemination which then leads to the development of abscesses in the subligamentous region (underneath the anterior longitudinal ligament) of the spine. These abscesses usually ensue in the absence of classical inflammatory signs and are, hence, termed as "cold." Cold abscesses, the most predominant feature of spinal tuberculosis, are directly correlated to the compression of adjacent bundles of spinal nerves [5].

27.3.2 Spine Deformities

Tuberculosis preferentially involves the anterior segment of the vertebrae. As the anterior vertebral column becomes heavily devastated, the healthy vertebrae lying immediately superior to the site of lesion, descend to establish contact with the lower degenerating vertebrae [5, 6]. This results in kyphotic deformity of the spine which is classically termed as "gibbus," and is usually recognized in the late stages of spinal TB. Such deformities are most commonly encountered in the lumbar, thoracic, and thoracolumbar regions. Vertebral instability and deformity are prevalent in 21% and 16% cases of spinal tuberculosis, respectively. Moreover, spine intervention is itself known to result in kyphosis in at least 11% of the population [7].

27.3.3 Neurological Deficit

The neurological features mostly occur due to mass effects exerted by cold abscesses or granulomatous debris. Rarely, the spinal cord is infected which in turn, becomes edematous enough to lead to neurological compression. Additionally, the spinal dura may undergo fibrosis, thereby leading to nerve compression. Above all, it is possible that the kyphotic deformity of the spine causes a direct compression of the spinal cord. Neurological manifestations occur in around 20% of spinal TB cases. This complication mostly affects the cervicothoracic region and causes excruciating regional pain, as well as sensorimotor deficit. In severe cases, the disease may progress to paraparesis, paraplegia, or even quadriplegia [5, 8].

27.3.4 Diagnostic Modalities

A careful diagnosis of spinal involvement in tuberculosis is mainly twofold. Firstly, there are laboratory investigations which can confirm the presence of secondary or reactivation TB, e.g., Mantoux test, T-SPOT TB, QuantiFERON TB, and interferon gamma release assay (IGRA). Secondly, a series of imaging investigations can unveil the characteristic spinal findings of TB. Furthermore, tissue histopathology is also considered a "gold standard" in this regard [9].

27.3.5 Radiography

A radiographic picture of the TB spine is usually undertaken as the principal imaging investigation. It can clearly reveal the following classical signs of vertebral destruction endured during the course of chronic TB disease [10]:

1. Gibbus formation; anterior collapse of the vertebrae overlying the Pott's lesion which produces a kyphotic spine.
2. Paravertebral abscess formation, usually in the form of a spindle-shaped lesion. This sign is called "bird-nest appearance."
3. Narrowing of the intervertebral disc space.
4. Swelling of the vertebral bodies.
5. Reduced vertical height of the spine.

27.3.6 Radiographic Danger Signs

Table 27.1 depicts a few characteristic radiographic findings [10, 11] which refer to the "high-risk features" of spinal deformity.

27.3.7 Magnetic Resonance Imaging (MRI)

MRI can be used as a highly specific investigation for revealing the overall magnitude of soft tissue involvement in Pott's disease. Therefore, contrast-enhanced MRI is very helpful in localizing the multifocal collections of pus, which include epidural, paravertebral, and prevertebral cold abscesses. Other important features that can be looked for include intervertebral disc lesions, damage of the vertebral bodies as well as the endplates, and vertebral swelling. Moreover, MRI also provides diagnostic evidence in the events of dural invasion, and spinal cord compression. It can also help achieve a reliable differentiation between tuberculous and pyogenic forms of spondylitis. TB involving the sacroiliac joint (sacroiliitis) can also be detected through MRI [10, 12].

27.3.8 Computed Tomography (CT) Scan

A CT scan can provide an elaborate view of the damaged vertebral column in spinal TB. In line with plain radiography, it can be highly effective in judging the overall extent of Pott's disease while it is also extremely useful in

Table 27.1 High-risk features of TB spine

Involvement of thoracic and/or upper lumbar spine
Complete vertebral collapse
Loss of vertebral column height equivalent to at least 1.5 vertebral bodies
Dislocation of vertebral facet joints
Posterior and/or lateral displacement of the vertebral body

determining the exact sites of spinal abscesses, osteolytic lesions, and disc or vertebral collapse. Most importantly, a CT scan is a useful tool for assessing the development of sequestrum and involucrum sites in the spine following Pott's degeneration [13].

27.4 Surgical Management of Spinal TB

Antitubercular therapy (ATT) remains the mainstay of an efficient management of spinal TB. Regardless, surgical intervention is still often required when a combination of these two treatment modalities offers the best outcome [14].

27.5 Surgical Methods

Surgical treatment of spinal tuberculosis has drastically evolved in the recent decades as the therapeutic goals, indications, and approaches for operative intervention have been entirely reformed. At present, surgery is largely aimed at preserving the integrity of the spine and minimizing the spinal deformities and neurological deficits. The following are some major indications of invasive surgery in spinal TB [4]:

1. Younger age (<11 years)
2. Presence of spinal abscesses that are resistant to conservative management
3. Deteriorating neurological deficit (grade 4 paraplegia)
4. Gradually worsening kyphosis (>60°)
5. Large-scale disintegration of vertebral bodies

27.6 Major Surgical Procedures

27.6.1 Surgical Debridement

In the earlier years, a cautious debridement of the affected spinal region was the primary aim of surgical intervention. Removal of the abscess material and other granulomatous debris was generally associated with an improved neurological prognosis.

27.6.2 Spine Fusion Surgery

27.6.2.1 Posterior Fusion

Posterior spinal fusion was pioneered by Hibbs and Albee [15]. Although this arthrodesis approach was partially successful in correcting the deformity in spine curvature through posterior immobilization, it was not appropriate for clearing out the more anteriorly located abscesses.

27.6.2.2 Anterior Fusion

Hodgson et al. initiated a modified operative approach which allowed a wider anterior exposure of the diseased area as well as an adequate excision of the devitalized tissues. The dorsally located spine was approached via transoral (cervical), transthoracic, transsternal, transpleural (thoracic), or transperitoneal approach (lumbar). The debridement was followed by the placement of a fibular graft that bridged the healthy vertebral bodies and provided vertebral stability [16]. Hodgson and colleagues conducted a long-term follow-up of their patients which resulted in a successful spinal fusion in up to 93% cases while 74% of the patients were relieved of their paraplegia [17].

27.6.2.3 Anterolateral Approach

For thoracic spine, an extrapleural or anterolateral approach could be preferred in event of a severely declining pulmonary capacity. Thus, spinal decompression can be performed without compromising the posterior vertebral elements [16].

27.6.3 Advanced Posterior Stabilization Technique

Posterior spinal stabilization has been redefined in the present era, especially after the introduction of modern operative equipment. Therefore, a number of spine surgeons now tend to prefer the utilization of anterior spinal debridement and decompression, coupled with posterior stabilization surgery. This technique offers a major advantage over the anterior approach since it refrains from penetrating the thoracoabdominal cavities.

27.6.3.1 Comparative Data

Evidence suggests that the posterior surgical approach parallels the anterior approach in terms of operative outcome. This can be justified with the help of a comparable improvement seen in terms of kyphotic deformity, pain intensity, and neurological manifestations, while other operative parameters (e.g., timing of surgery and hemorrhage risk) also seem to be identical [18, 19]. Additionally, an exhaustive analysis of the postoperative drainage fluid shows an equivalent effectiveness of both approaches in eliminating the tuberculous bacteria from the affected spinal segments [20]. Thus, it is still debatable as to which approach offers a relatively better prospect of improvement.

By intervening lumbosacral TB via a posterior transforaminal approach, [21] spine surgeons can achieve a considerable reduction in sensorimotor deficit in up to 90% of individuals. In addition, thoracic spine TB with kyphosis can be efficiently managed with the aid of transpedicular decompression combined with posterior vertebral instrumentation and fusion [22].

27.6.4 4. Minimally Invasive Spine Surgery (MISS) in TB

In the recent years, minimally invasive surgery has entirely transformed the course of management in several pathologies pertinent to the spine. Undoubtedly, this is going to shape the future of TB spine surgery in the developing countries.

27.6.4.1 Anterior Spine Intervention via Video Assisted Thoracoscopic Surgery (VATS)

One form of MISS is an improved, alternative version of the conventional open thoracotomy approach. VATS only utilizes two incisions, one smaller incision for introducing the thoracoscope device and a second larger one for operating on the anterior spine. This is mostly used for debridement of the anteriorly localized spinal TB lesions. Moreover, this procedure is rarely associated with any major complications [16, 23].

27.6.4.2 Posterior Spine Instrumentation

This variety of MISS is of pivotal importance in the debridement, fusion, and stabilization of the posterior spinal column. Authors have reported that it not only helps achieve a drastic improvement in neurological symptoms but it also halts the deterioration of kyphotic spine. No significant complications have been reported in this regard while it also leads to a shorter hospital stay, and an earlier postoperative recovery [24].

27.6.5 Intraoperative Monitoring

Intraoperative imaging tools, such as MRI, are becoming increasingly common in spine surgery as they help the surgeons conduct a much safer and far effective correction of an anomaly. For TB spine, MRI studies allow for an accurate detection of the spatial relationships of the lesion in question, which assists in an indiscriminate removal of the devitalized soft tissues. In addition, intraoperative somatosensory and motor-evoked potentials have a proven efficacy in spine surgery as they help avoid an unwarranted and disastrous severance of spinal nerves [25]. Perioperative monitoring of the patient can be performed by comparing the concentration of tuberculous bacteria at the site of lesion and in the postoperative drainage fluid which can quickly assess the overall quality of spine surgery [20].

27.6.5.1 Surgical Outcome and Patient Prognosis

Spinal tuberculosis is a fairly treatable condition, and when an adequate anti-tuberculous chemotherapy is combined with a timely surgical debridement and repair, patient outcome can be remarkably improved. Older data indicate that up to 75% of TB patients observe either a complete or partial recovery while the remaining population either remains unchanged or deteriorates further [26]. However, recent data show that >95% of the population can undergo a full symptomatic recovery following a careful operation [27].

Surgery-related outcome can be determined by the following prognostic factors [28]:

1. Multidrug resistant/extensive drug-resistant (MDR/XDR) TB
2. Demographic factors, e.g., patient age, etc.
3. Patient comorbidities, e.g., diabetes, etc.
4. Permanent paralysis of the lower extremities
5. Number of vertebrae damaged by Pott's lesion
6. Duration and severity of spinal symptoms

27.7 Conclusion

The surgical management of spinal TB has evolved over the years as the advent of new imaging modalities and interventional therapies have advanced. Nonetheless, perhaps the biggest advancement in the management of spinal TB would be the eradication of the disease as a whole in third-world countries through proper hygiene, screening, treatment, and public awareness.

This research received no specific grant from any funding agency in the public, commercial, or not-for-profit sectors.Competing Interests StatementThe authors have no personal or institutional interest with regard to the authorship and/or publication of this manuscript.

Contributorship Statement All authors were involved in the design and conception of this manuscript.

Data Sharing All data pertaining to this research article are included within the manuscript as written.

References

1. Dunn RN, Ben HM. Spinal tuberculosis: review of current management. Bone Joint J. 2018;100-b(4):425–31.
2. Gautam MP, Karki P, Rijal S, Singh R. Pott's spine and paraplegia. JNMA J Nepal Med Assoc. 2005;44(159):106–15.
3. Tuli SM. Tuberculosis of the spine: a historical review. Clin Orthop Relat Res. 2007;460:29–38.
4. Tuli SM. Historical aspects of Pott's disease (spinal tuberculosis) management. Eur Spine J Off Publ Eur Spine Soc Eur Spinal Deformity Soc Eur Sect Cervical Spine Res Soc. 2013;22(Suppl 4):529–38.
5. Khanna K, Sabharwal S. Spinal tuberculosis: a comprehensive review for the modern spine surgeon. Spine J Off J N Am Spine Soc. 2019;19(11):1858–70.
6. Rajasekaran S. The problem of deformity in spinal tuberculosis. Clin Orthop Relat Res. 2002;398:85–92.
7. Batirel A, Erdem H, Sengoz G, et al. The course of spinal tuberculosis (Pott disease): results of the multinational, multicentre Backbone-2 study. Clin Microbiol Infect. 2015;21(11):1008.e1009–18.
8. Kumar K. Spinal tuberculosis, natural history of disease, classifications and principles of management with historical perspective. Eur J Orthop Surg Traumatol Orthop Traumatol. 2016;26(6):551–8.
9. Esteves S, Catarino I, Lopes D, Sousa C. Spinal tuberculosis: rethinking an old disease. J Spine. 2017;6(1):358.
10. Ansari S, Amanullah MF, Ahmad K, Rauniyar RK. Pott's spine: diagnostic imaging modalities and technology advancements. N Am J Med Sci. 2013;5(7):404–11.
11. Rajasekaran S, Soundararajan DCR, Shetty AP, Kanna RM. Spinal tuberculosis: current concepts. Global Spine J. 2018;8(4 Suppl):96s–108s.
12. Kilborn T, Janse van Rensburg P, Candy S. Pediatric and adult spinal tuberculosis: imaging and pathophysiology. Neuroimaging Clin N Am. 2015;25(2):209–31.
13. Shanley DJ. Tuberculosis of the spine: imaging features. AJR Am J Roentgenol. 1995;164(3):659–64.
14. Muralidharan V, Nair BR, Rajshekhar V. Changing trends of presentation of central nervous system tuberculosis: Relative prevalence of cranial and spinal tuberculosis and drug resistance patterns. Neurol India. 2019;67(3):792–6.
15. Young CS. Tuberculosis of the spine and scoliosis: an improved technic for arthrodesis of the vertebral joints. J Am Med Assoc. 1936;107(25):2035–9.
16. Kandwal P, Vijayaraghavan G, Jayaswal A. Management of tuberculous infection of the spine. Asian Spine J. 2016;10(4):792–800.
17. Hodgson AR, Stock FE, Fang HS, Ong GB. Anterior spinal fusion. The operative approach and pathological findings in 412 patients with Pott's disease of the spine. Br J Surg. 1960;48:172–8.

18. Liu H, Luo J, Wang X, Dong X, Hao D. Efficacy of surgery via the single anterior and single posterior approaches for treatment of thoracic spinal tuberculosis. J Int Med Res. 2020;48(1):300060519896743.
19. Huang Y, Lin J, Chen X, Lin J, Lin Y, Zhang H. A posterior versus anterior debridement in combination with bone graft and internal fixation for lumbar and thoracic tuberculosis. J Orthop Surg Res. 2017;12(1):150.
20. Zhao C, Pu X, Zhou Q, et al. Can a posterior approach effectively heal thoracic and lumbar tuberculosis? microbiology outcomes of the operative area. J Orthop Surg Res. 2019;14(1):24.
21. Pang X, Wu P, Shen X, Li D, Luo C, Wang X. One-stage posterior transforaminal lumbar debridement, 360° interbody fusion, and posterior instrumentation in treating lumbosacral spinal tuberculosis. Arch Orthop Trauma Surg. 2013;133(8):1033–9.
22. Luo C, Wang X, Wu P, Ge L, Zhang H, Hu J. Single-stage transpedicular decompression, debridement, posterior instrumentation, and fusion for thoracic tuberculosis with kyphosis and spinal cord compression in aged individuals. Spine J Off J N Am Spine Soc. 2016;16(2):154–62.
23. Huang TJ, Hsu RW, Chen SH, Liu HP. Video-assisted thoracoscopic surgery in managing tuberculous spondylitis. Clin Orthop Relat Res. 2000;379:143–53.
24. Xiong W, Yu B, Zhang Y, et al. Minimally invasive far lateral debridement combined with posterior instrumentation for thoracic and lumbar tuberculosis without severe kyphosis. J Orthop Surg Res. 2020;15(1):221.
25. Feng B, Qiu G, Shen J, et al. Impact of multimodal intraoperative monitoring during surgery for spine deformity and potential risk factors for neurological monitoring changes. J Spinal Disord Tech. 2012;25(4):E108–14.
26. Turgut M. Spinal tuberculosis (Pott's disease): its clinical presentation, surgical management, and outcome. A survey study on 694 patients. Neurosurg Rev. 2001;24(1):8–13.
27. Ma YZ, Cui X, Li HW, Chen X, Cai XJ, Bai YB. Outcomes of anterior and posterior instrumentation under different surgical procedures for treating thoracic and lumbar spinal tuberculosis in adults. Int Orthop. 2012;36(2):299–305.
28. Yao Y, Zhang H, Liu M, et al. Prognostic factors for recovery of patients after surgery for thoracic spinal tuberculosis. World Neurosurg. 2017;105:327–31.

Chapter 28
End Point of Chemotherapy for TB Spine?

Abhay Nene and Munjal Shah

Abstract Tuberculosis is a major health problem in developing countries, and India is considered endemic for the disease. The management of spinal tuberculosis has come to a full circle. It has evolved drastically from an era of conservative treatment due to lack of good surgical techniques to an era of aggressive surgery with anterior reconstructions and now back to conservative treatment with better availability of diagnostic methods and superior understanding of the microbiology of the bug and the pharmacology of drugs.

Spinal tuberculosis is essentially a medical disease. Successful outcome of spinal tuberculosis relies on accurate histopathological and microbiological diagnosis, appropriate chemotherapeutic regimens, and optimum monitoring.

Though the chemotherapeutic regimen for sensitive TB is largely accepted, no consensus has been reached on appropriate duration of anti-tubercular drugs, as there has been no accepted definition of "healed status" in spinal TB.

In most studies, the duration of chemotherapy varies from 6 months to 12 months.

The end point of treatment is based on combination of clinical, radiological, and laboratory parameters, but the lack of hard criteria to define healed spinal TB keep the controversy about the duration of AKT alive.

Keywords Spinal tuberculosis · Diagnosis · Anti-tubercular drugs · End point

28.1 Introduction

Tuberculosis constitutes 85–90% of primary spinal infections in endemic areas and developing countries [1]. Spine still remains the leading cause of non-traumatic paraplegia in developing nations [2, 3]. According to the WHO global TB report from 2019, extrapulmonary TB was reported in 15% of new incident TB cases in

A. Nene (✉) · M. Shah
WeareSpine, Lilavati Hospital and Research Centre, Mumbai, India
e-mail: abhaynene@yahoo.com

S. S. Dhatt, V. Kumar (eds.), *Tuberculosis of the Spine*,
https://doi.org/10.1007/978-981-16-9495-0_28

2018. Osteoarticular TB has been reported to account for 11.3% of extrapulmonary sites with spinal TB accounting for the vast majority, reported to be up to 50% [4–6]. In the late 1980s, the medical fraternity seemed to be on its way to achieving control over tuberculosis (TB), one of the most dreaded infectious diseases of the twentieth century. However, a rising worldwide incidence of diabetes mellitus and human immunodeficiency virus (HIV) marked a dramatic comeback by this "millennium bug" [7].

Neurological complications incidence in TB spine patients varies from 10% to 43% [8]. Early diagnosis and treatment in TB spine is necessary to prevent permanent neurological disability, and minimize spinal deformity [7, 9].

Treatment of tuberculosis of spine has varied since time of Hippocrates. It has always remained controversial. The evolution of treatment of tuberculosis of spine has passed through different phases. It seems that treatment of TB spine has come to full circle from conservative resulting from lack of appropriate techniques, through aggressive surgical debridement and reconstruction for "disease control" and drug resistance, with availability of modern spinal instrumentation, and now relearning non-operative care, with a better understanding of drug-resistant TB and the natural history of spinal TB. Thus it is important to make an early diagnosis to prevent complications and morbidity.

Fundamentally, the treatment of tuberculosis is by chemotherapy and surgery attempts only to eliminate the complications arising from the disease process. Hence, all uncomplicated cases of spinal TB merit medical rather than surgical treatment.

28.2 Clinical Presentation

The presentation of the spinal tuberculosis depends upon the stage of disease, the region of the spine affected, and the development of complications such as neurologic deficits, abscesses, or the sinus tracts. The reported average duration of symptoms at diagnosis is 4 months but can be considerably longer due to nonspecific presentation of chronic back pain in some of the patients.

The commonest presenting symptom is progressive local back pain for weeks to months, with or without associated muscle spasm [10]. Constitutional symptoms like malaise, loss of feeling of wellbeing, loss of appetite and weight loss, and evening rise of the temperature with occasional night sweats are seldom present.

28.2.1 Diagnosis

Early diagnosis of spinal tuberculosis is essential in order to initiate appropriate treatment and prevent potentially horrendous morbidity and sequelae arising due to missing the same.

Though the initial suspicion of spinal tuberculosis relies on clinic-radiological diagnosis, a confirmation by tissue biopsy for histopathology and microbiological examination of the tissue becomes mandatory today.

Plain radiograph, MRI spine, and CT scan are useful as imaging diagnostic tools, while the role of Radionuclide (FDG PET Scan) is under evaluation.

Various hematological tests like Erythrocyte sedimentation rate, C-reactive protein, and complete blood count are the initial investigations used as corroborative evidence for diagnosis of spinal infections. ESR is more of a prognostic tool rather than diagnostic. Decreasing trend in ESR suggest that medication is effective. CRP, though being non-specific inflammatory marker, is elevated in 75% cases of spinal tuberculosis [11].

28.2.2 Treatment

Treatment of tuberculosis is by chemotherapy and surgery aims to eliminate the complications arising from the disease process. Indications of non-operative and operative have been well defined now in literature.

Anti-tubercular therapy is the mainstay of treatment of spinal tuberculosis. Proper drug regimen, drug dosage, and drug duration and monitoring of ATT is the key to success for spinal tuberculosis.

28.2.3 Determining End Point of Treatment of Spinal Tuberculosis

The biggest problem in spinal TB is the lack of strict criteria to determine "healed status." Hence, the end point for stopping anti-tuberculous drugs is not well defined.

Repeat tissue biopsy and culture conversion—the "gold standard" in pulmonary TB, is not pursued to determine end point of treatment in spinal TB, as aside of it being an invasive, cumbersome and hence impractical approach, it has very low yield due to the paucibacillary nature of TB spine.

Also there is no known methodology to measure the total body burden of *M. tuberculosis* or to predict clinical outcomes.

Thus clinical improvement, laboratory markers, and radiological assessment remains the trilogy to help determine "healed" status corroboratively.

28.3 Clinical Criteria for Healing in TB Spine

Since spinal tuberculosis is often a localized infection, systemic symptoms of disease like fever, loss of appetite, weight loss, etc. are present in rather small percentage of patients, precluding using these to monitor recovery.

The clinical signs of spinal tuberculosis are local back pain, deformity, and/or neurology. An improvement in these is used by clinicians to gauge the extent of recovery.

28.3.1 Pain

Though the majority of healing spinal TB patients report improvement in pain, it cannot be an absolute criteria, as sources of back pain can be multiple, and more importantly, healing can occur without solid bony fusion leading to persistent pain due to spinal instability despite disease healing (Fig. 28.1). Besides this, pain remains a subjective criteria that doesn't have a true metric to document its intensity.

28.3.2 Deformity

The same holds true for spinal deformity, as in most adults the deformity persists or worsens as the disease heals with collapse (Fig. 28.1).

28.3.3 Neurology

Though reduction in the diseased soft tissue compressing the neural elements leads to improvement in the patient's neurology, in a select group of patients neurology can persist despite disease healing due to persistent bony compression of the neural structures, or irreversible functional damage to the nerve cells.

28.3.4 Laboratory Markers

Inflammatory markers—ESR and CRP—are used by most clinicians as aids to assess recovery in spinal TB. Both are non-specific markers and can be used at best as a comparison to the index reading during the course of treatment.

28.3.5 Erythrocyte Sedimentation Rate (ESR)

ESR is elevated generally in most cases. It is used to monitor the response to treatment. Failure to normalize after treatment should arouse suspicion regarding primary drug resistance or alternative etiology.

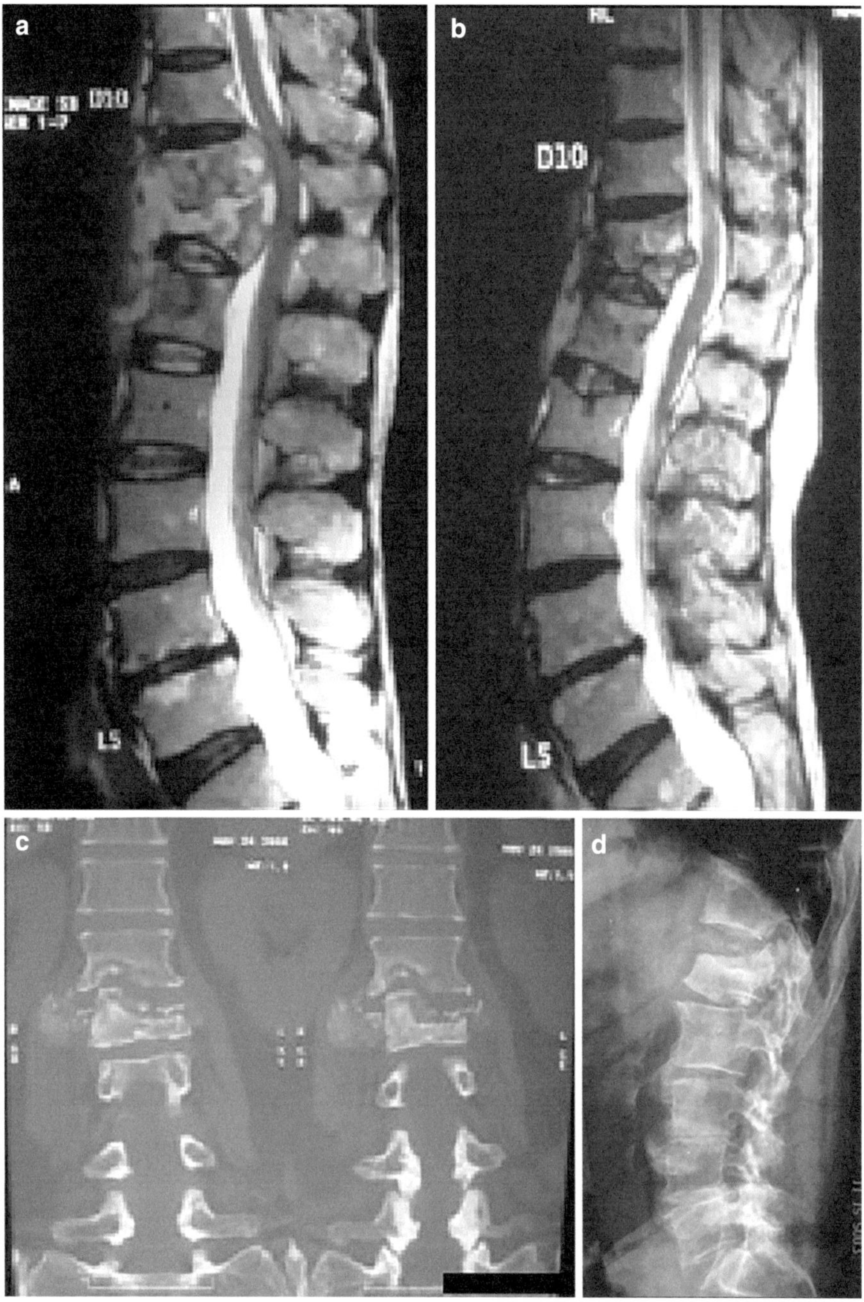

Fig. 28.1 Shows improvement in MRI after giving conservative treatment for 12 months in biopsy proven case of Tb spine (**a**) and (**b**). Though pain and deformity still persisted clinically (**c**) and (**d**) even after resolution in MRI

28.3.6 C-Reactive Protein (CRP)

C-Reactive protein has been found to be elevated in spinal tuberculosis up to 75% [11]. It is more specific for infectious and inflammatory lesions. It takes 2 weeks while erythrocyte sedimentation rate takes about 4 weeks to register a change and thus has a more value in monitoring the treatment response.

Other laboratory investigations like the TB IgG/IgM, TB "gold" test, and the Mantoux test have no role in determining the presence or absence of spinal TB, especially in endemic regions.

28.4 Radiological Criteria for Healing in TB Spine

MRI remains the gold standard radiological investigation for the diagnosis and status assessment of spinal TB.

Generally, healing is suggested by MRI evidence of complete resolution of pre- and paravertebral collections, resolution of vertebral body marrow edema, and replacement of marrow edema by fat or calcification. Number of studies have now shown utility of MRI scans in demonstrating serial changes in improvement in patients responding to ATT [12, 13].

However, there are several well-known lacunae in using the above as "hard criteria" to determine healing in spinal TB.

1. MRI can continue to show soft tissues and even sterile abscesses after complete eradication of infection (Fig. 28.2).
2. MRI generally lags behind clinical improvement by up to 3 months.
3. The MRI can be over sensitive if used as a stand-alone proof to judge the severity of present infection, inflammatory edema, active disease pus, and sterile residual soft tissue can't be well differentiated in all cases (Fig. 28.2).
   Hence, although the MRI is useful in tracking disease healing, its utility in determining the end point of ATT is still debatable.

   However, it's value in judging disease worsening remains critical.

   Appearance of new lesions while on treatment, worsening of existing lesions/marrow edema, and new bony destruction/abscess are all indicative of poor disease control, especially if accompanied by clinical worsening.

   In this scenario, a repeat biopsy for culture/drug sensitivity and/or a change in the drug regimen should be considered.

   Another challenging scenario is one where the patient shows clinical improvement with a worsening in MRI. Here the following differentials should be considered: (1) reactive inflammatory tissue, (2) MRI done too early on treatment, and (3) inadequate dosage of drugs or drug-resistance.

Jain et al. [14] have shown that there is MRI evidence of healing at the end of 8 months of combination drug therapy occurred only in about one third of the cases, but the criteria used for "healed status" on MRI were not standardized/universally accepted.

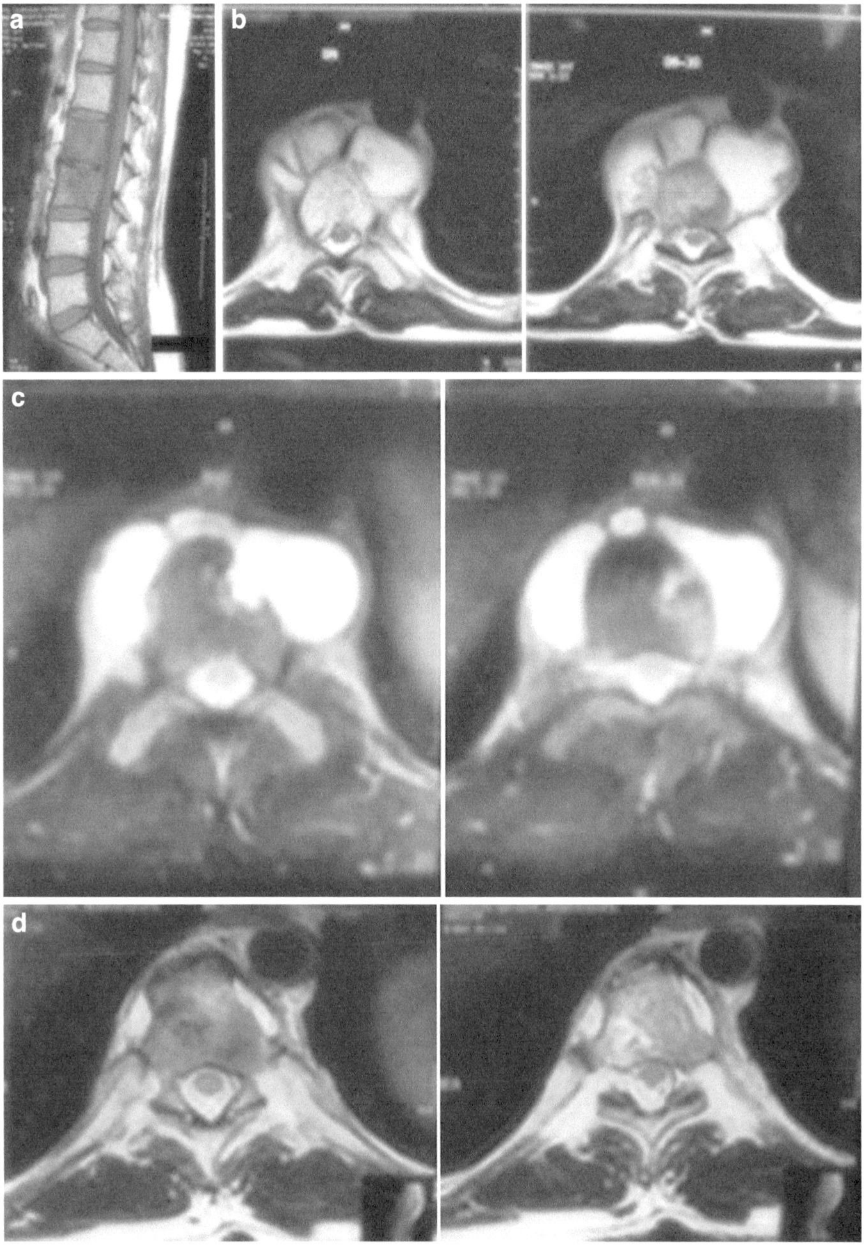

Fig. 28.2 (**a**) MRI LS spine showing worsening at 2 months after starting primary AKT for biopsy proven TB spine despite of clinical improvement. (**b**) MRI LS spine showing paravertebral abscess at 6 months after starting primary AKT despite patient clinically healed. (**c**) MRI LS spine showing paravertebral abscess at 12 months after starting primary AKT despite patient clinically healed at 6 months of treatment. (**d**) Twelve months after AKT stopped despite above MRI

On the other hand, Nene et al. [15] showed that the rate of recurrence of spinal TB after stopping chemotherapy at 6 months, regardless of the MRI reading, remained acceptably low.

28.4.1 Role of X-Ray and CT Scan

Bony reconstitution on X-ray or CT scan is an unequivocal sign of healing.

Additionally, spine surgeons often look for sclerosis on the above two investigations to settle a disputed "edema" on MRI scan.

28.5 PET Scan in Healing in TB Spine

Recently, there has been considerable interest in the use of 18F-fluorodeoxyglucose (18F-FDG) PET to differentiate active from inactive disease in patients with TB [16].

Though this is potentially an important clinical application in some patients, there is no convincing evidence on the utility of the PET scan in infections as there is in malignancy.

There is overlap in the standardized uptake values of TB and malignant lesions on 18F-FDG PET, which limits its usefulness in distinguishing them (Fig. 28.3).

There is a lack of consensus regarding the ideal duration of multidrug chemotherapy for spinal TB. WHO recommends 9 months of treatment for TB of bones and joints (2HREZ + 7 HR) because of the serious risk of disability in addition to difficulties in assessing treatment response. British Thoracic Society (BTS) recommends 6 months (2HREZ + 4 HR) of chemotherapy. American Thoracic Society (ATS) recommends 6 months of chemotherapy in adults and 12 months in children for spinal TB. Inadequate or unessential, prolonged duration of treatment should be avoided. Generally ATT is given for 6–12 months on case to case basis.

In 2016, Central Tuberculosis Division of India came out with a new set of recommendations specifically pertaining to spinal TB [17] where end points are decided on a case by case basis.

Thus clinical improvement, laboratory markers, and radiological assessment help us to determine "healed" status and in constitutional symptoms, normalization of ESR, CRP and improving trend on MRI and bony healing on X-ray are generally used as end point of treatment of ATT.

Tuberculosis of spine is paucibacillary and has dormant mycobacteria which are harder to kill and retain viability despite chemotherapy. Exogenous reinfection can cause recurrence in highly endemic countries of TB like India [18, 19]. It is also due to inadequate killing of endogenous TB bacteria which can lead to relapse of TB [19–21].

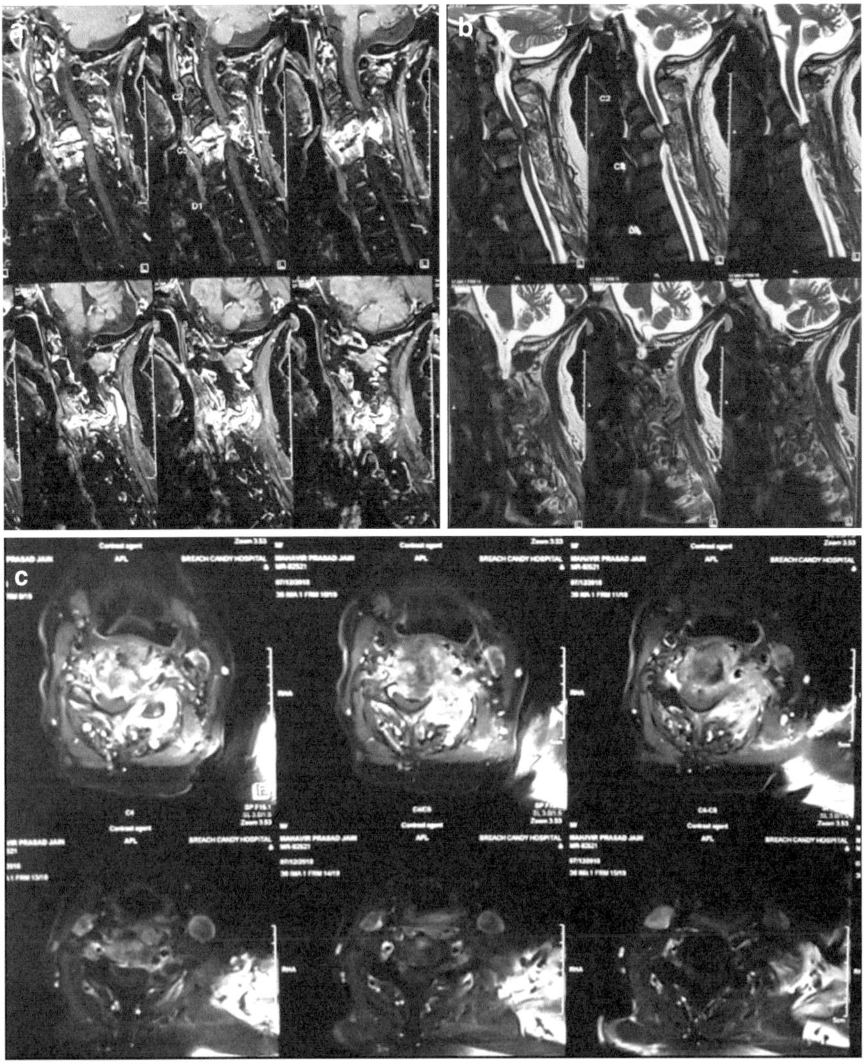

Fig. 28.3 A 75-year-old male presented with progressive quadriparesis for more than a month. Rest pain and weight loss was significant. MRI was showing permeative lesion with collapse in C5 body with rest of spine screening was clean (**a**–**d**). X-ray showed C5 body collapse (**e**). CT scan showed C5 body collapse (**f**). PET scan showed multifocal uptake in cervical lymph nodes, shaft of humerus, right scapula, and right sphenoid sinus. And were not able to comment on it being neoplastic or infective (**g**). Post op X-ray after posterior decompression and fixation (**h**). Biopsy from the site showed it to be drug-sensitive tuberculosis. Thus PET scan still not sensitive enough to differentiate TB from malignancy

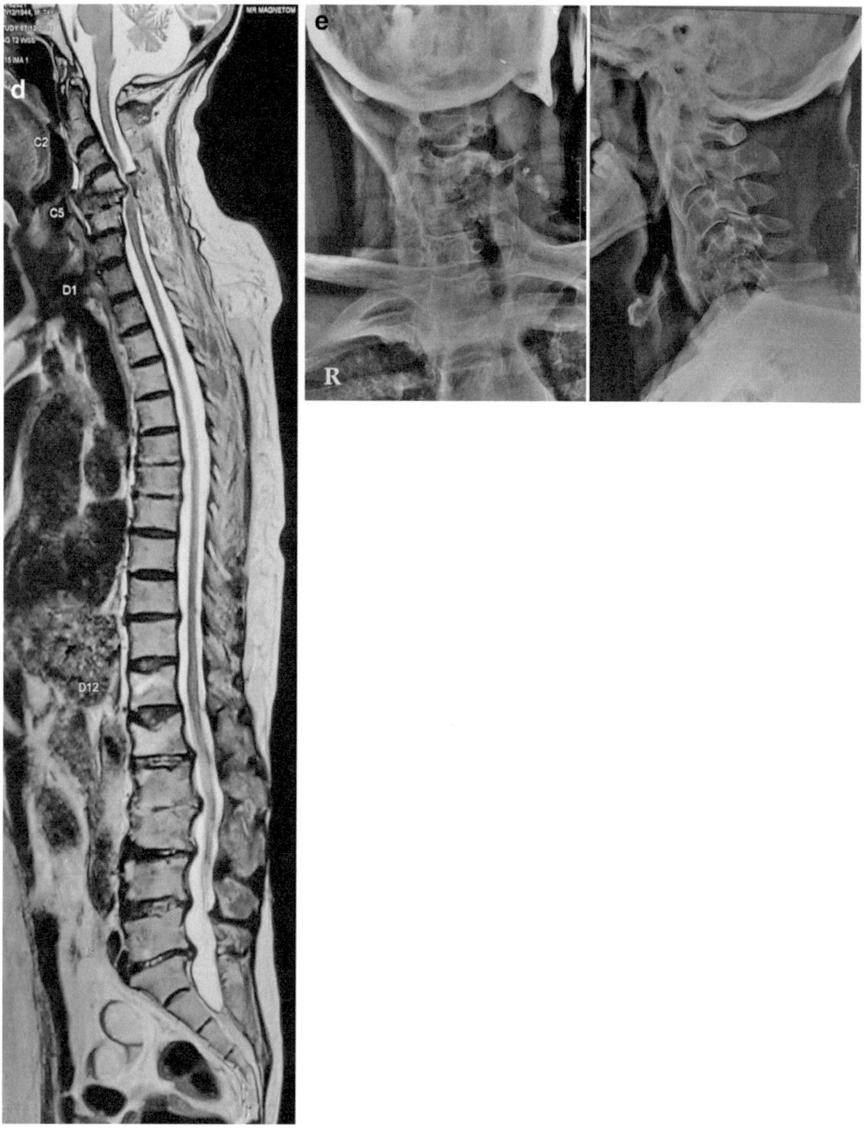

Fig. 28.3 (continued)

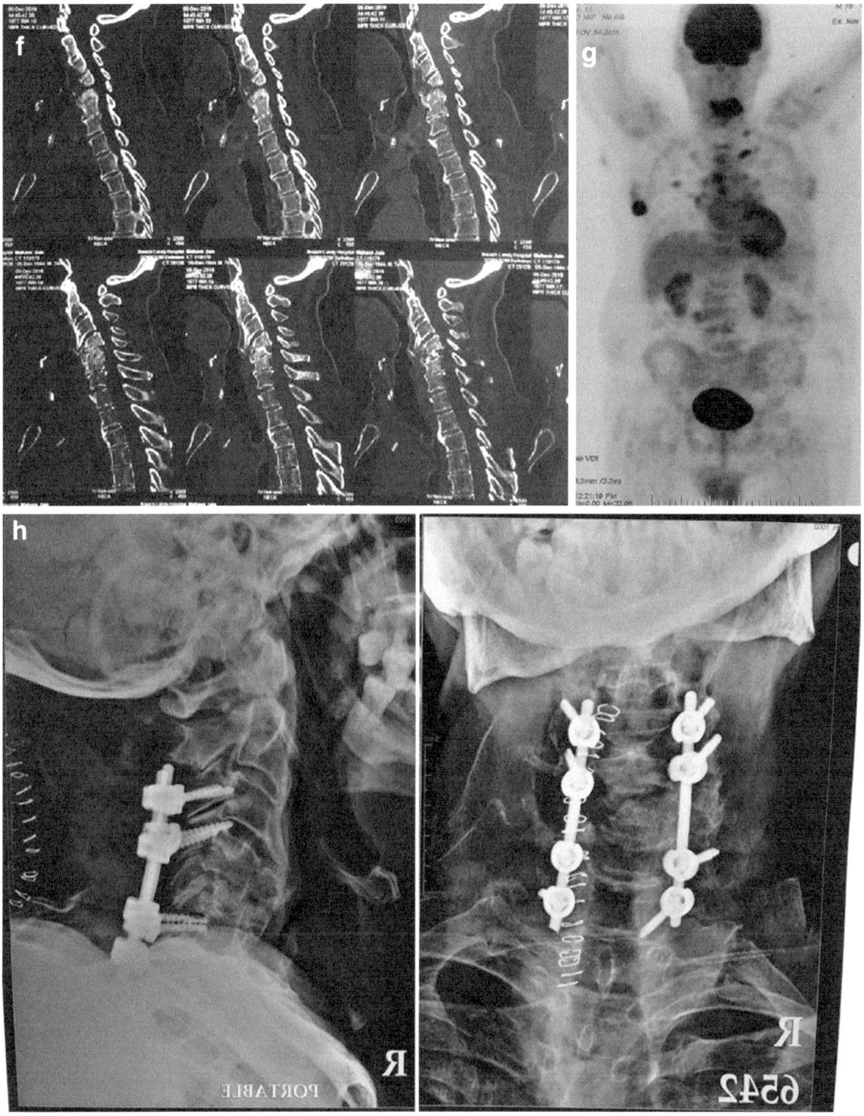

Fig. 28.3 (continued)

28.5.1 Follow-Up After Stopping AKT

To prevent relapse and recurrence of disease, patient should be followed up regularly. The authors recommend patient should be followed up clinically and with blood markers at 6 monthly and 1 year after stopping AKT. And 1 yearly after that for a period of 5 years. We ask for MRI yearly for first 2 years and then at 5 years, though with no evidence either way.

Relapse, recurrence, or reinfection of tuberculosis strongly points towards drug-resistant TB.

28.5.2 New Avenues to Determine End Point in TB Spine

28.5.2.1 PET Scan

Use of positron emission tomography-computed tomography (PET-CT) in Tb spine is being studied now. MRI is not useful in differentiating active or healing disease. So role of PET scan in follow-up modality in TB spine is being explored. Some researchers have suggested the role of PET scan to differentiate relapsed from resolved TB spine [22–25]. Current research is underway to determine usefulness of PET/CT to know resolution in spinal TB.

28.5.2.2 Biomarkers

Hope exists for biomarkers to be a surrogate end point and for customization of treatment regimen and tailoring of duration for individual patients. That would in turn potentially solve the problem of long duration of treatment that makes conducting clinical trials with good follow-up extremely challenging in extrapulmonary TB.

In addition to biomarkers, the diagnostics to quantify the total body burden of mycobacteria is also non-existent. There is a growing need for such tests which could ultimately help with prognosis as well as personalization of various aspects of treatment in extrapulmonary TB.

Biomarker discovery and application in TB diagnostics would particularly change the existing paradigm in these extrapulmonary patients by avoiding delay in diagnosis and treatment initiation and prevention of subsequent complications that in turn occur from such a delay.

References

1. Global Tuberculosis report 2017: World Health Organisation.
2. Rajasekaran S, Prasad Shetty A, Dheenadhayalan J, Shashidhar Reddy J, Naresh-Babu J, Kishen T. Morphological changes during growth in healed childhood spinal tuberculosis a 15-year prospective study of 61 children treated with ambulatory chemotherapy. J Pediatr Orthop. 2006;26(6):716–24.
3. Teo H, Peh W. Skeletal tuberculosis in children. Pediatr Radiol. 2004;34(11):853–60.
4. Peto HM, Pratt RH, Harrington TA, LoBue PA, Armstrong LR. Epidemiology of extrapulmonary tuberculosis in the United States, 1993–2006. Clin Infect Dis. 2009;49:1350–7.
5. Naim-ur-Rahman. Atypical forms of spinal tuberculosis. J Bone Joint Surg Br. 1980;62-B:162–5.
6. Talbot JC, Bismil Q, Saralaya D, Newton D, Frizzel RM, Shaw DL. Musculoskeletal tuberculosis in bradford – a 6-year review. Ann R Coll Surg Engl. 2007;89:405–9.

7. Jain AK. Tuberculosis of the spine: a fresh look at an old disease. J Bone Joint Surg Br. 2010;92:905–13.
8. Kiran N, Vaishya S, Kale S, Sharma B, Mahapatra A. Surgical results in patients with tuberculosis of the spine and severe lower-extremity motor deficits: a retrospective study of 48 patients. J Neurosurg Spine. 2007;6(4):320–6.
9. Jain A, Dhammi I. Tuberculosis of the spine. Clin Orthop Relat Res. 2007;460:39–4.
10. Tuli S. Tuberculosis of the skeletal system. New Delhi: Jaypee Brothers Medical Publishers; 2010. p. 4.
11. Thelander U, Larsson S. Quantitation of C-reactive protein and Erythrocyte sedimentation rate after spinal surgery. Spine. 1992;17(4):400–4.
12. Singh R, Magu NK, Rohilla RK. Clinicoradiologic profile of involvement and healing in tuberculosis of the spine. Ann Med Health Sci Res. 2016;6(5):311–27.
13. Antonio RG, Silvana SE, Carme TO, et al. Imaging findings of Pott's disease. Eur Spine J. 2013;22(Suppl 4):567–78.
14. Jain AK, Srivastava A, Saini NS, Dhammi IK, Sreenivasan R, Kumar S. Efficacy of extended dots category i chemotherapy in spinal tuberculosis based on MRI-based healed status. Indian J Orthop. 2012;46:633–9.
15. Nene AM, Patil S, Kathare AP, Nagad P, Nene A, Kapadia F. Six vs twelve months of anti-tubercular therapy in patients with biopsy proven spinal tuberculosis. A single centre, open labelled, prospective randomized clinical trial - a pilot study. Spine (Phila Pa 1976). 2019;44(1):E1–E6.
16. Ohtori S, Suzuki M, Koshi T, Yamashita M, Yamauchi K, Inoue G, et al. 18F- fluorodeoxyglucose-PET for patients with suspected spondylitis showing modic change. Spine (Phila Pa 1976). 2010;35:E1599–603.
17. INDEX-TB guidelines - guidelines on extra-pulmonary tuberculosis for India. 2016. http://tbcindia.nic.in/showfile.php?lid=3245. Accessed 4 Apr 2017.
18. Alland D, Kalkut GE, Moss AR, McAdam RA, Hahn JA, Bosworth W. Transmission of tuberculosis in new york city. an analysis by DNA fingerprinting and conventional epidemiologic methods. N Engl J Med. 1994;330:1710–6.
19. Small PM, Hopewell PC, Singh SP, Paz A, Parsonnet J, Ruston DC. The epidemiology of tuberculosis in San Francisco – a population-based study using conventional and molecular methods. N Engl J Med. 1994;330:1703–9.
20. Sahadevan R, Narayanan S, Paramasivan CN, Prabhakar R, Narayanan PR. Restriction fragment length polymorphism typing of clinical isolates of mycobacterium tuberculosis from patients with pulmonary tuberculosis in madras, India, by use of direct-repeat probe. J Clin Microbiol. 1995;33:3037–9.
21. Das S, Chan SL, Allen BW, Mitchison DA, Lowrie DB. Application of DNA fingerprinting with IS986 to sequential mycobacterial isolates obtained from pulmonary tuberculosis patients in Hong Kong before, during and after short-course chemotherapy. Tuber Lung Dis. 1993;74:47–51.
22. Rivas-Garcia A, Sarria-Estrada S, Torrents-Odin C, Casas-Gomila L, Franquet E. Imaging findings of Pott's disease. Eur Spine J. 2013;22(Suppl 4):567–78.
23. Kim S-J, Kim I-J, Suh KT, Kim Y-K, Lee JS. Prediction of residual disease of spine infection using F-18 FDG pet/ct. Spine. 2009;34:2424–30.
24. Vorster M, Sathekge MM, Bomanji J. Advances in imaging of tuberculosis: the role of ^{18}F-FDG pet and pet/ct. Curr Opin Pulm Med. 2014;20:287–93.
25. Grigolato D, Del Rizzo M, Cucca M, Zuffante M, Concia E, Ferdeghini M. 18F-FDG PET/CT in tuberculosis: a single hospital experience. J Nucl Med. 2016;57:1742.

MIX
Papier aus verantwortungsvollen Quellen
Paper from responsible sources
FSC® C105338

If you have any concerns about our products,
you can contact us on
ProductSafety@springernature.com

In case Publisher is established outside the EU,
the EU authorized representative is:
Springer Nature Customer Service Center GmbH
Europaplatz 3, 69115 Heidelberg, Germany

Printed by Libri Plureos GmbH
in Hamburg, Germany